Contemporary Endocrinology

Series Editor
Leonid Poretsky
Division of Endocrinology
Lenox Hill Hospital
New York, NY, USA

Contemporary Endocrinology offers an array of titles covering clinical as well as bench research topics of interest to practicing endocrinologists and researchers. Topics include obesity management, androgen excess disorders, stem cells in endocrinology, evidence-based endocrinology, diabetes, genomics and endocrinology, as well as others. Series Editor Leonid Poretsky, MD, is Chief of the Division of Endocrinology and Associate Chairman for Research at Lenox Hill Hospital, and Professor of Medicine at Hofstra North Shore-LIJ School of Medicine.

More information about this series at http://link.springer.com/series/7680

Marcella Donovan Walker

Editor

Hypercalcemia

Clinical Diagnosis and Management

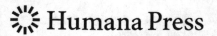 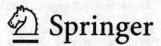

Editor
Marcella Donovan Walker
Division of Endocrinology
Columbia University Irving Medical Center
New York, NY, USA

ISSN 2523-3785   ISSN 2523-3793   (electronic)
Contemporary Endocrinology

ISBN 978-3-030-93184-1   ISBN 978-3-030-93182-7   (eBook)
https://doi.org/10.1007/978-3-030-93182-7

This Humana imprint is published by the registered company Springer Nature Switzerland AG
The registered company address is: Gewerbestrasse 11, 6330 Cham, Switzerland

To my parents, Ryan and Grant, for their unwavering support

Series Editor's Foreword

Calcium, as pointed out by the authors of this book, is the most abundant mineral in the human body. It is central to a myriad of physiological functions on both cellular and organ levels and its concentration in the serum is tightly regulated. If calcium regulatory mechanisms fail, a life-threatening condition may develop.

I vividly remember how, as a medical resident, I would frequently consult the legendary *Washington Manual of Medical Therapeutics* (which most house officers at that time faithfully carried in their uniform's pocket—imagine, no Internet!) on management of hypercalcemia. Indeed, most hospital-based physicians are proficient in treating acute hypercalcemia. It is usually left to endocrinologists, however, to make a definitive diagnosis and to recommend appropriate medical or surgical therapy.

In this regard, the volume edited by Dr. Marcella Walker provides invaluable information. Classic in its structure and encyclopedic in its content, the book is authored by experts on all topics related to hypercalcemia. Many authors, including the book's editor, work at the world-renowned calcium and bone metabolism center at Columbia University. The Columbia crew is joined by an equally renowned international group of authorities addressing both normal physiology and pathophysiology of calcium regulation, and covering, among other areas, pediatrics, genetics, cancer, and other common and rare causes of hypercalcemia.

Once in possession of this book, there is no longer a need to consult the *Washington Manual* (either in print or online) on hypercalcemia, since all necessary information is now compiled in a single volume. The editor and the authors are to be congratulated on this remarkable accomplishment.

New York, NY, USA   Leonid Poretsky

Preface

My interest in calcium metabolism and metabolic bone disease began as a second-year medical student. I found that endocrine pathophysiology, particularly that related to hypercalcemia, appealed to me because of the elegance of the endocrine system. While the complexity of endocrinology presented an intellectual challenge, there were guiding principles that served to unify the discipline. As a medical student, I found endocrine feedback loops to be inherently logical and the clinical evaluation of hormonal disorders uniquely satisfying. Over 20 years later, as an academic endocrinologist and metabolic bone specialist, the thrill of investigating the etiology of hypercalcemia and other endocrine disorders persists. While our knowledge of the pathophysiology and genetics of many of the conditions that cause hypercalcemia has advanced, the core principles guiding evaluation and treatment of patients with hypercalcemia largely endure.

This book is intended to convey the logical approach to the diagnosis, etiology, and management of hypercalcemia introduced to me as a medical student and refined by world-renowned mentors at Johns Hopkins and Columbia, distinguished colleagues (many of whom have contributed to this work), and clinical practice. My hope is that this book simultaneously conveys a comprehensive but accessible approach to the diagnosis and management of hypercalcemia. It is intended for endocrinologists, internists, medical residents, and medical students. This work provides both basic guidance on the etiology, diagnostic evaluation, and treatment of hypercalcemia, while also offering an in-depth, detailed, and state-of-the-art review of the individual causes by prominent experts in the field. Where applicable, some chapters include illustrative cases to complement theoretical matter with real-world applications to the practice of medicine. By integrating an evidence-based framework along with an up-to-date, research-based summary of each cause of hypercalcemia, my hope is that this text is useful for both the expert and student and that it leads to enhanced patient care.

New York, NY, USA   Marcella Donovan Walker

Contents

Contributors

Ejigayehu G. Abate Department of Internal Medicine and the Division of Endocrinology, Mayo Clinic, Jacksonville, FL, USA

Robert A. Adler Endocrinology and Metabolism Section, Central Virginia Veterans Affairs Health Care System, Richmond, VA, USA

Division of Endocrinology, Metabolism, and Diabetes Mellitus, Virginia Commonwealth University, Richmond, VA, USA

Divaya Bhutani Division of Hematology Oncology, Columbia University Irving Medical Center, New York, NY, USA

John P. Bilezikian Division of Endocrinology, Department of Medicine, Vagelos College of Physicians and Surgeons, Columbia University, New York, NY, USA

Maria Luisa Brandi F.I.R.M.O. Foundation, Florence, Italy

Angela L. Carrelli Division of Endocrinology, Columbia University Irving Medical Center, New York, NY, USA

Rajshekhar Chakraborty Division of Hematology Oncology, Columbia University Irving Medical Center, New York, NY, USA

Lena Fan Division of Endocrinology, Columbia University Irving Medical Center, New York, NY, USA

Azeez Farooki Division of Endocrinology, Memorial Sloan Kettering Cancer Center, New York, NY, USA

Abdallah S. Geara Renal, Electrolyte and Hypertension Division, University of Pennsylvania, Philadelphia, PA, USA

Hoang-Long C. Huynh Division of Endocrinology, Columbia University Irving Medical Center, New York, NY, USA

Ananya Kondapalli Division of Endocrinology, Department of Medicine, Columbia University Irving Medical Center, New York, NY, USA

Salila Kurra Division of Endocrinology, Department of Medicine, Columbia University Irving Medical Center, New York, NY, USA

Suzanne Lentzsch Division of Hematology Oncology, Columbia University Irving Medical Center, New York, NY, USA

Michael A. Levine Division of Endocrinology and Diabetes and the Center for Bone Health, The Children's Hospital of Philadelphia, Philadelphia, PA, USA

Department of Pediatrics, University of Pennsylvania Perelman School of Medicine, Philadelphia, PA, USA

Naim M. Maalouf Division of Endocrinology, Department of Internal Medicine and the Charles and Jane Pak Center of Mineral Metabolism and Clinical Research, University of Texas Southwestern Medical Center, Dallas, TX, USA

Alyyah Malick Columbia University, Vagelos College of Physicians and Surgeons, New York, NY, USA

Francesca Marini Department of Clinical and Experimental Biochemical Sciences, University of Florence, Florence, Italy

Hannah McMullen Columbia University, Vagelos College of Physicians and Surgeons, New York, NY, USA

Sajal Patel Endocrinology and Metabolism Section, Central Virginia Veterans Affairs Health Care System, Richmond, VA, USA

Division of Endocrinology, Metabolism, and Diabetes Mellitus, Virginia Commonwealth University, Richmond, VA, USA

Beatriz Martinez Quintero Endocrinology and Metabolism Section, Central Virginia Veterans Affairs Health Care System, Richmond, VA, USA

Division of Endocrinology, Metabolism, and Diabetes Mellitus, Virginia Commonwealth University, Richmond, VA, USA

Mishaela R. Rubin Metabolic Bone Disease Unit, Columbia University, New York, NY, USA

Elizabeth Shane Division of Endocrinology, Columbia University Irving Medical Center, New York, NY, USA

Susan Shey Division of Endocrinology and Metabolism, University of California, San Francisco, CA, USA

Dolores Shoback Division of Endocrinology and Metabolism, University of California, San Francisco, CA, USA

Endocrine Research Unit, Department of Veterans Affairs Medical Center, San Francisco, CA, USA

Shonni Silverberg Division of Endocrinology, Columbia University Irving Medical Center, New York, NY, USA

Li Song Division of Endocrinology, Department of Internal Medicine and the Charles and Jane Pak Center of Mineral Metabolism and Clinical Research, University of Texas Southwestern Medical Center, Dallas, TX, USA

Ryan Spiardi Renal, Electrolyte and Hypertension Division, University of Pennsylvania, Philadelphia, PA, USA

Marcella Donovan Walker Division of Endocrinology, Columbia University Irving Medical Center, New York, NY, USA

David R. Weber Division of Endocrinology and Diabetes and the Center for Bone Health, The Children's Hospital of Philadelphia, Philadelphia, PA, USA

Department of Pediatrics, University of Pennsylvania Perelman School of Medicine, Philadelphia, PA, USA

Robert A. Wermers Department of Internal Medicine and the Division of Endocrinology, Diabetes, Nutrition, and Metabolism, Mayo Clinic, Rochester, MN, USA

Mayo College of Medicine, Rochester, MN, USA

Chapter 1
Normal Regulation of Serum Calcium

Ryan Spiardi and Abdallah S. Geara

Abbreviations

1,25-OH VitD$_3$	1,25-dihydroxycholecalciferol
25-OH VitD$_3$	25-hydroxycholecalciferol
CaSR	calcium sensing receptor
CYP	cytochrome p450
dL	deciliter
eGFR	estimated glomerular filtration rate
FGF23	fibroblast growth factor 23
FGFR	fibroblast growth factor receptor
iPTH	intact PTH
kDa	kilodaltons
L	liter
meq	milliequivalent
mg	milligram
NaPi	sodium phosphate cotransport
NCX	sodium calcium exchanger
NKCC2	sodium potassium 2 chloride channel
PiT-2	inorganic phosphate transporter
PMCA1b	plasma membrane calcium ATPase
PTH	parathyroid hormone
PTHrP	parathyroid related protein

R. Spiardi · A. S. Geara (✉)
Renal, Electrolyte and Hypertension Division, University of Pennsylvania,
Philadelphia, PA, USA
e-mail: Ryan.Spiardi@Pennmedicine.upenn.edu; abdallah.geara@pennmedicine.upenn.edu

© The Author(s), under exclusive license to Springer Nature
Switzerland AG 2022
M. D. Walker (ed.), *Hypercalcemia*, Contemporary Endocrinology,
https://doi.org/10.1007/978-3-030-93182-7_1

RXR	retinoic X receptor
TRPV	transient receptor potential family, vanilloid subgroup
VDR	vitamin D receptor

Introduction

Calcium, a ubiquitous and primarily extracellular divalent cation, is integrally involved in a variety of physiologic processes. It is the most abundant mineral in the human body constituting 1 kg of the adult total body weight. Calcium plays an important role in muscular contraction of both smooth and skeletal muscle and perhaps most importantly in cardiac muscle. Additionally, calcium functions in the clotting cascade, mineralization of the skeleton, secretion of hormones, and nervous system impulse transmission. The regulation of the serum calcium level is tightly controlled by a variety of hormones and is closely linked to control of other ions such as magnesium and phosphorus [1].

Calcium Distribution

Calcium Distribution: Daily Homeostasis

Calcium takes different forms depending on its distribution throughout the body. Initially, calcium is ingested in the diet through a variety of calcium-rich foods. While dairy foods account for up to 75% of dietary calcium intake, calcium can also be found in fish, calcium-fortified food, or dark leafy greens. The bioavailability of dietary calcium varies depending on host factors such as individual health state, vitamin D status, and genetic polymorphisms of the vitamin D receptor (VDR). This can also vary based on different absorption patterns; for example, dark leafy greens not only are abundant in calcium but also contain oxalate and phytic acid, which bind calcium in the gut and prevent meaningful absorption.

On average, humans ingest approximately 1000 mg of calcium daily. Intestinal calcium absorption utilizes both vitamin D-dependent transcellular active transport in the duodenum and proximal jejunum and passive paracellular transport throughout the small intestine. Around 350–400 mg is absorbed by the gastrointestinal system, with assistance by active vitamin D. Since around 200 mg of calcium is shed in intestinal secretions daily, the net absorption is truly somewhere around 150–200 mg daily. Excretion of calcium takes place via feces (approximately 800 mg daily) and urine (approximately 200 mg daily) [2]. While endocrine negative feedback loops predominantly control the absorption of calcium, local factors and autocrine and paracrine mechanisms also play a role. Ingestion of glucose, galactose, and amino acids increases calcium absorption. Absorption is also upregulated in chronically low calcium diets. Conversely, iron and fructose, as well as high luminal calcium, can decrease calcium absorption [3].

Calcium Distribution: Extracellular and Intracellular Calcium Distribution

Once absorbed into the bloodstream, calcium can take several forms: protein-bound, nonprotein-bound, and free. While this calcium is tightly regulated and maintained, it is important to note that extracellular calcium represents approximately 0.1% of all calcium stores in the body. The cytoplasmic calcium concentration is several magnitudes lower than extracellular calcium concentration, but notably, the concentrations inside specific intracellular organelles such as mitochondria and the endoplasmic reticulum is high. In total, intracellular calcium constitutes about 1% of total body calcium. Protein-bound calcium in serum is predominantly complexed with albumin, a 66.5 kDa plasma protein with remarkable capacity for binding and buffering; each molecule of albumin has ~30 calcium binding sites [4]. This form represents anywhere from 41% to 46% of total serum calcium [1, 2]. While albumin is the most dominant plasma protein capable of binding calcium, this does also occur with other globulins. This form of calcium, much like most of the proteins they are bound to, is typically not freely filtered by the renal glomerulus.

Nonprotein bound calcium in the serum represents 7–9% of all serum calcium and is usually complexed with anions, such as citrate and phosphate [1, 2]. Since this calcium is not protein-bound, it can be freely filtered by the kidney.

A final fate of calcium in the blood is free or ionized calcium. "Ionized" is technically incorrect, given all calcium within the body is ionized, and the more correct term is "free" calcium [5]. However, "ionized" is still widely used by clinicians and laboratories alike. Regardless, this calcium is free within the serum and can freely diffuse across cell membranes. This is the largest proportion of calcium in the serum, representing somewhere between approximately 48% and 50% of all serum calcium [1, 2].

When measuring serum calcium, the total serum calcium is reported by laboratories – this includes all free or ionized calcium and protein-bound and complexed calcium. Depending on the laboratory, the typical normal level for serum total calcium level is 8.5–10.5 mg/dL. Of greater physiologic importance, however, is free "ionized" calcium level. As noted above, free calcium can be altered by the ability of plasma proteins, predominantly albumin, to bind calcium. Further, the ability of albumin to bind calcium can be influenced by pH or other drug binding. Since hydrogen ions are also bound to albumin, when abundant, as with lower pH, the affinity to bind free calcium is lower, thus increasing the fraction of ionized calcium. The converse is also true. With alkalemia, less hydrogen ions are bound to albumin, increasing affinity for free calcium and therefore lowering the fraction of free calcium. This scenario with alkalemia can lead to life-threatening hypocalcemia, if prolonged or severe.

One strategy to more accurately estimate serum calcium is by "correcting" serum total calcium levels for serum albumin levels. This practice is based on the assumption that albumin binds calcium in a fixed manner when serum pH is normal – when albumin levels are lower, the total calcium as measured by the lab is underestimated due to reduced total calcium that is bound to albumin. To correct this, we often use the formula below:

$$\text{Corrected calcium} = \text{measured serum total calcium} + 0.8\left[4 - \text{albumin in g / dL}\right]$$

Another strategy for more accurate assessment of free, physiologically active calcium is the direct measurement of ionized calcium by the laboratory. The typical normal value for free "ionized" calcium is around 1.2 mmol/L, or 2.4 meq/L [1].

Calcium Distribution: Bone Is the Main Body Reservoir for Calcium

The main reservoirs for calcium in the human body are bones and teeth, comprising an estimated 99% of total body calcium [1, 2]. To understand calcium homeostasis and metabolism in the bone, first it is important to understand the basics surrounding bone structure. Human bones are predominantly composed of a matrix and organic calcium salts. Within the matrix is collagen, important for tensile strength, and ground substance, which is a combination of chondroitin sulfate and hyaluronic acid that is secreted by osteoblasts. Interspersed with matrix are the calcium salts – these can either be crystalline or amorphous. The amorphous salts comprise approximately 1% of all salts in bone and represent an easily "digestible" portion of calcium to quickly be released to the serum to maintain a tight physiologic range of calcium. The crystalline portion, however, represents a much larger proportion, approximately 99%. This is hydroxyapatite, represented by the chemical formula $Ca_{10}(PO_4)_6(OH)_2$ [1]. Figure 1.1 summarizes the calcium distribution across the different compartments.

Hormonal Calcium Regulation

As mentioned earlier, blood calcium level is very tightly regulated in the range of 8.5–10.5 mg/dL, depending on individual laboratories. This complex interplay involves a variety of hormones and electrolytes including parathyroid hormone (PTH), calcitonin, vitamin D, phosphorus, magnesium, and fibroblast growth factor 23 (FGF23). The major factors are summarized in Table 1.1.

Parathyroid Hormone

Parathyroid hormone (PTH) is an 84 amino acid polypeptide hormone that serves as the major regulator of free calcium in the blood. This is released from the chief cells of parathyroid glands – four almond-shaped glands on the posterior aspect of the

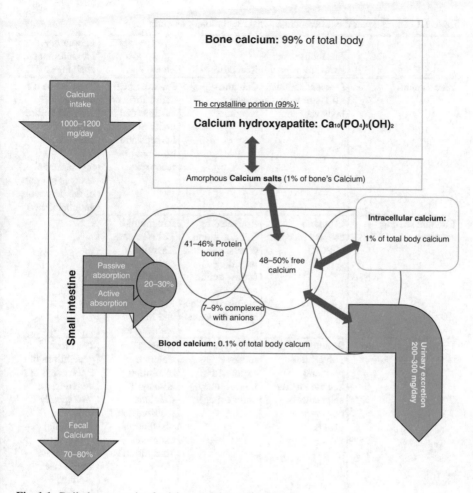

Bone calcium: 99% of total body

The crystalline portion (99%):

Calcium hydroxyapatite: Ca₁₀(PO₄)₆(OH)₂

Amorphous **Calcium salts** (1% of bone's Calcium)

Calcium intake

1000–1200 mg/day

Intracellular calcium:

1% of total body calcium

41–46% Protein bound

48–50% free calcium

Passive absorption

20–30%

Active absorption

Small intestine

7–9% complexed with anions

Blood calcium: 0.1% of total body calcum

Fecal Calcium

70–80%

Urinary excretion 200–300 mg/day

Fig. 1.1 Daily homeostasis of calcium and tissue distribution

thyroid gland. PTH release functions in a negative feedback manner, whereas lower calcium level stimulates PTH release, which is more vigorous during sudden drops in serum calcium [6]. PTH binds to the PTH receptor, a G-protein-coupled receptor that signals through both adenylate cyclase and phospholipase C. This binding predominantly occurs through the N-terminus, with high affinity for the receptor in the first 34 amino acids of the PTH molecule. Within minutes of PTH binding to its receptor, the receptor is desensitized, and the receptor is internalized [7].

The extracellular calcium-sensing receptor (CaSR) acts as a free calcium sensor and is expressed in a multitude of tissues. Its expression at the level of the parathyroid cells, C cells of the thyroid, and in the thick ascending limb of the kidney allows the CaSR to play a central role in calcium homeostasis. Other divalent cations are potential receptor agonists for CaSR, notably magnesium. In the parathyroid gland, elevated levels of free calcium activate intracellular pathways leading to

Table 1.1 Summary of the different hormonal regulation of calcium

	Metabolism and structure	Receptor	Functions	Laboratory measurement challenges
Free calcium	Divalent cation <0.1% of total body calcium	Calcium-sensing receptors	Physiological active form of calcium that is under different homeostatic hormonal feedback	The sample can undergo pH changes before iCa measurement iCa measurement assay is not part of the laboratory automated line
Calcium sensing receptor	G protein–coupled receptor (GPCR)	Activated by free Ca2+ and other cations including Mg2+, amino acids, aminoglycoside and polyamines	Parathyroid: ↓PTH release Thyroid C cells: ↑calcitonin release Kidney: ↓Ca and Mg reabsorption	
Parathyroid hormone	84 amino acid polypeptide hormone Secreted by the chief cells of parathyroid glands	PTH type 1 receptor expressed in bone, kidney and cartilages	Bone: ↑ Calcium resorption Kidney: ↑ Calcium reabsorption, ↑ phosphorus excretion, ↑ 1α-hydroxylase	The recent generations of PTH assays are targeting the biologically active N-terminal epitope Variation in assays can produce interlaboratory variation
1,25-dihydroxyvitamin D	Liver: 25-hydroxylation Kidney: 1-hydroxylation	Nuclear receptor VDR/RXR	Intestine: ↑calcium absorption Kidney: ↑ calcium reabsorption Bone: Resorption or mineralization depending on the calcium balance, ↑ FGF23 expression by osteocytes (extraskeletal effects in immunity and carcinogenesis)	1,25-OH VitD3 is normal to elevated in hypovitaminosis D 25-OH VitD3 used to assess vitamin D status

Table 1.1 (continued)

	Metabolism and structure	Receptor	Functions	Laboratory measurement challenges
Calcitonin	Peptide secreted by parathyroid C-cells		Bone: ↓ osteoclastic activity Kidney: ↓ calcium reabsoprtion	Calcitonin levels are measured in the assessment of thyroid nodule to screen for medullary thyroid cancer

inhibition of PTH release and PTH-gene expression. At the level of the thyroid C cells, activation of the CaSR leads to exocytosis of calcitonin. In the kidney, the best known function of CaSR is at the level of the thick ascending loop of Henle, where activation of CaSR decreases reabsorption of both calcium and magnesium.

In the circulation, in addition to the 84-amino acid peptide intact form, several fragments of the hormone are present. The inactive C-terminal region of PTH is also present, which has a longer half-life, especially in the setting of kidney disease. The half-life of intact PTH (iPTH) is between 2 and 4 minutes. The laboratory measurements of PTH have undergone several improvements, with the more recent generations of PTH assays being directed against the biologically active N-terminal end. Thus, it is, in theory, important when comparing PTH levels to use the same assay every time as these can vary between labs. Today, most commercial labs employ the second generation iPTH assay. This assay measures the whole molecule (PTH 1–84) and larger fragments (example PTH 7–84). Whole PTH assays, which measure PTH 1–84 exclusively, are available but less commonly used.

PTH has a multitude of functions to raise a decreased serum calcium level back to a physiologic range: first, it acts on bone to stimulate secretion of citric and lactic acid from osteoclasts to help dissolve bone calcium salts, which serve as an immediate source of calcium to release into the bloodstream. It also stimulates preosteo-clastic differentiation and downregulates osteoprotegerin, an inhibitor that usually serves to prevent bone dissolution [1]. Both of these actions promote further bone dissolution to release calcium salts in the blood. Longer-term solutions to increase serum calcium are achieved by PTH actions in the kidney. Here, PTH acts to [1] increase 1-alpha hydroxylase activity in proximal tubule cells and enhance activation of vitamin D to secondarily increase calcium absorption in the gastrointestinal tract and [2] increase calcium absorption within the kidney primarily in the proximal tubule and thick ascending limb of Henle [2]. PTH secretion is also enhanced by dopamine, catecholamines, and prostaglandin E_2 [2]. Severe hypomagnesemia (<0.8 meq/L) is associated with hypoparathyroidism through inhibition of release of PTH from the parathyroid gland and inhibition of its action on target organs.

Vitamin D

Acting in concert with PTH, vitamin D is a hormone that plays an integral role in the regulation of serum calcium. 1,25-dihydroxycholecalciferol, or active vitamin D, is needed for active physiological effects on calcium levels. Vitamin D is a cholesterol-based hormone that can either be activated in the skin from ultraviolet (UV) light, or ingested in multiple forms in the diet. In the skin, 7-dehydrocholesterol is converted to cholecalciferol (vitamin D_3), a reaction that is catalyzed by UVB rays. Vitamin D can also be ingested in the diet, either in plant form (ergocalciferol, vitamin D_2) or in animal form (cholecalciferol). From there, inactive vitamin D is bound to its binding protein (vitamin D binding protein) in the blood and carried to the liver for the first of several hydroxylation reactions – this first hydroxylation, by many cytochrome P-450 enzymes (CYPs) including CYP2R1, CYP27A1, and CYP2D25, forms 25-hydroxyvitamin D_3 (25-OH VitD_3 or 25-hydroxycholecalciferol) [9, 18]. 25-OH VitD_3 is the major circulating form of vitamin D and is measured clinically as a biomarker of the vitamin D status. 25-OH VitD_3 is transported next to the kidney where the 1-α-hydroxylase catalyzes the second hydroxylation, forming 1,25-dihydroxyvitamin D (1,25-OH VitD_3 or 1,25-dihydroxycholecalciferol) in the proximal tubule, which is considered the physiologically active form of vitamin D. The uptake of 25-OH VitD_3 by the renal tubules utilizes megalin-assisted endocytic internalization [18].

1,25-OH VitD_3 has an intranuclear receptor, VDR, and forms a 1,25-OH VitD_3-activated vitamin D receptor/retinoic X receptor (VDR/RXR) heterodimeric complex in cellular nuclei. The VDR/RXR complex binds to multiple sequences of DNA to either facilitate or suppress expression of vitamin D target genes [18]. 1,25-OH VitD_3 is the active form of vitamin D and can act on the gut to increase calcium absorption along the gastrointestinal tract and increase calcium reabsorption in the kidney. At the level of the bone, 1,25-OH VitD_3 accelerates bone resorption when the patient is in a negative calcium balance. Active vitamin D's role to achieve a positive calcium balance is not clear, but it is thought to act as a facilitator for bone mineralization.

In a negative feedback fashion, increasing levels of 1,25-OH VitD_3 decrease 1-alpha hydroxylase activity and increase 24-alpha hydroxylase activity, which in turn catalyzes the reaction to 24,25-hydroxyvitamin D_3, an inactive metabolite [2]. 1,25-OH VitD_3 increases expression of FGF23 by osteocytes, leading to an increase in phosphaturia and suppression of PTH secretion at the level of the parathyroid gland. Measurement of serum 1,25-OH VitD_3 does not correlate with vitamin D status since hypovitaminosis D leads to a secondary hyperparathyroidism, thereby increasing 1-α-hydroxylation and subsequently normal levels of 1,25-OH VitD_3.

Calcitonin

In contrast to PTH, calcitonin is a hormone released from the C cells of the thyroid in response to elevated serum calcium levels [6]. Calcitonin has actions both in the bone and kidney to assert its effects on calcium. In the bone, calcitonin exerts swift action to decrease osteoclastic activity and differentiation [6]. This leads to reduced breakdown of bone matrix and reduced release of calcium into the bloodstream [8]. In the kidney, calcitonin is thought to act in both the proximal tubule and thick ascending limb of Henle to reduce calcium reabsorption via active, transcellular mechanisms [2]. The physiological role of calcitonin in normal calcium homeostasis, however, remains unclear as "calcitonin deficiency" in patients who have had a total thyroidectomy does not affect serum calcium.

PTH-Related Peptide

PTH-related peptide, or PTHrP, was initially discovered in relation to hypercalcemia of malignancy and is encoded on chromosome 12. The amino termini of PTH and PTHrP share 8 of 13 of the same amino acids and likely explains its ability to bind to the PTH receptor and exert similar physiologic actions as PTH. Under normal physiologic conditions, PTHrP is described to function in cell growth. In pathologic processes, such as cancers of the upper gastrointestinal tract, head and neck, lymphomas, and female reproductive system, PTHrP can act as an agonist on the PTH receptor and produce hypercalcemia that is not regulated via a negative feedback mechanism [17].

Phosphorus Regulation

Phosphorus plays an important role in energy metabolism throughout the body, and its regulation and homeostatic mechanisms are intimately intertwined with calcium metabolism. Phosphorus is involved in energy production through adenosine triphosphate generation, cell membrane integrity, buffering, transcriptive processes, and cellular signaling [2, 10, 11]. The intake of phosphorus can be via inorganic phosphate or organic phosphate. Inorganic sources tend to be those with additives or preservatives and are much more readily absorbed. Conversely, organic phosphates come primarily from dairy or meat sources and are less readily absorbed [11]. Depending on diet, daily phosphorus intake ranges between 700 and 2000 mg, with absorption varying depending on intake level and source [2, 11]. Phosphorus in plasma can either be in the form of esters, phospholipids, or inorganic phosphate. Inorganic phosphate is the commonly measured laboratory value, with normal laboratory values ranging between 2.5 and 4.0 mg/dL. This represents the circulating ionized phosphate, which can either be HPO_4^{2-} or $H_2PO_4^-$, which is present at 4:1 ratio in serum when pH is in the normal physiologic range [12]. Despite clinical measurement of extracellular phosphate, this represents less than 1% of total body phosphorus, whereas most of this resides in the skeleton in the form of hydroxyapatite [2, 10].

Similarly to calcium, phosphorus regulation is an interplay between the gastrointestinal system, bone, and kidney and is regulated via negative feedback mechanisms and under hormonal control. As mentioned, phosphorus absorption in the gut is dependent on the form ingested, as well as 1,25-OH VitD$_3$ level, which upregulates phosphorus absorption here. This primarily occurs in the duodenum and jejunum, through sodium-phosphate cotransport type 2b (NaPi 2b), similar to type 2a and type 2c found in the kidney, with additional passive transport occurring paracellularly [2, 9].

The kidney is the primary regulator of serum phosphorus level in the body. Given its low molecular weight, phosphorus is freely filtered at the glomerulus and reabsorbed primarily in the proximal tubule. There are several transporters involved in phosphorus reabsorption here: NaPi 2a (exchanges three sodium for one divalent phosphate/HPO$_4{}^{2-}$), NaPi 2c (exchanges two sodium for one divalent phosphate/HPO$_4{}^{2-}$), and PiT-2 (exchanges two sodium for one monovalent phosphate/H$_2$PO$_4{}^{-}$). All transporters in the proximal tubule require two conditions for transport: energy and sodium. Transporters and subsequently renal phosphorus handling are affected by a variety of hormones and physiologic conditions. For example, 1,25-OH VitD$_3$, metabolic alkalosis, and triiodothyronine all increase phosphate reabsorption in the proximal tubule. PTH, estrogen, dopamine, metabolic acidosis, glucocorticoids, and acute episodes of hypertension all increase phosphate wasting in the proximal tubule [2]. The most prominent hormone involved in phosphorus regulation, however, is fibroblast growth factor 23, or FGF23.

Fibroblast Growth Factor 23 (FGF23)

FGF23 is a 32 kDa glycoprotein secreted by osteocytes and osteoblasts in response to changes of phosphorus intake; it is a central hormone in maintaining phosphorus homeostasis. In healthy human subjects with phosphorus serum levels within the physiologic range, FGF23 serum concentration varies in response to changes of dietary phosphorus intake. FGF receptors (FGFR1–4) are FGF23 receptors and are ubiquitously expressed on different tissues. The extra-skeletal role of FGF23 is poorly understood; it is believed that FGF23's main physiologic role is phosphorus regulation in the kidney and the bone. In addition to FGFR in target organs, the membrane coexpression of the protease α-klotho determines the effect of FGF23 on target organs. A deficiency of α-klotho will present with a phenotype similar to FGF23 deficiency.

In the kidney, FGF23/Klotho complexes with the FGFR to produce a phosphaturic effect by decreasing expression of NaPi 2a and NaPi 2c in the proximal tubular cells and thus inhibition of phosphorus reabsorption. A secondary effect of FGF23/Klotho complex is to decrease 1-alpha hydroxylase activity, thereby decreasing the formation of active vitamin D [13]. The FGF23 hormonal axis is of particular importance and interest in bone mineral metabolism in chronic kidney disease. As glomerular filtration rate decreases, (Fig. 1.2) the total nephron mass decreases, but

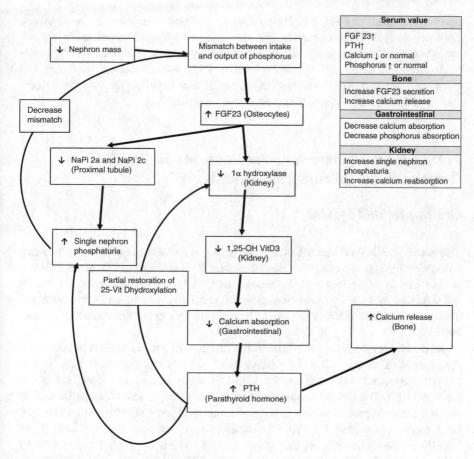

Fig. 1.2 Adaptive response to kidney disease

the kidney's ability to maintain phosphorus homeostasis is restored by the increase in secretion of FGF23 by bone and consequent increase in single nephron phosphaturia. This is an adaptive mechanism to restore phosphorus homeostasis and match the total intake of phosphorus to the output of phosphorus in early stages of kidney disease. This compensatory mechanism, however, will be overwhelmed in late stages of kidney disease.

An additional effect of the high circulating levels of FGF23 in chronic kidney disease is the reduction of 1-α hydroxylase activity and thus decreased conversion of 25-OH VitD$_3$ to 1,25-OH VitD$_3$. A low 1,25-OH VitD$_3$ state leads to decreased serum calcium levels by reduction of gastrointestinal absorption and secondary hyperparathyroidism. The net result is restoration of phosphorus level by: (a) increased phosphaturia mediated by both high level of PTH and FGF23 and (b) decreased absorption of phosphorus mediated by low 1,25-OH VitD$_3$. The hypocalcemia induced by reduced gastrointestinal absorption is combated by PTH-mediated increased calcium release from bone. However, with chronic kidney disease, bone becomes resistant to PTH, and higher levels are required to have the same effect. This vicious cycle continues as chronic kidney disease progresses and leads to commonly seen lab parameters with advanced kidney disease, including rising phosphate, hypocalcemia, and grossly elevated PTH levels. Recent literature has associated elevated FGF23 levels with left ventricular hypertrophy, vascular calcification, and both cardiovascular and all-cause mortality [14].

Putting It All Together: The Feedback Mechanisms Responsible for Calcium Homeostasis

Gastrointestinal System

The gastrointestinal system maintains calcium and phosphorus balance by primary absorption through the diet, which is altered by PTH and vitamin D. Here, calcium is absorbed by two primary mechanisms: paracellularly via tight junctions, which are regulated by a family of membrane proteins called claudins, and transcellularly. The process across the cell is similar in both the gut epithelium and renal tubular cells.

Regarding paracellular mechanisms, the driving force is via electrochemical gradients, with calcium moving in a passive mechanism across tight junctions. This is partially regulated and increased by 1,25-OH VitD$_3$ and occurs along the entire intestinal tract. The active transport mechanism that occurs across epithelial cells is much more intricate and occurs in the duodenum and jejunum primarily. Here, cellular entry is mediated by TRPV5 (transient receptor potential vanilloid 5) or TRVP6 calcium channels on the apical surface, which are highly influenced by active vitamin D levels to increase cellular entry. Most studies show that TRPV6 is predominantly expressed in the duodenum and jejunum [15]. After cellular entry, calcium ions need to be shuttled to the basal membrane. Calcium ions can be bound to calcium-binding proteins, called calbindin, or encapsulated in vesicles to be transported throughout the cytosol. Prior to vesicular transport, calcium binds with calmodulin, a protein associated with myosin. Once bound, calcium is packaged within vesicles and moved through the cytosol via a microtubular network. Activated vitamin D also increases nuclear synthesis of calmodulin to help increase cellular transport. Once reaching the basal aspect of the cell, calcium is extruded either via the NCX1 (sodium-calcium exchanger) or an ATP-dependent exchanger, PMCA1b. The NCX1 exchanger moves three sodium molecules intracellularly in exchange for extrusion of one calcium molecule [2, 15]. Similar to calcium absorption, phosphate is absorbed to the greatest extent in the duodenum and jejunum. As previously mentioned, this is regulated by NaPi 2b transporters in a transcellular fashion, which are upregulated by both increased active vitamin D levels and increased phosphate ingestion [2].

Kidneys

The kidneys play a crucial role in reabsorption of both calcium and phosphorus along the length of the tubule (Table 1.2). Here, approximately 8 g of calcium are filtered daily, with over 98% reabsorbed from the filtrate. As with phosphorus, the majority of calcium is reabsorbed in the proximal tubule and is estimated to account for around 70% of total reabsorbed calcium. The majority of this is a passive, paracellular mechanism, although some may occur via transcellular mechanism with similar cellular mechanics as described in the bowel. PTH has an effect on the proximal tubule to increase calcium reabsorption here.

Moving along the nephron, it should be noted that there is no meaningful calcium reabsorption along the descending or thin ascending loop of Henle. At the thick ascending loop of Henle, calcium reabsorption begins again – this accounts for about 20% of calcium reabsorption total and is primarily paracellular. An important consideration here is the development of an electrochemical gradient across the

Table 1.2 Calcium and phosphorus transport in the different kidney segments

	Calcium		Phosphorus	
	Transport/transporters	Regulatory factors	Transport/ transporters	Regulatory factors
Glomerulus	Free "ionized" calcium and other calcium-containing salts are freely filtered		Serum inorganic phosphorus (iP) is freely filtered	
Proximal tubule	Reabsorbs 60–70% of filtered calcium Passive paracellular transport	Follows sodium reabsorption PTH inhibits Na+/H+ exchanger	80% of filtered iP is reabsorbed Active transcellular using NaPi 2a and 2c for HPO$_4^{2-}$, PiT-2 for H2PO$_4^-$	Follows sodium reabsorption 1,25-OH VitD3 ↑phosphate reabsorption PTH ↓phosphate reabsorption FGF23 ↓phosphate reabsorption
Thick ascending limb of the loop of Henle	Reabsorbs 15% of filtered calcium	Passive paracellular CaSR when activated inhibits calcium reabsorption		
Distal convoluted tubule and connecting tubules	10–15% of reabsorption TRPV5, TRPV6 are calcium channels on the apical membrane regulating active transcellular transport	Active transcellular Main sites of PTH and 1,25-OH VitD3 action	80% of filtered iP is reabsorbed Active transcellular	

tubule toward the interstitium by the sodium potassium 2-chloride channel (NKCC2) and the renal outer medullary potassium (ROMK) channel. The NKCC2 channel, a target of loop diuretics, functions to reabsorb one sodium, one potassium, and two chloride ions. In isolation, this would be considered electroneutral. However, the ROMK channel is an outwardly rectifying potassium channel that allows one potassium ion to pass back into the lumen. This creates an overall positive charge luminally, with a negative charge across the cellular membrane to the interstitium. This generation of electrochemical gradient drives positively charged ion reabsorption, namely calcium and magnesium, via a paracellular route. Regulation here is augmented by the CaSR, which is found on the basolateral membrane. With increasing calcium level on the basolateral side, the calcium and magnesium reabsorption is slowed in the thick ascending limb by modulating claudin expression in the tight junctions [2, 15]. PTH can act here as well to increase absorption transcellularly, similar to actions in the proximal tubule.

The distal tubule and collecting duct, however, primarily regulate calcium reabsorption via the active, transcellular pathway and account for about 15% of total reabsoprtion [15]. Here, the active transport replicates the same process as seen in epithelial cells in the bowel. Again, the active apical transporter is of the TRPV family, predominantly TRPV5, which transports calcium against its electrochemical gradient and is activated by Klotho. Similar cystosolic transport occurs, and the NCX1 and ATP-dependent calcium channels exist on the basolateral membrane to extrude calcium from the tubular cell into the blood. TRPV5 and TRPV6 both increase activity with stimulation via active vitamin D and PTH, thereby increasing calcium transport across the cellular gradient [15, 16]. Additionally, active vitamin D, as in the bowel, increases replication of transport mechanisms in the cytosol to increase calcium transport capacity [12, 15].

Case 1

A 45-year-old woman with Crohn's disease presents for persistent diarrhea. Her evaluation shows signs of volume depletion with orthostatic hypotension and acute renal failure on initial laboratory evaluation.

Labs: Sodium 135 mEq/L; potassium 5.3 mEq/L; chloride 118 mEq/L; bicarbonate 7 mEq/L; creatinine 2.0 mg/dL; total calcium 6.8 mg/dL; and albumin 3.0 g/dL. The patient has acidosis with serum pH of 7.2.

When approaching this patient, the first step is assessing the calcium level corrected for albumin. This can be done using the following formula:

$$\text{Corrected calcium} = \text{measured serum total calcium}$$
$$+ 0.8\left[4 - \text{albumin in g / dL}\right]$$

The patient's total corrected serum calcium is 7.6 mg/dL, which is still below the normal range of 8.5–10.5 mg/dL. There are likely to be several compensatory mechanisms at play to counteract the hypocalcemia. The etiology of low calcium could be decreased intake of calcium due to illness but is more likely secondary to chronic malabsorption and steatorrhea leading to vitamin D deficiency and decreased intestinal absorption. We would expect an elevated PTH that would act to (1) increase osteoclastic activity in the skeleton to release physiologically active calcium, (2) increase calcium reabsorption in the proximal tubule and thick ascending limb of the nephron, and (3) increase 1-alpha hydroxylase activity in the proximal tubule to increase conversion of 25-OH VitD$_3$ to 1,25-OH VitD$_3$.

Since the patient is acidotic (normal anion gap metabolic acidosis), volume expansion with bicarbonate containing solution will be required to replete the excessive bicarbonate loss from the diarrhea. One should, however, be very careful when correcting this patient's acidosis with bicarbonate solution since the alkali therapy will free the negatively charged albumin leading to an increase of calcium binding to albumin. The patient's total calcium will not be affected, but the free calcium will decrease. Since it is the physiologically active form of calcium, the patient will become symptomatic.

Case 2

A 54-year-old male patient with chronic kidney disease stage 3b (eGFR of 42 ml/min/1.73m [2]) presents with the following labs: total calcium: 8.7 mg/dL; phosphorus 4.9; and albumin of 4.0 g/dL.

Assume the patient eats a nonrenal diet with daily intake of calcium of 1200 mg per day and daily phosphorus intake of 1600 mg. This patient has lost more than 50% of the nephron function, and since the patient did not modify his intake of phosphorus, he will need to increase the single nephron phosphaturia to restore phosphorus homeostasis. The main hormonal regulator of serum phosphorus level is FGF-23. With a mismatch between intake and output of phosphorus, FGF-23 is elevated, which increases phosphaturia by reducing NaPi 2a and NaPi 2c transporter expression in the proximal tubule in the kidney. Additionally, FGF-23 decreases 1-alpha hydroxylase activity, decreases conversion of 25-OH VitD$_3$ to 1,25-OH VitD$_3$, and reduces phosphate absorption in the gut primarily by reducing NaPi 2b transporters. This has an additional consequence of decreasing calcium absorption in the gut. Finally, FGF23 increases 24-alpha hydroxylase activity to increase conversion within the kidney to the inactive vitamin D metabolite, 24,25-OH vitamin D (Fig. 1.2).

Case 3

A 76-year-old woman presents to the hospital with muscle cramps, fatigue, and mild dyspnea. Her serum phosphorus is 1.5 mg/dL. Her medical team believes that the cause of her hypophosphatemia is due to reduced intake; this is verified by a low fractional excretion of phosphate, calculated at 3%.

There are several hormonal mechanisms that reduce urinary phosphate excretion in this setting. In the case of reduced phosphorus in diet, both FGF23 and PTH are downregulated. The reduction of FGF23 will increase NaPi 2a and NaPi 2c transporters in the luminal surface of the tubular cells in the proximal tubule, increase phosphorus reabsorption in the proximal tubule, and therefore reduce phosphorus excretion in the urine. This mechanism, however, is usually quite effective at preventing profound hypophosphatemia, and other causes should be examined in this patient.

References

1. Hall JE, Guyton A. Guyton and hall textbook of medical physiology. Philadelphia: Saunders/Elsevier; 2011.
2. Blaine J, Chonchol M, Levi M. Renal control of calcium, phosphate, and magnesium homeostasis. Clin J Am Soc Nephrol. 2014;10(7):1257–72. https://doi.org/10.2215/cjn.09750913.
3. Wongdee K, Rodrat M, Teerapornpuntakit J, Krishnamra N, Charoenphandhu N. Factors inhibiting intestinal calcium absorption: hormones and luminal factors that prevent excessive calcium uptake. J Physiol Sci. 2019;69(5):683–96. https://doi.org/10.1007/s12576-019-00688-3.
4. Rabbani G, Ahn S. Structure, enzymatic activities, glycation and therapeutic potential of human serum albumin: A natural cargo. Int J Biol Macromol. 2019;123:979–90. https://doi.org/10.1016/j.ijbiomac.2018.11.053.
5. Baird GS. Ionized calcium. Clinica Chimica Acta. 2011;412(9–10):696–701. https://doi.org/10.1016/j.cca.2011.01.004.
6. F, Demay M, Kronenberg H. Williams textbook of endocrinology. 17th ed. Philadelpha: Elsevier; 2020. p. 1196–1255.
7. Gardella TJ, Jüppner H. Molecular properties of the PTH/PTHrP receptor. Trends Endocrinol Metab. 2001;12(5):210–7. https://doi.org/10.1016/s1043-2760(01)00409-x.
8. Naot D, Musson D, Cornish J. The activity of peptides of the calcitonin family in bone. Physiol Rev. 2019;99(1):781–805. https://doi.org/10.1152/physrev.00066.2017.
9. Yu ASL, Chertow G, Luyckx V, Marsden P, Skorecki K, Taal M. Brenner & Rector's the kidney. 11th ed. Philadelphia: Elsevier. p. 1805–37.
10. Berndt T, Kumar R. Novel mechanisms in the regulation of phosphorus homeostasis. Physiology. 2009;24(1):17–25. https://doi.org/10.1152/physiol.00034.2008.
11. Calvo MS, Lamberg-Allardt C. Phosphorus. Adv Nutr. 2015;6(6):860–2. https://doi.org/10.3945/an.115.008516.
12. Rose BD, Post T. Clinical physiology of acid-base and electrolyte disorders. New York: McGraw Hill Professional; 2011.
13. Jüppner H. Phosphate and FGF-23. Kidney Int. 2011;79(Suppl 121):S24–7.
14. Batra J, Buttar R, Kaur P, Kreimerman J, Melamed M. FGF-23 and cardiovascular disease. Curr Opin Endocrinol Diabet Obesity. 2016;23(6):423–9. https://doi.org/10.1097/med.0000000000000294.

15. Hoenderop JGJ, Nilius B, Bindels R. Calcium absorption across epithelia. Physiol Rev. 2005;85(1):373–422. https://doi.org/10.1152/physrev.00003.2004.
16. Subramanya AR, Ellison DH. Distal convoluted tubule. Clin J Am Soc Nephrol. 2014;9(12):2147–63. https://doi.org/10.2215/cjn.05920613.
17. D. *Endotext*. South Dartmouth: MDText.com, Inc; 2019.
18. Dhawan S, Dhawan P, Verstuyf A, Verlinden L, Carmeliet G. Vitamin D: metabolism, molecular mechanism of action, and pleiotropic effects. Physiol Rev. 2016;96(1):365–408. https://doi.org/10.1152/physrev.00014.2015.

Chapter 2
Pathophysiology, Causes, and Clinical Manifestations of Hypercalcemia

Mishaela R. Rubin

Introduction

The ionized calcium concentration is maintained within a tight range in the extracellular fluid. This regulation is critical because of the key role that calcium plays in multiple cellular functions, particularly those involved in protein secretion, muscle contraction, neuronal excitability, and signal transduction. In the blood, total calcium concentration is normally approximately 8.5–10.5 mg/dL (2.2–2.6 mmol/L), of which approximately 45% is ionized and biologically functional. The remaining 45% is bound ionically to negatively charged proteins (principally albumin and immunoglobulins) in a pH-dependent manner, while 10% is loosely complexed with phosphate, carbonate, citrate, sulfate, or other anions [1].

Prior to commencing a diagnostic evaluation, the presence of true hypercalcemia and not a false-positive laboratory test should be confirmed. A false-positive diagnosis of hypercalcemia is usually the result of unintended hemoconcentration during blood collection or an elevation in albumin. Changes in serum albumin concentration directly affect the total blood calcium concentration even if the ionized calcium concentration remains normal. As a result, the total serum calcium concentration will change correspondingly with the albumin concentration and may not correctly reflect the physiologically active ionized calcium concentration. A calculation to correct for protein adjusts the total serum calcium (in mg/dL) upward by 0.8 times the deficit in serum albumin (g/dL) or by 0.5 times the deficit in serum immunoglobulin (in g/dL). However, such corrections provide only approximations of actual free calcium concentrations and may be unreliable, particularly during acute illness. Notably, acidosis alters ionized calcium by reducing its association with proteins.

M. R. Rubin (✉)
Metabolic Bone Disease Unit, Columbia University, New York, NY, USA
e-mail: Mrr6@columbia.edu

© The Author(s), under exclusive license to Springer Nature Switzerland AG 2022
M. D. Walker (ed.), *Hypercalcemia*, Contemporary Endocrinology, https://doi.org/10.1007/978-3-030-93182-7_2

Hypercalcemia is a fairly common clinical problem. Persistent hypercalcemia has been reported to occur in up to 1% of individuals in the general population [2]. It is defined as a serum calcium greater than two standard deviations above the normal mean in a given laboratory, frequently 10.6 mg/dl (2.65 mmol/L) for total serum calcium and 1.25 mmol/L for ionized serum calcium. There is no recognized grading scale for defining the severity of hypercalcemia. Nevertheless, serum calcium concentrations less than 12 mg/dl (3.00 mmol/L) can be categorized as mild, those between 12 and 14 mg/dl (3.00–3.50 mmol/L) as moderate, and those above 14 mg/dl (3.50 mmol/L) as severe.

Calcium Homeostasis: Roles of the Skeleton, Intestine, and Kidney

While an in-depth description of normal calcium regulation is provided in Chap. 1, this chapter provides a brief overview of the salient mechanisms. As noted, the serum calcium concentration is tightly regulated by the flux of serum ionized calcium to and from three physiologic compartments: the skeleton, intestine, and kidney.

Skeleton

The skeleton is a storage site of about 1–2 kg of Ca or 99% of the calcium normally present in the adult human. Generally, in the setting of normal bone turnover, roughly 500 mg of Ca is released daily from bone, and a comparable amount is accreted each day. The high daily rates of similar fluxes of calcium out of and into bone (~250–500 mg each) are mediated by coupled osteoclastic and osteoblastic activity. An additional 1% of skeletal calcium is in chemical equilibrium with the calcium in the extracellular fluid. The skeleton is thus a major reservoir for extracellular fluid calcium concentration.

Intestine

Typical dietary calcium intake in the United States fluctuates widely, ranging from 400 to 1500 mg per day. A National Academy of Medicine analysis endorses a daily allowance of 1000–1200 mg for most adults [3]. As described in Chap. 1, intestinal absorption of calcium involves both active and passive pathways. Passive calcium absorption is not saturable and approaches 5% of daily calcium intake, while active absorption typically ranges from 20% to 70%, occurring with calcium entry via ion channels controlled by 1,25-dihydroxyvitamin D ($1,25(OH)_2D$). Active calcium transport occurs mainly in the duodenum and proximal jejunum, although some active calcium absorption occurs in other areas of the small intestine. Maximal rates of calcium absorption occur in the presence of gastric acid. Overall, despite large differences in daily dietary calcium intake, intestinal absorption leads to a rather constant daily net calcium absorption of approximately 200–400 mg per day. Thus, in a typical person, if 1000 mg of daily calcium is consumed, roughly 200 mg will be absorbed.

Kidney

Approximately 8–10 g per day of calcium is filtered by the glomeruli, of which most will be reabsorbed, with only 2–3% being excreted in the urine. Most filtered calcium (65%) is reabsorbed in the proximal tubules via a passive mechanism that is coupled to simultaneous NaCl reabsorption. The cortical thick ascending limb of Henle absorbs approximately another 20% of filtered calcium. Calcium reabsorption in the cortical thick ascending limb of Henle is inhibited by increased blood concentrations of calcium or magnesium, acting via the calcium sensing receptor (CaSR), which is present on basolateral membranes. Finally, approximately 10% of filtered calcium is reabsorbed in the distal convoluted tubules. The normal 24-hour excretion of calcium varies between 100 and 300 mg per day.

Hormonal Regulation

Ca-sensitive cells modulate the production of hormones that act on cells in the bone, intestine, and kidney [4–7]. Accordingly, a decrease in extracellular fluid calcium stimulates the release of PTH from the parathyroids (Fig. 2.1). PTH then activates bone resorption and releases both calcium and phosphorus from the skeleton. PTH also enhances the release of the phosphaturic hormone, FGF23, from osteocytes [8]. At the same time, PTH increases calcium reabsorption in the kidney and reduces phosphate reabsorption, leading to phosphaturia. PTH additionally stimulates the conversion of inactive vitamin D, 25-hydroxyvitamin D (25OHD), to the active metabolite $1,25(OH)_2D$ [9], which subsequently augments intestinal calcium absorption, and to a lesser extent reabsorption of renal phosphorous. The collective effect of the release of calcium from bone, the augmented absorption of calcium from the gut, and the enhanced reabsorption of filtered calcium along the nephron is to increase the extracellular fluid calcium concentration.

Hypercalcemia results from an abnormality in calcium flux between the extracellular fluid and either the skeleton, intestine or kidney, or a combination of these compartments. Hence, when there is accelerated bone resorption, excessive gastrointestinal absorption, or decreased renal excretion of calcium, the entry of calcium

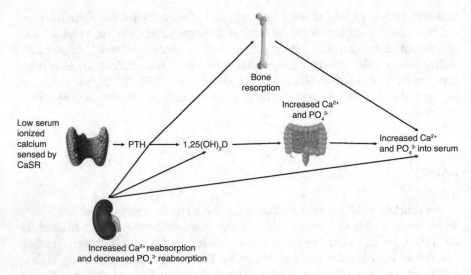

Fig. 2.1 Regulation of calcium homeostasis. Decreased ionized Ca $^{2+}$ leads to PTH release from the parathyroids by the calcium sensing receptor (CaSR). The rise in PTH at the kidney stimulates renal calcium reabsorption while blocking phosphorous reabsorption. PTH also enhances bone resorption, leading to increased mobilization of calcium and phosphorus. In addition, PTH stimulates renal conversion of 25OHD to 1,25(OH)$_2$D, which will in turn increase intestinal absorption of calcium and phosphorous

Table 2.1 Symptoms and signs of hypercalcemia

Gastrointestinal	Nausea, constipation, anorexia, pancreatitis, peptic ulcer disease
Renal	Polyuria, polydipsia, renal insufficiency, nephrocalcinosis, nephrolithiasis, renal failure
Neuropsychiatric	Fatigue, lethargy, confusion, obtundation
Musculoskeletal	Weakness
Cardiovascular	Shortened QT interval, vascular calcification

into the circulation exceeds the excretion of calcium into the urine or deposition into bone. Importantly, multiple mechanism may be involved. For example, in primary hyperparathyroidism, there is stimulation of bone resorption, renal calcium reabsorption, synthesis of 1,25(OH)$_2$D, and intestinal calcium absorption.

Symptoms and Signs of Hypercalcemia

General

Patients with mild hypercalcemia (calcium <12 mg/dL [3.00 mmol/L]) may be asymptomatic or have symptoms such as fatigue and constipation. Serum calcium in the range of 12–14 mg/dL (3.00–3.50 mmol/L) may be well tolerated if it is chronic. However, a rapid increase in this range may cause a range of symptoms (Table 2.1). In patients with calcium >14 mg/dL (3.50 mmol/L), obtundation or coma may occur if the onset is acute [10]. The symptoms and signs associated with hypercalcemia are typically independent of the etiology.

Gastrointestinal

Constipation, nausea, and anorexia are frequent. Constipation may be related to altered autonomic or smooth muscle function. Pancreatitis and peptic ulcer disease occur infrequently [11–13]. Peptic ulcer disease may be caused by calcium-induced increases in gastrin secretion.

Renal

Hypercalcemia acts directly at the nephron to prevent reabsorption of water, leading to a functional nephrogenic diabetes and polyuria in up to 20% of patients. This may lead to prerenal azotemia, thirst, and dehydration, which further exacerbates the hypercalcemia, in a "vicious cycle." Hypercalcemia may also cause precipitation of calcium phosphate salts in the renal interstitium, leading to necrosis of tubular cells with interstitial fibrosis in over one-half of hypercalcemic patients, with possible development of renal insufficiency. Moreover, hypercalcemia can precipitate renal failure as a result of obstructive uropathy, nephrolithiasis (particularly with primary hyperparathyroidism and sarcoidosis), or nephrocalcinosis. Renal failure can furthermore develop from prerenal causes, including a natriuresis-induced volume contraction and a reversible component of direct hypercalcemia-induced afferent arteriolar vasoconstriction [14, 15]. Chronic hypercalcemia also infrequently causes type 1 (distal) renal tubular acidosis [16].

Neuropsychiatric

Hypercalcemia increases the electrical potential difference across cell membranes and raises the depolarization threshold. This can present as a variety of neurological symptoms ranging from fatigue to lethargy, confusion, or with severe acute onset hypercalcemia, to obtundation or coma. In patients with primary hyperparathyroidism, anxiety, depression, and cognitive dysfunction have been observed [17]. There is no specific serum calcium level that leads to compromised neurologic function. Rather, the neurologic symptoms depend on the rate of rise of the calcium level, the age, and the baseline neurological functioning of the patient.

Musculoskeletal

The effect of hypercalcemia to raise the depolarization threshold causes skeletal and smooth muscle to become more resistant to neuronal stimulation. Consequent reductions in muscle contraction present as constipation and skeletal muscle weakness.

Cardiovascular

Hypercalcemia can lead to electrocardiographic abnormalities by shortening of the myocardial action potential, which is reflected in a shortened QT interval [18]. Arrhythmia has been described in patients with severe hypercalcemia [19, 20]. ST segment elevation with hypercalcemia can also imitate myocardial infarction [21]. Additionally, chronic hypercalcemia can lead to deposition of calcium phosphate salts in the heart valves, vasculature (including coronary arteries) and cardiac conduction system, and cardiomyopathy.

Physical Exam Findings

There are few physical findings related to hypercalcemia per se, other than dehydration. A rare finding is band keratopathy, resulting in corneal calcium phosphate deposition, detected by slit-lamp examination.

Causes of Hypercalcemia

Hypercalcemia can be a sign of a serious disease such as malignancy or can be discovered incidentally by laboratory testing in an asymptomatic individual. There are many causes of hypercalcemia (Table 2.2), but primary hyperparathyroidism (PHPT) and malignancy account for over 90% of all cases. An overview of the main causes of hypercalcemia is reviewed here. Further detailed information on each of the major conditions is provided in subsequent chapters. The diagnostic approach to determining the etiology of hypercalcemia in adults and children can be found in Chaps. 3 and 4, respectively.

Table 2.2 Causes of hypercalcemia

Parathyroid- related	Primary hyperparathyroidism	Adenoma
		Multiple endocrine neoplasia syndromes
		Hyperparathyroidism-jaw tumor syndrome
		Carcinoma
	Lithium therapy	
	Familial hypocalciuric hypercalcemia	
	Metaphyseal chondrodysplasia	
	PTH-therapy related	
Malignancy-related	Local osteolysis	
	PTHrP	
	Increased calcitriol production	
Vitamin D–related	Vitamin D intoxication	
	Increased 1,25(OH)$_2$D	
Associated with high bone turnover	Hyperthyroidism	
	Immobilization	
	Thiazides	
	Vitamin A intoxication	
Associated with renal failure	Severe secondary hyperparathyroidism	
	Aluminum intoxication	
	Milk-alkali syndrome	
	Rhabdomyolysis	
Miscellaneous	Pheochromocytoma, adrenal insufficiency, theophylline toxicity	

Parathyroid Related

Primary Hyperparathyroidism

Hypercalcemia in an asymptomatic individual is typically caused by PHPT. PHPT is a disorder of calcium, phosphate, and bone metabolism, resulting from excess PTH secretion, with the elevated PTH leading to hypercalcemia and hypophosphatemia. The diagnosis is generally made by finding an elevated immunoreactive PTH level in an individual with asymptomatic hypercalcemia [22]. Patients usually have only mild elevations in serum calcium concentrations (< 11 mg/dL [2.75 mmol/L]), and some patients have mostly high-normal values with only intermittent hypercalcemia. Serum phosphate is usually low, although if renal failure is present it can be normal. The parathyroid tumor is generally an isolated adenoma without the presence of other endocrinopathy.

The manifestations of PHPT are widely variable. Patients may develop numerous signs and symptoms, including nephrolithiasis, mental changes, and bone resorption. However, with wider use in recent decades of multichannel autoanalyzer tests that include measurement of the blood calcium, the diagnosis is frequently made in patients who have no symptoms and minimal, if any, signs of the disease other than hypercalcemia and elevated levels of PTH. This milder form of the disease is termed "asymptomatic PHPT." "Normocalcemic PHPT" is a variant of the more common presentation of PHPT with hypercalcemia, in which serum calcium is normal without there being a secondary cause for PTH elevation [22]. Occasionally, patients with PHPT have more severe hypercalcemia with levels over 12 mg/dL (3.00 mmol/L). Rarely, PHPT develops or worsens suddenly as a "parathyroid crisis" and causes serious complications such as severe dehydration and coma. The diagnosis of a multiple endocrine neoplasia syndrome should be considered in a patient who is young and has a familial history of PHPT or multi-gland involvement [23]. Parathyroid carcinoma is a rare cause of primary hyperparathyroidism, which is usually caused by a parathyroid adenoma. Parathyroid carcinoma patients, as compared with patients with parathyroid adenomas, are more likely to have symptoms, a neck mass, bone and kidney disease, marked hypercalcemia, and very elevated parathyroid hormone concentrations. Chapter 6 provides further information regarding PHPT.

Lithium Therapy

Lithium, used in the management of psychiatric disorders, causes hypercalcemia in ~10% of treated patients [24]. It is most likely due to increased secretion of PTH because of an increase in the set point at which calcium suppresses PTH release [25]. The hypercalcemia is generally dependent on continued lithium treatment, remitting when lithium is stopped. Parathyroid adenomas have been reported in some hypercalcemic patients treated with lithium therapy. Lithium may unmask previously unrecognized mild hyperparathyroidism. Although most patients have normalization of serum calcium when lithium is stopped, long-standing stimulation of parathyroid cell replication by lithium might prompt development of adenomas. See Chap. 14 for a detailed description of medication-induced hypercalcemia.

Familial Hypocalciuric Hypercalcemia

Familial hypocalciuric hypercalcemia (FHH), also known as familial benign hypercalcemia, is a rare autosomal dominant disorder characterized by mild hypercalcemia, normal to slightly increased serum PTH levels and hypocalciuria [26]. Affected individuals are discovered because of asymptomatic hypercalcemia. The key defect in this disorder is most commonly an inactivating mutation in a single allele of the

CaSR on the parathyroid cells and in the kidneys leading to inappropriate secretion of PTH and excessive reabsorption of calcium in the distal renal tubules. In contrast to PHPT, hypercalcemia is often detectable in affected members of the kindreds in the first decade of life, and most patients have >99% renal calcium reabsorption. Importantly, patients with FHH require no therapy, and parathyroidectomy does not correct the hypercalcemia. A rare acquired form of hypocalciuric hypercalcemia due to autoantibodies directed against the CaSR has also been described [27]. See Chaps. 7 and 8 for a further detailed discussion of FHH.

Metaphyseal Chondrodysplasia

Jansen-type metaphyseal chondrodysplasia is a rare form of dwarfism that is associated with hypercalcemia and hypophosphatemia. The defect is a mutation in the PTH-parathyroid hormone-related protein (PTHrP) receptor gene, leading to constitutive activation of the receptor at low levels of PTH [28]. Serum PTH and PTHrP concentrations are normal or low. See Chap. 4 for further discussion and review of the clinical features.

PTH Therapy Related

When parathyroid hormone or parathyroid hormone analogs are used as treatment for osteoporosis, they can be associated with hypercalcemia in a small minority of patients. In general, it is mild and requires no treatment or a decrease in the dose of PTH or supplemental calcium.

Malignancy Related

Hypercalcemia due to malignancy is not infrequent, occurring in up to 20% of cancer patients [28]. Typically, symptoms of malignancy bring the patient to medical attention, and hypercalcemia is then uncovered during the evaluation. Serum calcium levels are generally higher with malignancy than with PHPT, the other most common cause of hypercalcemia. In patients with hypercalcemia of malignancy, the time between detection of hypercalcemia and death is often less than 6 months, especially in the absence of aggressive treatment.

The mechanisms by which hypercalcemia of malignancy occurs are threefold [29]. The first mechanism is local osteolysis by the tumor, in which tumor cells produce cytokines, which stimulate osteoclast differentiation and action [30]. Examples include breast cancer or multiple myeloma, which release or alter levels of osteoclast activating factors such as receptor activator of nuclear factor kappa B ligand

(RANKL) and interleukin-6, consequently increasing bone resorption. Chapter 10 reviews hypercalcemia related to multiple myeloma. The second mechanism is secretion of PTHrP by the tumor, also known as humoral hypercalcemia of malignancy (see Chap. 9) [31]. Tumoral secretion of PTHrP leads to an uncoupling of bone formation from resorption, by suppressing bone formation and activating bone resorption. Consequently, up to 1 g of calcium a day can become mobilized from the skeleton, causing hypercalcemia. Moreover, renal calcium clearance is reduced by the anti-calciuric effects of PTHrP, further exacerbating the hypercalcemia. Notably, with PTHrP secretion, there is typically a reduction in circulating calcitriol levels, in contrast to the increase in calcitriol that occurs with PTH secretion. PTHrP secretion is the most common cause of hypercalcemia in patients with nonmetastatic solid tumors such as squamous cell carcinomas (such as lung, head, and neck), renal, bladder, breast, or ovarian carcinomas. The third mechanism for hypercalcemia of malignancy is tumor production of calcitriol. In this scenario, there is extrarenal PTH-independent production of calcitriol from calcidiol by activated mononuclear cells, particularly macrophages, leading to hypercalcemia. This mechanism is most common in patients with Hodgkin and non-Hodgkin lymphoma [32]. Chapter 11 provides further information regarding malignancy-associated production of calcitriol.

Vitamin D Related

Vitamin D Intoxication

Vitamin D–mediated hypercalcemia can result from an excessive intake of vitamin D analogs. Elevated serum concentrations of 25-hydroxyvitamin D [25(OH)D] or $1,25(OH)_2D$ (calcitriol) will increase calcium absorption and bone resorption and thus cause hypercalcemia. Intestinal transport of calcium is mainly controlled by $1,25(OH)_2D$, which has greater biological activity than 25(OH)D. Nevertheless, hypercalcemia can develop in individuals with significantly elevated serum 25(OH)D concentrations, for example, in patients who ingest high doses of vitamin D. Notably, chronic ingestion of 40–100 times the physiologic requirement of vitamin D (i.e., >40,000–100,000 IU/d) generally causes hypercalcemia in a healthy person. There have been reports of excess vitamin D intake being unknown to the patients because milk was unintentionally fortified with extra vitamin D [33]. Ingestion of "over-the-counter" supplements that contain very large doses of vitamin D can also lead to intoxication [34], as can be the use of topical calcipotriol, a vitamin D analog used for skin disease disorders [35]. The diagnosis is confirmed by levels of 25(OH)D > 100 ng/mL. Importantly, vitamin D stores in fat may be considerable, and the intoxication may continue for weeks after vitamin D intake has ceased. A further review of vitamin D intoxication can be found in Chap. 12.

Increased 1,25(OH)₂D

Vitamin D metabolism is carefully controlled, predominantly by the activity of renal 1-α-hydroxylase, the enzyme that stimulates conversion of 25(OH)D to its active form, 1,25(OH)2D. Abnormal metabolism of vitamin D is typically acquired in association with a widespread granulomatous disorder. The most common disorder is sarcoidosis, but elevated 1,25(OH)2D levels have been reported with tuberculosis, berylliosis, histiocytosis X, histoplasmosis, *Pneumocystis*, coccidiomycosis, inflammatory bowel disease, foreign body granulomas, and granulomatous leprosy [36, 37]. The mechanism is the excess production of 1,25(OH)₂ D by the granulomas, due to increased activity of 1-α-hydroxylase [38], which leads to increased intestinal absorption of calcium, hypercalciuria, and eventually hypercalcemia. The extrarenal source of 1,25(OH)2D has been confirmed by reports of anephric patients with sarcoidosis and elevated 1,25(OH)2D levels [39]. Interestingly, there is a positive relationship in patients with sarcoidosis between 25(OH)D levels (reflecting vitamin D intake) and the level of 1,25(OH)2D, while normally there is no increase in 1,25(OH)2D with rising 25(OH)D levels due to various feedback controls on renal 1α-hydroxylase. A separate cause of increased 1,25(OH)2D levels can be a deficiency of 24-hydroxylase [40], the enzyme which degrades 1,25(OH)2D, leading to impaired 1,25(OH)₂D metabolism and hypercalcemia [40]. Chapter 13 provides a further review of hypercalcemia caused by the production of calcitriol from granulomatous disease and other benign causes.

Associated with High Bone Turnover

Hyperthyroidism

As many as 20% of thyrotoxic patients have mild hypercalcemia, with hypercalciuria being even more frequent. The hypercalcemia is due to a thyroid-mediated increase in bone turnover, with bone resorption exceeding bone formation [41]. A severe increase in calcium levels is unusual and if present may suggest the presence of attendant PHPT. Chapter 15 provides a detailed review of hypercalcemia related to thyrotoxicosis.

Immobilization

Immobilization is an infrequent cause of hypercalcemia in adults in the absence of an associated disease of high bone turnover (e.g., hyperparathyroidism, myeloma or breast cancer with bone metastases, and Paget's disease). However, it may cause hypercalcemia in children and adolescents, especially after spinal cord injury and paralysis [42]. The mechanism is uncoupling of bone turnover, with suppression of bone formation and a marked increase in bone resorption [43]. Further information regarding immobilization-induced hypercalcemia can be found in Chap. 16.

Thiazides

Administration of thiazides can lead to hypercalcemia in patients with high rates of bone turnover [44]. Usually, thiazides are associated with exacerbation of hypercalcemia in underlying PHPT. Chronic thiazide administration leads to a decrease in urinary calcium; the hypocalciuria is due to the augmentation of proximal tubular resorption of calcium and sodium in response to sodium reduction.

Vitamin A Intoxication

Vitamin A intoxication is a rare cause of hypercalcemia and is most commonly a side effect of excess supplemental intake. Calcium levels can be elevated after the intake of more than 50,000 units of vitamin A daily (10–20 times the minimum daily requirement) [45]. Characteristic features include fatigue, anorexia, and, in some, marked bone and muscle pain. Excess vitamin A intake is thought to increase bone resorption, possibly by increasing serum interleukin-6 concentrations [46]. Further information on medication-induced hypercalcemia is found in Chap. 14.

Associated with Renal Failure

Severe Secondary Hyperparathyroidism

Patients with secondary hyperparathyroidism accompanying advanced chronic kidney disease frequently have parathyroid hyperplasia and low serum calcium levels. Hypercalcemia is generally prevented by coexistent hyperphosphatemia and decreased calcitriol levels. However, with prolonged disease, some patients may develop hypercalcemia. The rise in plasma calcium may be due to attendant adynamic bone disease and reduced bone turnover, which leads to a reduction in the bone deposition of calcium after calcium administration. This can occur when calcium carbonate or calcium acetate is used as a phosphate binder to treat hyperphosphatemia, or with the use of vitamin D analogs to prevent secondary hyperparathyroidism [47]. In some patients with protracted renal failure, parathyroid hyperplasia may slowly progress to autonomous overproduction of PTH. In this situation, elevated serum PTH levels are associated with hypercalcemia, a condition known as tertiary hyperparathyroidism.

Aluminum Intoxication

Aluminum intoxication used to be a complication in patients on chronic dialysis as a result of exposure to aluminum in dialysis fluid, leading to osteomalacia. Hypercalcemia would develop when these patients were treated with vitamin D or calcitriol because of impaired skeletal responsiveness. Nowadays, aluminum is removed from water used for dialysis, making aluminum toxicity rare.

Milk-Alkali Syndrome

The milk-alkali syndrome typically occurs in the setting of excess calcium carbonate supplementation to treat dyspepsia, leading to hypercalcemia, metabolic alkalosis, and renal insufficiency [48]. The metabolic alkalosis exacerbates the hypercalcemia by directly stimulating calcium reabsorption in the distal tubule, thereby reducing calcium excretion [49]. A calcium-induced reduction in renal function, due to renal vasoconstriction and, with chronic hypercalcemia, structural damage, can also exacerbate the incapacity to excrete the excess calcium. Renal function usually returns to baseline after cessation of milk or calcium carbonate intake, but irreversible injury (Burnett's syndrome) can occur in patients who have prolonged hypercalcemia. The milk-alkali syndrome is much less frequent since proton-pump inhibitors became available for gastric reflux. Chapter 14 provides further information on milk-alkali syndrome.

Rhabdomyolysis

The recovery phase from acute renal failure caused by rhabdomyolysis has been linked to hypercalcemia [50]. Generally, this follows an incident of marked hyperphosphatemia and hypocalcemia in the acute, oliguric phase, accompanied by secondary hyperparathyroidism. It has been attributed to lingering effects of PTH on bone turnover, in addition to release of calcium phosphate precipitated into skeletal muscle during the early hyperphosphatemic hypocalcemic phase. A detailed discussion of hypercalcemia related to rhabdomyolysis can be found in Chap. 16.

Miscellaneous Causes and Medications

Patients with pheochromocytoma can rarely have hypercalcemia [51]. It can be due to the pheochromocytoma producing PTHrP [52] or to coexisting hyperparathyroidism with multiple endocrine neoplasia syndromes. Addisonian crisis has been reported to cause hypercalcemia [53]. The cause is unknown, but it may be due to the associated volume contraction with hemoconcentration. (See Chap. 15 for a discussion of Non-Parathyroid Endocrine-Mediated causes of Hypercalcemia). There have been reports of medications associated with hypercalcemia, including aminophylline and theophylline [54] when used in supratherapeutic doses, estrogens in women with breast cancer and widespread skeletal metastatic disease [55], and Foscarnet, an antiviral human immunodeficiency virus (HIV) treatment agent used in HIV and acquired immunodeficiency syndrome [56]. Further information on medication-induced hypercalcemia is found in Chap. 14.

References

1. Walser M. Ion association. VI. Interactions between calcium, magnesium, inorganic phosphate, citrate and protein in normal human plasma. J Clin Invest. 1961;40:723–30.
2. Palmer M, Jakobsson S, Akerstrom G, Ljunghall S. Prevalence of hypercalcaemia in a health survey: a 14-year follow-up study of serum calcium values. Eur J Clin Investig. 1988;18(1):39–46.
3. Ross AC, Manson JE, Abrams SA, Aloia JF, Brannon PM, Clinton SK, et al. The 2011 report on dietary reference intakes for calcium and vitamin D from the Institute of Medicine: what clinicians need to know. J Clin Endocrinol Metab. 2011;96(1):53–8.
4. Parfitt A, Kleerekoper M. Clinical disorders of calcium, phosphorus and magnesium metabolism. In: Clinical disorders of fluid and electrolyte metabolism. 3rd ed. New York: McGraw-Hill; 1980. p. 947.
5. Stewart A, Broadus A. Mineral metabolism. Endocrinology and metabolism. 2nd ed. New York: McGraw-Hill; 1987. p. 1317.
6. Bringhurst F, Demay M, Kronenberg H. Hormones and disorders of mineral metabolism. In: Williams Textbook of Endocrinology. Philadelphia: Saunders; 1998. p. 1155.
7. Brown E. Physiology of calcium homeostasis. The parathyroids: basic and clinical concepts. 2nd ed. San Diego: Academic Press; 2001. p. 167.
8. Lavi-Moshayoff V, Wasserman G, Meir T, Silver J, Naveh-Many T. PTH increases FGF23 gene expression and mediates the high-FGF23 levels of experimental kidney failure: a bone parathyroid feedback loop. Am J Physiol Renal Physiol. 2010;299(4):F882–9.
9. Fraser DR, Kodicek E. Regulation of 25-hydroxycholecalciferol-1-hydroxylase activity in kidney by parathyroid hormone. Nat New Biol. 1973;241(110):163–6.
10. Inzucchi SE. Understanding hypercalcemia. Its metabolic basis, signs, and symptoms. Postgrad Med. 2004;115(4):69–70. 3-6
11. Gardner EC Jr, Hersh T. Primary hyperparathyroidism and the gastrointestinal tract. South Med J. 1981;74(2):197–9.
12. Carnaille B, Oudar C, Pattou F, Combemale F, Rocha J, Proye C. Pancreatitis and primary hyperparathyroidism: forty cases. Aust N Z J Surg. 1998;68(2):117–9.
13. Wynn D, Everett GD, Boothby RA. Small cell carcinoma of the ovary with hypercalcemia causes severe pancreatitis and altered mental status. Gynecol Oncol. 2004;95(3):716–8.

14. Levi M, Ellis MA, Berl T. Control of renal hemodynamics and glomerular filtration rate in chronic hypercalcemia. Role of prostaglandins, renin-angiotensin system, and calcium. J Clin Invest. 1983;71(6):1624–32.
15. Lins LE. Reversible renal failure caused by hypercalcemia. A retrospective study. Acta Med Scand. 1978;203(4):309–14.
16. Caruana RJ, Buckalew VM Jr. The syndrome of distal (type 1) renal tubular acidosis. Clinical and laboratory findings in 58 cases. Medicine (Baltimore). 1988;67(2):84–99.
17. Walker MD, McMahon DJ, Inabnet WB, Lazar RM, Brown I, Vardy S, et al. Neuropsychological features in primary hyperparathyroidism: a prospective study. J Clin Endocrinol Metab. 2009;94(6):1951–8.
18. Ahmed R, Hashiba K. Reliability of QT intervals as indicators of clinical hypercalcemia. Clin Cardiol. 1988;11(6):395–400.
19. Kiewiet RM, Ponssen HH, Janssens EN, Fels PW. Ventricular fibrillation in hypercalcaemic crisis due to primary hyperparathyroidism. Neth J Med. 2004;62(3):94–6.
20. Diercks DB, Shumaik GM, Harrigan RA, Brady WJ, Chan TC. Electrocardiographic manifestations: electrolyte abnormalities. J Emerg Med. 2004;27(2):153–60.
21. Nishi SP, Barbagelata NA, Atar S, Birnbaum Y, Tuero E. Hypercalcemia-induced ST-segment elevation mimicking acute myocardial infarction. J Electrocardiol. 2006;39(3):298–300.
22. Eastell R, Brandi ML, Costa AG, D'Amour P, Shoback DM, Thakker RV. Diagnosis of asymptomatic primary hyperparathyroidism: proceedings of the Fourth International Workshop. J Clin Endocrinol Metab. 2014;99(10):3570–9.
23. McKnight RF, Adida M, Budge K, Stockton S, Goodwin GM, Geddes JR. Lithium toxicity profile: a systematic review and meta-analysis. Lancet. 2012;379(9817):721–8.
24. Haden ST, Stoll AL, McCormick S, Scott J, Fuleihan G-H. Alterations in parathyroid dynamics in lithium-treated subjects. J Clin Endocrinol Metab. 1997;82(9):2844–8.
25. Law WM Jr, Heath H 3rd. Familial benign hypercalcemia (hypocalciuric hypercalcemia). Clinical and pathogenetic studies in 21 families. Ann Intern Med. 1985;102(4):511–9.
26. Pallais JC, Kifor O, Chen YB, Slovik D, Brown EM. Acquired hypocalciuric hypercalcemia due to autoantibodies against the calcium-sensing receptor. N Engl J Med. 2004;351(4):362–9.
27. Schipani E, Langman CB, Parfitt AM, Jensen GS, Kikuchi S, Kooh SW, et al. Constitutively activated receptors for parathyroid hormone and parathyroid hormone-related peptide in Jansen's metaphyseal chondrodysplasia. N Engl J Med. 1996;335(10):708–14.
28. Stewart AF. Clinical practice. Hypercalcemia associated with cancer. N Engl J Med. 2005;352(4):373–9.
29. Clines GA, Guise TA. Hypercalcaemia of malignancy and basic research on mechanisms responsible for osteolytic and osteoblastic metastasis to bone. Endocr Relat Cancer. 2005;12(3):549–83.
30. Roodman GD. Mechanisms of bone metastasis. N Engl J Med. 2004;350(16):1655–64.
31. Burtis WJ, Brady TG, Orloff JJ, Ersbak JB, Warrell RP Jr, Olson BR, et al. Immunochemical characterization of circulating parathyroid hormone-related protein in patients with humoral hypercalcemia of cancer. N Engl J Med. 1990;322(16):1106–12.
32. Roodman GD. Mechanisms of bone lesions in multiple myeloma and lymphoma. Cancer. 1997;80(8 Suppl):1557–63.
33. Jacobus CH, Holick MF, Shao Q, Chen TC, Holm IA, Kolodny JM, et al. Hypervitaminosis D associated with drinking milk. N Engl J Med. 1992;326(18):1173–7.
34. Lowe H, Cusano NE, Binkley N, Blaner WS, Bilezikian JP. Vitamin D toxicity due to a commonly available "over the counter" remedy from the Dominican Republic. J Clin Endocrinol Metab. 2011;96(2):291–5.
35. Hoeck HC, Laurberg G, Laurberg P. Hypercalcaemic crisis after excessive topical use of a vitamin D derivative. J Intern Med. 1994;235(3):281–2.
36. Parker MS, Dokoh S, Woolfenden JM, Buchsbaum HW. Hypercalcemia in coccidioidomycosis. Am J Med. 1984;76(2):341–4.
37. Gkonos PJ, London R, Hendler ED. Hypercalcemia and elevated 1,25-dihydroxyvitamin D levels in a patient with end-stage renal disease and active tuberculosis. N Engl J Med. 1984;311(26):1683–5.

38. Adams JS, Gacad MA. Characterization of 1 alpha-hydroxylation of vitamin D3 sterols by cultured alveolar macrophages from patients with sarcoidosis. J Exp Med. 1985;161(4):755–65.
39. Barbour GL, Coburn JW, Slatopolsky E, Norman AW, Horst RL. Hypercalcemia in an anephric patient with sarcoidosis: evidence for extrarenal generation of 1,25-dihydroxyvitamin D. N Engl J Med. 1981;305(8):440–3.
40. Molin A, Baudoin R, Kaufmann M, Souberbielle JC, Ryckewaert A, Vantyghem MC, et al. CYP24A1 mutations in a cohort of hypercalcemic patients: evidence for a recessive trait. J Clin Endocrinol Metab. 2015;100(10):E1343–52.
41. Burman KD, Monchik JM, Earll JM, Wartofsky L. Ionized and total serum calcium and parathyroid hormone in hyperthyroidism. Ann Intern Med. 1976;84(6):668–71.
42. Bergstrom WH. Hypercalciuria and hypercalcemia complicating immobilization. Am J Dis Child. 1978;132(6):553–4.
43. Stewart AF, Adler M, Byers CM, Segre GV, Broadus AE. Calcium homeostasis in immobilization: an example of resorptive hypercalciuria. N Engl J Med. 1982;306(19):1136–40.
44. Wermers RA, Kearns AE, Jenkins GD, Melton LJ 3rd. Incidence and clinical spectrum of thiazide-associated hypercalcemia. Am J Med. 2007;120(10):911 e9–15.
45. Bhalla K, Ennis DM, Ennis ED. Hypercalcemia caused by iatrogenic hypervitaminosis a. J Am Diet Assoc. 2005;105(1):119–21.
46. Niesvizky R, Siegel DS, Busquets X, Nichols G, Muindi J, Warrell RP Jr, et al. Hypercalcaemia and increased serum interleukin-6 levels induced by all-trans retinoic acid in patients with multiple myeloma. Br J Haematol. 1995;89(1):217–8.
47. Meric F, Yap P, Bia MJ. Etiology of hypercalcemia in hemodialysis patients on calcium carbonate therapy. Am J Kidney Dis. 1990;16(5):459–64.
48. Beall DP, Scofield RH. Milk-alkali syndrome associated with calcium carbonate consumption. Report of 7 patients with parathyroid hormone levels and an estimate of prevalence among patients hospitalized with hypercalcemia. Medicine (Baltimore). 1995;74(2):89–96.
49. Orwoll ES. The milk-alkali syndrome: current concepts. Ann Intern Med. 1982;97(2):242–8.
50. Llach F, Felsenfeld AJ, Haussler MR. The pathophysiology of altered calcium metabolism in rhabdomyolysis-induced acute renal failure. Interactions of parathyroid hormone, 25-hydroxycholecalciferol, and 1,25-dihydroxycholecalciferol. N Engl J Med. 1981;305(3):117–23.
51. Stewart AF, Hoecker JL, Mallette LE, Segre GV, Amatruda TT Jr, Vignery A. Hypercalcemia in pheochromocytoma. Evidence for a novel mechanism. Ann Intern Med. 1985;102(6):776–9.
52. Kimura S, Nishimura Y, Yamaguchi K, Nagasaki K, Shimada K, Uchida H. A case of pheochromocytoma producing parathyroid hormone-related protein and presenting with hypercalcemia. J Clin Endocrinol Metab. 1990;70(6):1559–63.
53. Muls E, Bouillon R, Boelaert J, Lamberigts G, Van Imschoot S, Daneels R, et al. Etiology of hypercalcemia in a patient with Addison's disease. Calcif Tissue Int. 1982;34(6):523–6.
54. McPherson ML, Prince SR, Atamer ER, Maxwell DB, Ross-Clunis H, Estep HL. Theophylline-induced hypercalcemia. Ann Intern Med. 1986;105(1):52–4.
55. Ellis MJ, Gao F, Dehdashti F, Jeffe DB, Marcom PK, Carey LA, et al. Lower-dose vs high-dose oral estradiol therapy of hormone receptor-positive, aromatase inhibitor-resistant advanced breast cancer: a phase 2 randomized study. JAMA. 2009;302(7):774–80.
56. Gayet S, Ville E, Durand JM, Mars ME, Morange S, Kaplanski G, et al. Foscarnet-induced hypercalcaemia in AIDS. AIDS. 1997;11(8):1068–70.

Chapter 3
Diagnostic Approach to the Adult Patient with Hypercalcemia

Lena Fan, Hoang-Long C. Huynh, Shonni Silverberg, and Marcella Donovan Walker

Introduction and Epidemiology

Calcium plays an integral role in numerous physiological processes and is the most abundant cation found in the human body. The serum calcium level is normally tightly controlled, primarily by PTH, due to its importance in many cellular processes. Disruptions in the regulation of calcium can, however, lead to hypercalcemia. Hypercalcemia refers to a state of elevated serum calcium above the upper limit of the laboratory normal reference range. It occurs when the entry of calcium into the serum is greater than its renal excretion through the urine or the deposition of calcium into the bone. Hypercalcemia is a relatively common clinical condition. Prevalence and incidence rates vary between different global populations due to differences in screening rates [1].The prevalence of hypercalcemia is estimated to be 1.4–3% in the general North American hospitalized and ambulatory populations [2].

While there are numerous causes of hypercalcemia (Table 3.1), the majority of cases are related to either PHPT or malignancy. Together, these two causes encompass over 90% of cases, with the incidence of PHPT ranging up to 21.6 cases per 100,000 person-years [3, 4]. Thus, the diagnostic evaluation of hypercalcemia focuses initially upon discriminating between PHPT and malignancy. These two etiologies can typically be readily distinguished due to differences in their clinical and biochemical presentation. PHPT is responsible for the majority of cases of hypercalcemia in well-appearing outpatients, whereas hypercalcemia of malignancy is the

$Lena Fan and Hoang-Long C. Huynh contributed equally to this work.

L. Fan · H.-L. C. Huynh · S. Silverberg · M. D. Walker (✉)
Division of Endocrinology, Columbia University Irving Medical Center, New York, NY, USA
e-mail: hh2823@cumc.columbia.edu; sjs5@columbia.edu; mad2037@columbia.edu

Table 3.1 Major causes of hypercalcemia by primary mechanism in adults [20]

	Non-PTH mediated	PTH mediated

Increased bone resorption	**Malignancy**
	 Humoral hypercalcemia of malignancy
	 Osteolytic metastases
	 Immobilization
	 Vitamin A toxicity
	 Hyperthyroidism
	 Drugs – teriparatide, abaloparatide
		Primary hyperparathyroidism
		 Sporadic
		 Familial/inherited
		     Multiple endocrine neoplasia
		     Familial isolated
		     hyperparathyroidism
		     Hyperparathyroidism-jaw
		     tumor syndrome
		     Parathyroid cancer
		 Tertiary hyperparathyroidism
		 (renal failure)
		 Drugs – Lithium
		 Malignancy – Ectopic PTH production

Increased gastrointestinal absorption	Malignancy - increased calcitriol by activation of extrarenal 1-alpha-hydroxylase (i.e. lymphoma)
	 Drugs
	     Cholecalciferol or ergocalciferol
	     intoxication
	     Calcipotriene topical use
	     Calcitriol ingestion
	 Granulomatous disorders (TB, sarcoid, Wegner's, Crohn's, silicosis, etc.)
	 CYP24A1 mutation
	 Catch scratch fever
	 Crohn's disease
	 BCG therapy
	 8-cl-cAMP therapy
	 Lipoid pneumonia	

Reduced renal clearance	Drugs – thiazides Milk-alkali syndrome Rare presentations (oyster shell calcium in betel nut chewing, overdose with buffered aspirin, massive cheese ingestion, Munchausen's syndrome) Acute renal failure	
Other	Acromegaly Pheochromocytoma Adrenal insufficiency Drugs –theophylline Rhabdomyolysis	Familial hypocalciuric hypercalcemia Neonatal severe hyperparathyroidism (inactivating CaSR mutation)

most common cause in ill-appearing inpatients. Patients with hypercalcemia of malignancy typically have severe and symptomatic hypercalcemia and advanced cancers that are clinically obvious. On the other hand, in PHPT, most patients are asymptomatic, and the serum calcium level is typically mildly elevated. These two causes are biochemically discriminated by the serum PTH level. PHPT is characterized by an elevated or inappropriately normal PTH level. The other major cause of hypercalcemia, malignancy, is typified by suppressed PTH level. Thus, the conceptual framework of considering etiologies as either PTH-mediated or non-PTH-mediated guides the evaluation of hypercalcemia. This chapter focuses on the diagnostic approach to hypercalcemia in the adult patient.

Normal Regulation of Serum Calcium

The normal reference range for serum calcium varies between different laboratories by as much as 0.5 mg/dl, but usually ranges approximately between 8.5 and 10.5 mg/dl. Ionized calcium is the physiologically active form. Most laboratory assays recognize an ionized calcium level (at a serum pH of 7.4) between 1.10 and 1.35 mmol /L as normal [5, 6]. While the normal regulation of serum calcium is reviewed in depth in Chap. 1, this chapter provides a brief overview. Calcium homeostasis is regulated primarily by two key hormones – PTH and vitamin D. PTH is an 84 amino-acid polypeptide hormone secreted by the parathyroid glands. Slight changes in ionized calcium trigger a rapid change in PTH level (Fig. 3.1) [7]. When ionized calcium levels fall, this change is detected by the calcium sensing receptor located on the plasma membrane of the parathyroid chief cells, leading to a rapid increase in the release of PTH [8]. Conversely, elevated serum ionized calcium leads to a decrease in the release of PTH and the serum PTH level. PTH exerts its effect on the major organs responsible for calcium homeostasis – the kidneys, gastrointestinal tract, and skeleton – to restore ionized calcium to normal.

In the setting of calcium deficiency, PTH has direct and indirect actions that serve to increase serum calcium to maintain normal levels. In the kidney, PTH directly increases serum ionized calcium by increasing urinary calcium reabsorption via its effect to increase expression of calbindin (calcium-binding protein), the sodium calcium exchanger (NCX), the plasma membrane calcium ATPase (PMCA), and the transient receptor potential cation channel (TRPV5) in the distal nephron [9, 10].

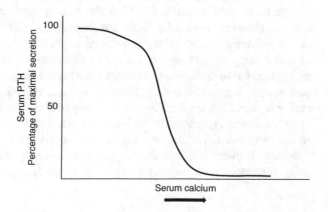

Fig. 3.1 Schematic of effect of ionized calcium on PTH level [7–11]. (Adapted from Walker et al. [7])

PTH also acts indirectly to stimulate the transcription of the renal 1-α-hydroxylase (CYP27B1), which converts 25-hydroxyvitamin D to its active form, 1,25-dihydroxyvitamin D. In the gastrointestinal tract, 1,25-dihydroxyvitamin D acts as a transcription factor, enhancing the transcription of transient receptor potential vanilloid channel type 6 and the plasma membrane calcium ATPase, which facilitate the active absorption of calcium [11]. In the skeleton, PTH binds to its receptor on osteoblasts and has multiple actions including increasing the production of receptor activator of nuclear factor kappa-B ligand (RANKL). RANKL increases osteoclast differentiation, activity, and bone resorption, leading to the release of ionized calcium into the plasma.

Under normal circumstances, when ionized calcium rises, the reverse sequence of events serves to decrease and restore serum calcium to normal. The decline in PTH facilitates the renal excretion of calcium. Calcium excess or sufficiency along with suppressed PTH leads to the preferential formation of 24,25-dihydroxyvitamin D (an inactive metabolite), rather than 1,25-dihydroxyvitamin D, thereby limiting gastrointestinal absorption. The decrease in PTH also reduces bone resorption.

Pathophysiology, Differential Diagnosis, and Overview of Causes of Hypercalcemia

Hypercalcemia may occur via PTH-mediated or non-PTH-mediated pathophysiological processes (Table 3.1). In all cases, hypercalcemia results from either increased bone resorption, reduced renal excretion, increased gastrointestinal absorption, or a combination [3]. Hypercalcemia leads to renal salt and water loss, volume contraction, and reduced filtration and excretion of calcium, which tend to further exacerbate the hypercalcemia. This is often compounded by nausea and vomiting, thus setting off a vicious cycle by which hypercalcemia worsens and sustains itself.

The major causes of hypercalcemia are shown in Table 3.1 according to their major mechanism. Many causes act via multiple mechanisms. For example, the predominant mechanism in PHPT is the excess production of PTH, leading to increased bone resorption, but increased gastrointestinal absorption also plays a role due to enhanced expression of the 1-α-hydroxylase by PTH [7, 12]. Hypercalcemia of malignancy may occur via multiple mechanisms. The most common is bone resorption due to osteolytic metastases (most often from multiple myeloma, breast cancer, melanoma, renal cell carcinoma, non-small cell lung cancer, and thyroid cancer) or humoral hypercalcemia of malignancy (HHM), while 1,25-dihydroxyvitamin D production by lymphoma is relatively rare [13–17]. Less common causes of hypercalcemia include thyrotoxicosis, vitamin toxicity (A or D), medications (e.g., lithium and thiazide diuretics), milk-alkali syndrome, granulomatous disease (e.g., sarcoidosis, mycobacterium infection, and tuberculosis), prolonged immobilization, familial hypocalciuric hypercalcemia, and primary adrenal insufficiency (see Chap. 2 for a complete discussion of etiology) [16].

Diagnostic Approach

It is imperative to have a systematic approach to the diagnosis of hypercalcemia. This typically consists of confirming hypercalcemia and determining the etiology via history, physical examination, and a set algorithm of laboratory investigations that may be followed by more specific testing depending on the clinical circumstances (Fig. 3.2).

Confirm Hypercalcemia

When hypercalcemia is encountered, it is typically detected as an increase in serum total calcium. While total calcium is often reflective of ionized calcium, it is greatly influenced by serum albumin since approximately 40% of calcium is protein bound. Hyperalbuminemia results in a high total serum calcium due to an increase in calcium's protein-bound fraction, but the physiologically active ionized calcium level remains normal. Thus, the first step of the diagnostic evaluation is to confirm that hypercalcemia is present and that it is not a result of "pseudohypercalcemia" from hyperalbuminemia or, less commonly, hypergammaglobulinemia (as may be seen in multiple myeloma) [18, 19]. Pseudohypercalcemia occurs when there is an elevation in total serum calcium without an increase in ionized calcium. Conversely, serum total calcium may appear normal, causing hypercalcemia to go unrecognized, in the setting of hypoalbuminemia. Total calcium should be confirmed with repeat measurement along with measurement of albumin and/or measurement of ionized calcium. The following formula can be utilized as a correction for hypoalbuminemia:

$$\text{Corrected calcium} = \text{measured serum total calcium} + 0.8\left[4 - \text{albumin in g / dL}\right]$$

The opposite formula in which the albumin correction is subtracted from the measured serum total calcium can be used for hyperalbuminemia, but some authorities advocate using ionized calcium in this situation [20]. In complex clinical situations, such as the presence of acid-based disorders or retention of anions (e.g., critical illness and renal failure), measurement of ionized calcium is necessary since correction does not address the shift in albumin's affinity for calcium or its complexing with anions, respectively [21, 22]. In addition to confirming hypercalcemia, reviewing labs to ascertain the duration and degree of hypercalcemia are helpful in

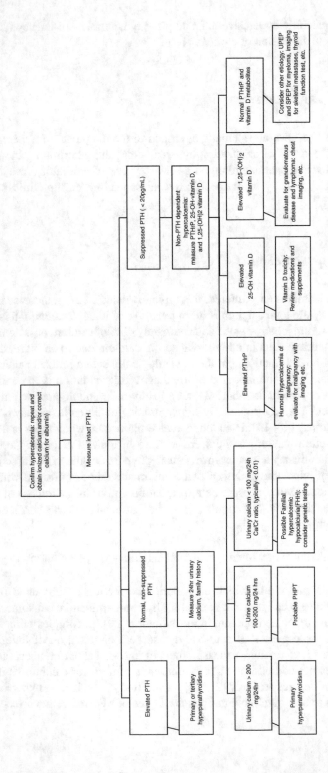

Fig. 3.2 Diagnostic evaluation of hypercalcemia

guiding diagnosis. Chronic hypercalcemia that is present for many years suggests a benign diagnosis (e.g., PHPT and sarcoid).

History and Physical Examination: Symptoms and Signs

Clinical clues to the etiology of hypercalcemia may be obvious from patient's presentation and history (Table 3.2). While the symptoms related to moderate to severe hypercalcemia (fatigue, nausea, vomiting, constipation, polyuria, polydipsia, confusion, etc.) are not specific to etiology, the presence of symptoms tends to indicate a more ominous, rapidly progressive condition. That is, a patient with severe and symptomatic hypercalcemia is more likely to have hypercalcemia of malignancy than PHPT. On the other hand, mild asymptomatic hypercalcemia that has been present for many years, particularly in healthy postmenopausal women, is most likely to be PHPT [12].

The history should elicit prior episodes of hypercalcemia, history of nephrolithiasis, osteoporosis and fractures, history of neck irradiation, cosmetic injections or procedures (e.g. silicone implants and injections), calcium and vitamin D intake from dietary sources and supplements, symptoms of hypercalcemia, prior medical history with careful attention to possible etiologies of hypercalcemia (e.g., sarcoid and hyperthyroidism), exposure to tuberculosis (and other granuloma-forming pathogens), review of medications (particularly thiazides, lithium, PTH analogs,

Table 3.2 Clinical features that may guide the diagnosis of hypercalcemia

	History	Physical
PHPT	Asymptomatic, kidney stones, osteoporosis, fragility fracture; lithium use	Well appearing/no physical signs
FHH	Family history, lifelong or longstanding hypercalcemia	None
Malignancy	Weight loss, fevers, anorexia, nausea, polyuria, polydipsia, constitutional symptoms; tobacco use	Ill appearance, thin body habitus, wasting; masses, lymphadenopathy; spinal tenderness in myeloma,
Sarcoid, TB	Cough, hemoptysis, fever, constitutional symptoms; history of TB exposure or positive PPD test	Thin body habitus, fever, respiratory findings, lymphadenopathy
Vitamin D intoxication	History of taking vitamin D supplements	None
Silicon-associated hypercalcemia	History of cosmetic injections	Exogenous material may be palpable overlying areas that have had cosmetic procedures
Milk-alkali syndrome	Zealous calcium supplement use, history of osteoporosis	None

and vitamin D), family history of hypercalcemia, tobacco use, whether age-appropriate cancer screening is current, and a review of prior laboratory work. A thorough review of systems that includes constitutional (fever, weight loss, diaphoresis, etc.) and other (cough, etc.) symptoms is helpful as it may point to undiagnosed systemic disorders such as malignancies, hyperthyroidism, sarcoid, and infectious etiologies.

There are few physical signs of hypercalcemia except those related to the consequences of recent onset moderate to severe hypercalcemia (i.e., signs of dehydration, altered mental status, lethargy, etc.), and they are not specific to etiology. Vital signs and general appearance are helpful in broadly guiding one toward the two major etiologies, PHPT versus malignancy. Band keratopathy (which describes the precipitation of calcium salt in a band-like distribution on the corneal surface) is uncommon and not specific to cause [23]. Certain findings may raise suspicion for specific diagnoses. For example, spinal tenderness, kyphosis, and vertebral fractures could indicate myeloma, whereas a breast mass may point to hypercalcemia of malignancy. QT shortening on the electrocardiogram may be observed with moderate to severe hypercalcemia but is not specific to cause [24]. Other EKG features of hypercalcemia include T wave inversion or flattening, mild prolongation of the PR interval, shortening of the ST interval, ST-elevation, and the presence of J wave at the end of the QRS complex [24].

Laboratory Testing

PTH

The next step in the diagnostic approach to assess the cause of hypercalcemia is to measure serum intact PTH to distinguish PTH-mediated from non-PTH mediated hypercalcemia. PTH is an 84-amino acid peptide that is produced by the parathyroid glands. PTH should be measured with an intact immunoradiometric (IRMA) or immunochemiluminometric (ICMA) second generation assay, which readily discriminates between PHPT and hypercalcemia of malignancy. In PHPT, PTH concentrations are usually frankly elevated. A minority of patients with PHPT may have PTH levels in the normal range, typically the upper half of the normal range. Such values, although within the normal range, are clearly abnormal in a hypercalcemic setting and consistent with PHPT. PTH levels that are lower but greater than 20 pg/ml are also consistent with PHPT, though in such cases it is often prudent to exclude other causes [25, 26]. In familial hypocalciuric hypercalcemia (FHH), a genetic condition characterized by hypercalcemia and mutations in the calcium sensing receptor (CASR), or GNA11 and AP2S1 genes, PTH levels tend to be in the high normal range [27, 28]. Given the rarity of this condition, a PTH level in this range is still most likely to be consistent with PHPT.

The other major cause of hypercalcemia, malignancy, is characterized by suppressed PTH level. For patients with suppressed PTH (non-PTH-mediated hypercalcemia), the next step involves measurement of parathyroid hormone-related peptide (PTHrP) and vitamin D metabolites. PTHrP does not cross-react in the PTH assay. Ectopic production of PTH by malignancies is extremely rare but has been reported occasionally in neuroendocrine tumors, lung, thymus, and ovarian cancers. There have also been cases reports of patients with neuroendocrine tumors that cosecrete both PTH and PTHrP [29]. However, when the PTH level is elevated in someone with a malignancy, it is more likely that the malignancy is present in association with PHPT rather than the elevation being due to a true ectopic PTH syndrome.

Parathyroid Hormone–Related Peptide and Other Testing for Malignancy

If PTH is suppressed, PTHrP should be measured. In the 1940s, Albright proposed a PTH-like factor to explain the syndrome of hypercalcemia of malignancy in a patient with renal cell carcinoma [30] . His hypothesis was based on similarities between the clinical presentation of his patient and that of PHPT. In the 1980s, PTHrP was eventually identified, and an assay was developed to measure it [30, 31]. PTHrP is a peptide with close homology to PTH in the N-terminal sequence. Circulating levels are negligible in the adult under normal circumstances, but production by malignancies can lead to "humoral hypercalcemia of malignancy" or HHM. Like PTH, its actions are mediated by its binding to the type 1 PTH receptor. HHM, in contrast to PHPT, however, typically has an abrupt, symptomatic onset and results in higher serum calcium levels. Most patients have advanced, clinically obvious malignancies at the time hypercalcemia develops. If, however, the patient has no known history, appropriate evaluation with imaging and sex- and age-specific screening should be undertaken. Another distinguishing features of HHM, in contrast to PHPT, includes 1,25-dihydroxyvitamin D levels that are typically, but not always, low normal due to suppressed PTH [32]. Phosphate is often low in HHM (depending on renal function) due to the phosphaturic effects of PTHrP, similar to those of PTH. HHM is associated with squamous cell carcinoma and other malignancies including renal cell and bladder carcinoma, breast and ovarian cancer, leukemia (e.g. CML), and some lymphomas (adult T-cell and HTLV1-associated adult T-cell lymphoma/leukemia) [14–17, 33]. Hypercalcemia is particularly frequent and can be very severe in HTLV1-associated adult T-cell lymphoma/leukemia. In one series, 87% of patients with ATLL developed hypercalcemia at least once [34].

Malignancies may also cause hypercalcemia by multiple other mechanisms besides HHM, including osteolytic metastases and production of 1,25-dihydroxyvitamin D (see below and Chap. 11). Thus, the absence of a detectable PTHrP level does not exclude malignancy. In the case of osteolytic metastases, hypercalcemia is the result of locally activated bone destruction, rather than circulating PTHrP. Tumor cells at the site of metastasis increase osteoclast activity and inhibit osteoblasts through the release of cytokines including interleukins 1 and 6, macrophage colony stimulating factor, and macrophage inflammatory protein 1 α [35]. Hypercalcemia caused by osteolytic metastases is a late-stage manifestation of solid malignancies, such as breast, lung, prostate, and kidney [36]. Thus, this type of hypercalcemia is not usually a diagnostic dilemma. Extremely rarely, hypercalcemia related to osteolytic metastases will be the presenting manifestation of an undiagnosed late-stage cancer that may be discovered via imaging or other testing. In multiple myeloma, hypercalcemia is also caused by the release of local factors and cytokines (receptor activator of nuclear factor-kB ligand (RANKL), macrophage inflammatory protein (MIP)-1alpha, and tumor necrosis factors) that activate osteoclasts [37, 38]. Hypercalcemia is present in approximately 13–20% of myeloma patients, and bone pain is the presenting symptom or sign in 58% of patients [39]. Screening with serum and urine electrophoresis and immunofixation identify 97% of patients with myeloma [39]. See Chap. 10.

Vitamin D Metabolites

Only 10% of cases of hypercalcemia are due to causes other than PHPT and malignancy. Vitamin D metabolites should be measured in the absence of elevated PTH. Vitamin D intoxication may be suspected based on history. Patients are, however, sometimes unknowingly ingesting supraphysiological quantities of vitamin D. An over-the-counter supplement, which contains 864,000 IU of vitamin D and vitamin A (predominantly retinyl palmitate 123,500 IU), has been associated with the development of hypercalcemia and is a popular "health tonic" in some communities [40]. A careful history and visual review of over-the-counter herbals and supplements is sometimes required to uncover the source of vitamin D ingestion. An elevated serum level of 25-hydroxyvitamin D confirms intake of vitamin D. The exact threshold of 25-hydroxyvitamin D needed to cause hypercalcemia is unclear, and in one case series, many who developed hypercalcemia, in the setting of excessive vitamin D intake, had an underlying condition predisposing to hypercalcemia [40]. Thus, the presence of "high" vitamin d level does not necessarily exclude other causes. One review indicated no cases of intoxication reported for daily intakes of <30,000 IU per day for extended periods or serum 25-hydroxyvitamin D levels <200 ng/ml [41]. Other experts define a 25-hydroxyvitamin D level > 100–150 ng/ml as consistent with vitamin D toxicity (see Chap. 12) [42]. In addition to supplements, repeated exposure to sunlight can raise serum 25-hydroxyvitamin D concentrations to as high as 79 ng per milliliter [43]. There has, however, never been a case of vitamin D toxicity reported due to sunlight exposure.

Elevated 1,25-dihydroxyvitamin D in the setting of hypercalcemia and a suppressed PTH is consistent with ectopic production of 1,25-dihydroxyvitamin D, calcitriol or calcitriol analog ingestion, or impaired 1,25-dihydroxyvitamin D metabolism. In all causes of 1,25-dihydroxyvitamin D-mediated hypercalcemia, the major mechanism is increased intestinal calcium absorption, though increased bone resorption plays a role as well. Serum phosphate is often high since 1,25-dihydroxyvitamin D mediates not only calcium but also phosphate absorption.

In patients with sarcoid, macrophages within granulomas are responsible for increased and unrestrained 1 α-hydroxylase activity and the increase in serum 1,25-dihydroxyvitamin D levels. Hypercalcemia related to sarcoid may be intermittent but is often long-standing, and hypercalciuria is also common. Hypercalcemia associated with elevated 1,25-dihydroxyvitamin D has been associated with numerous other granulomatous disorders, including tuberculosis, mycobacterium infection, fungal infections, and others (see Table 3.1). These etiologies are presumed to have a similar mechanism. Less common granulomatous disorders reported to result in hypercalcemia include silicone granulomatosis related to silicone injections and implants, Crohn's disease, Wegner's granulomatosis, and cat scratch fever [20]. Chest imaging can be helpful to assess for lymphadenopathy, malignancy, and the characteristic findings associated with pulmonary sarcoid or granulomatous infections. Biopsy with culture and flow-cytometry may be needed as well as testing for tuberculosis. Failure to identify the culprit diagnosis may require more extensive imaging and testing including positron emission tomography (PET)/computed tomography (CT), etc. Elevated circulating angiotensin converting enzyme (ACE) levels have been associated with various granulomatous disorders. Measurement of ACE levels is not necessarily recommended due to its limited sensitivity and specificity, though elevated levels may be supportive of a diagnosis of granulomatous disease [44].

Hodgkin's and non-Hodgkin's lymphoma can cause hypercalcemia due to malignant lymphocyte and/or neighboring macrophage unregulated expression of 1 α-hydroxylase, the enzyme responsible for converting 25-hydroxyvitamin D to 1, 25-dihydroxyvitamin D, similar to the mechanism seen in sarcoid [45]. Hypercalcemia due to this cause is relatively rare but when present can be marked and symptomatic. A more thorough discussion is included in Chap. 11. Overingestion of calcitriol can lead to elevated 1,25-dihydroxyvitamin D levels and hypercalcemia. Hypercalcemia related to this cause is similar to other 1,25-dihydroxyvitamin D-mediated causes. Calcipotriol, also known as calcipotriene, is a synthetic derivative of calcitriol that is commonly used for psoriasis. Hypercalcemia related to calcipotriol is dose-dependent and has been observed with doses of more than 5.6 g of calcipotriol (50 ug/g) ointment per kilogram of body weight per week [46, 47].

Other Tests and Timing of Tests

Other tests that are useful in the evaluation of hypercalcemia include measurement of serum phosphate, renal function, urinary calcium, serum magnesium, serum bone markers (particularly alkaline phosphatase), and bicarbonate and chloride. In fact, routine laboratories (serum phosphate, magnesium, renal function, and alkaline phosphatase) are often obtained early in the evaluation of an ill patient and available before more specific testing, such as serum PTH. While all such tests are not specifically in the "algorithm," their early evaluation is often critical in providing early clues to the etiology of hypercalcemia and the status of the patient. Because the phosphate level rapidly results, it, in particular, may provide helpful initial insight

Table 3.3 Biochemical patterns in hypercalcemia of various etiologies

Diagnosis	Calcium	Phosphorus	PTH	25OHD	1,25OHD
Primary hyperparathyroidism	↑	↓	↑/normal	Dependent on intake	↑/↔
Vitamin D toxicity/ingestion	↑	↑	↓	↑	↑/↔
Humoral hypercalcemia of malignancy (PTHrP mediated)	↑↑	↓	↓	Dependent on intake	↓
Osteolytic metastasis	↑↑	↔	↓	Dependent on intake	↓
Granulomatous disease and malignancies producing 1,25-dihydroxyvitamin D (1 α-hydroxylase mediated)	↑	↑	↓	Dependent on intake	↑
Familial hypocalciuric hypercalcemia	↑	↔ or ↓	Inappropriately normal	Dependent on intake	↔[a]

[a]1,25 OH D levels are increased when compared with those without FHH, but still within normal reference range [75]

into the etiology until such time PTH and vitamin D metabolites are available. As shown in Table 3.3, the biochemical patterns of serum calcium, PTH, phosphate, and vitamin D metabolites are helpful in determining the etiology. Various causes of hypercalcemia tend to have distinct patterns.

Evaluation of hypercalcemia is presented as a stepwise algorithm in this chapter, but in practice, the timing and order of testing may vary depending on the clinical situation. Serum PTH level is typically the best initial and most cost-effective specific test to address the etiology of hypercalcemia, particularly in healthy outpatients. In patients with moderate to severe hypercalcemia, particularly those that are hospitalized, however, it often makes sense to obtain much of the testing simultaneously.

Serum Phosphate Phosphate is typically low in PTH- or PTHrP-mediated hypercalcemia due to their phosphaturic effects on the kidney, though renal function affects phosphate levels (Table 3.3). On the other hand, in vitamin D-mediated hypercalcemia, serum phosphate levels tend to be elevated toward the high end of normal secondary to vitamin D's effect on the absorption of phosphate. Hypophosphatemia is also common in Milk-Alkali syndrome because calcium carbonate acts as a phosphate-binder in the gastrointestinal tract [48, 49].

Renal function The assessment of renal function is important in all causes of hypercalcemia to understand the impact of hypercalcemia on renal function. Acute renal dysfunction, particularly transient impairment due to dehydration, may be present in moderate to severe hypercalcemia of any etiology that has developed rapidly. Thus, the presence of acute renal impairment is not particularly useful in discriminating the cause other than to suggest the etiology is associated with a more rapidly progressive cause. Tertiary hyperparathyroidism is characterized by autonomous parathyroid function that develops in the setting of prolong secondary hyperparathyroidism, usually due to late- or end-stage kidney disease before or after kidney transplant. The diagnosis of tertiary hyperparathyroidism is usually obvious from the history.

Twenty-four-hour urinary calcium Urinary calcium excretion is usually increased in patients with hypercalcemia of most etiologies when renal function is intact due to the increased filtration of calcium. Hypercalciuria (defined as urinary calcium excretion >250 mg/day in women and > 300 mg/day in men) is present in some patients with PHPT [25, 50]. In PHPT, urinary calcium is, however, affected by dietary factors such as vitamin D. Urinary calcium may be low in patients on thiazides and in patients with vitamin D deficiency or renal insufficiency. Thus, excretion is variable. Urinary calcium may be useful in differentiating PHPT from FHH [2]. Calcium urinary excretion >200 mg/day makes FHH unlikely. Fractional excretion of calcium [(24-hour urine Ca × serum Cr) / (serum Ca × 24-hour urine Cr)] in PHPT is often >0.02, while in FHH, it is <0.01, but there is considerable overlap between the disorders [51]. Because of the rarity of FHH, patients with low urinary calcium are still more likely to have PHPT, rather than FHH. Genetic testing can be utilized to confirm FHH. Additionally, review of onset of hypercalcemia is helpful since in FHH, hypercalcemia should be present from birth, though it may not be discovered at that time. Family history also provides critical information. FHH is characterized by autosomal dominant inheritance and high penetrance.

Markers of bone turnover Markers of bone formation, such as alkaline phosphatase, and markers of bone resorption such as c-telopeptide of type 1 collagen or n-telopeptide can be helpful in supporting a diagnosis of hypercalcemia related to immobilization [52]. It is important to remember, however, that hypercalcemia of immobilization is a diagnosis of exclusion. Markers of bone turnover may also be elevated in patients with skeletal metastases, though uncoupling of resorption and formation may be present [53, 54]. The absence of elevation of markers does not, however, exclude metastatic disease, and thus, their use is only adjunctive.

Chloride and bicarbonate In milk alkali syndrome caused by ingestion of calcium carbonate, alkalosis and renal impairment are typically present. The maintenance of hypercalcemia is facilitated by an increase in renal reabsorption of calcium as a result of metabolic alkalosis and volume depletion. In most patients with milk alkali syndrome, serum chloride tends to be low [55, 56].

Serum magnesium Serum magnesium tends to be high normal in FHH due to increased reabsorption. Hypomagnesemia may be present in milk alkali syndrome due to reduced reabsorption in the kidney [48, 49].

Creatinine kinase Although hypocalcemia is often seen in patients with rhabdomyolysis and acute renal failure during the oliguric phase, hypercalcemia may be seen during the diuretic phase. This occurs in approximately 30% of patients due to the mobilization of calcium that had been deposited in the injured muscle and may be related to 1,25-dihydroxyvitamin D levels [57].

Other Etiologies

If testing for PTH, PTHrP, or vitamin D metabolites (25-hydroxyvitamin D and 1,25-dihydroxyvitamin D) is not revealing, less common etiologies such as hyperthyroidism, adrenal insufficiency, pheochromocytoma, and vitamin A toxicity, etc. should be ruled out with appropriate testing (TSH, cortisol, plasma metanephrines, etc.). These tests may be helpful earlier in the evaluation depending on clinical suspicion or the severity of illness of the patient. A rare cause of 1,25-dihydroxyvitamin D-mediated hypercalcemia is due to a mutation in the 1,25(OH)$_2$D-24-hydroxylase cytochrome P450 (CYP24A1) enzyme that is responsible for the inactivation of 1,25-dihydroxyvitamin D by its metabolism to 1,24,25-dihydroxvitamin D. In this case, however, hypercalcemia is presumably lifelong and often associated with nephrolithiasis [58]. There is variability in expression, onset, and severity and adult onset has been described. Homozygotes typically, but not always, present with more severe hypercalcemia in infancy. Family history can be helpful. Levels of circulating 24,25-(OH)$_2$D are low, and the circulating 25-OHD to 24,25-(OH)$_2$D ratio may be a useful screen [59]. A more complete discussion of rare causes of hypercalcemia is reviewed in Chaps. 15 and 16.

Pitfalls in Diagnosis and Other Considerations

Assay Interference

There are several publications that have reported falsely low PTH levels in patients with PHPT due to interference from biotin [60, 61]. Biotin is a B vitamin that has recently been marketed for hair, nail, and skin health. While adequate intake for biotin is reported to be 30 ug daily, over-the-counter supplements may contain as much as 10 mg [62, 63]. Immunoassay interference has not been reported in biotin doses up to 1 mg. However, high dose ingestion (e.g., > 5 mg) can interfere with commonly used immunoassays that utilize a biotin–streptavidin linkage (e.g., PTH). Excess biotin in the specimen allows biotin to bind to the streptavidin sites, blocking the biotinylated antibody and the binding of PTH. Other assays that utilize this methodology are also susceptible, and this phenomenon has been reported to interfere with the measurement of 25-hydroxyvitamin D, TSH, and other hormones. In 2017, the FDA published a safety alert regarding biotin interference [60, 62, 64, 65]. Biotin should be discontinued for 72 hours after which PTH can be remeasured [66].

Heterophile antibodies can interfere with PTH and PTHrP immunoassays [67]. When the clinical history is incongruent with the assay result, heterophile antibodies should be considered. For example, elevated PTHrP in women with long-standing, mild hypercalcemia and no history of malignancy may raise suspicion for this phenomenon. In these situations, running the specimen in a different assay, with dilution or with a heterophile blocking agent, may be helpful. Prevalence is of heterophile antibodies is low (0.2–3.7%) [68].

Effect of Renal Dysfunction on PTH and PTHrP Assays

While the "intact" PTH IRMA overestimates the concentration of biologically active PTH in renal failure, this does not typically interfere with distinguishing PTH-mediated and non-PTH-mediated causes. In 1998, Lepage demonstrated a large non-(1–84) PTH fragment that comigrated with a large aminoterminally truncated fragment (PTH[7–84]) and showed cross-reactivity in commercially available IRMAs [69]. This large, inactive moiety constituted 50% or greater of the immunoreactivity by IRMA for PTH in individuals with chronic renal failure. Recognition of this molecule led to the development of a newer IRMA using affinity-purified polyclonal antibodies to PTH(39–84) and to the extreme N-terminal amino acid regions, PTH(1–4)(1). This "whole PTH" or third generation assay detects only the full-length PTH molecule, PTH(1–84). Use of a third-generation assay does not increase the diagnostic sensitivity for distinguishing PHPT from other causes of hypercalcemia, however [7, 70].

Similarly, accumulation of carboxy-terminal PTHrP can be seen in severe renal insufficiency (typically creatinine clearance less than 20 ml/min), even in patients without cancer [71]. Thus, the presence of elevated PTHrP in the setting of hypercalcemia does not always indicate HHM [72]. N-terminal PTHrP may be helpful in distinguishing HHM in this circumstance because it is less affected by renal function.

Benign Production of PTHrP

Rarely, PTHrP may be produced via benign causes (see Chap. 16). In 1990, Khosla et al. described a case of hypercalcemia from the production of PTHrP by hypertrophied breast tissue that resolved after mastectomy, indicating that PTHrP-induced hypercalcemia is not limited to malignant disorders and can be seen in benign etiologies [73]. In one recent case series, benign causes accounted for 8.7% of cases of PTHrP-mediated hypercalcemia. Other unusual PTHrP-mediated hypercalcemic causes have been reported including HIV-associated lymphadenopathy, lymphedema of chest and pleural cavities, systemic lupus erythematous, benign tumors of ovary and kidney, and benign pheochromocytoma [20, 74].

Conclusion

Hypercalcemia is a common clinical problem. While the etiology is most often related to PHPT or malignancy, following a methodical approach that entails considering PTH-mediated and non-PTH-mediated causes facilitates accurate diagnosis and correct identification of the underlying disorder, particularly those that are less common. After confirming hypercalcemia, performing a history and physical examination, the first and most useful test is the measurement of serum intact PTH. This distinguishes PHPT from other causes. A limited number of other laboratory investigations that include PTHrP, vitamin D metabolites, TSH, electrophoresis, serum phosphate, and serum magnesium typically identify most other causes of hypercalcemia. Rare etiologies may require other testing. The accurate identification of hypercalcemia not only is gratifying for the clinician but also enables successful and definitive management.

Case

A 56-year-old healthy woman was found to have mild hypercalcemia (serum calcium 10.5 mg/dL; reference range 8.5–10.2 mg/dL) on routine blood work performed in the course of laboratory testing done at the time of her annual physical. Repeat testing indicated a calcium of 10.6 mg/dl with parathyroid hormone 16 pg/mL (normal 15–65 pg/mL), albumin of 4.0, and ionized calcium that was mildly elevated. She had menopause 6 years prior. She had no other medical history except for osteopenia. She had no history of nephrolithiasis or fracture. She consumed cholecalciferol 1000 IU orally daily and had no history of smoking. There was no family history of hypercalcemia. Review of systems was negative for fevers, weight loss, night sweats, nausea, vomiting, constipation, or any other symptoms except for thinning of her hair. On examination, she was a healthy appearing woman with normal body mass index and vital signs. She had no kyphosis or bony tenderness. Review of her prior serum calcium levels revealed no evidence of prior hypercalcemia.

Her physician was concerned about non-PTH-mediated causes of hypercalcemia, particularly malignancy. Evaluation for other causes of hypercalcemia was sent: serum calcium 10.3 mg/dl (normal 8.5–10.2 mg/dL), PTH 18 (normal 15–65 pg/mL), ionized calcium mildly elevated, PTHrP within normal, 25-hydroxyvitamin D 40 ng/ml, 1,25-dihydroxyvitamin D 37 pg/ml (18–72 pg/mL), creatinine 0.8 mg/dl, TSH 1.5 mIU/L (normal 0.5–4.5 mIU/L), phosphate 2.7 mg/dl (2.5–4.5 mg/dL), albumin 4.0 mg/dL, magnesium 1.9 mg/dL (normal 1.5–2 mg/dL), alkaline phosphatase 87 U/L (35–144 U/L), serum and urine protein electrophoresis normal, and 24 hour urine calcium 240 mg/24 hours.

She was referred to an endocrinologist for further evaluation of hypercalcemia. On further direct questioning, the patient reported taking biotin for her hair loss but states she forgot to include this in her history when her primary physician had asked her about medications. The patient was instructed to stop her biotin supplementation. Repeat laboratory work up 2 weeks later indicated serum calcium 10.4 mg/dl (normal 8.5–10.2 mg/dL) with PTH

69 pg/mL (normal 15–65 pg/mL). A diagnosis of primary hyperparathyroidism was made.

This case illustrates biotin interference with the PTH assay leading to a pattern that mimics non-PTH-mediated hypercalcemia. Recently, biotin has been marketed as beneficial for skin, hair, and nail growth, and the frequency of biotin supplementation by patients has increased in the United States. Ingestion of biotin can interfere with the performance of a number of immunoassays that utilize a biotin–streptavidin interaction, including the assay for parathyroid hormone. In such an assay, PTH is sandwiched between the signal antibody and the biotinylated antibody, which links the antibody–PTH "sandwich" to a streptavidin-coated solid phase. Without interference, the signal increases as the concentration of PTH increases. If there is excess biotin in the patient's sample related to biotin ingestion, biotin saturates streptavidin binding sites, thereby limiting adherence of the signal bound antibody–PTH complex. This creates a falsely lowered PTH level, which in the context of hypercalcemia, may cause the clinician to infer a non-PTH-mediated cause of hypercalcemia. Thus, in this setting, the physician should query patients regarding the ingestion of biotin. If biotin supplementation is reported, discontinuation and remeasurement of PTH after biotin clearance is usually definitive. Typically, measurement of biotin is not necessary.

References

1. Yeh MW, Ituarte PHG, Zhou HC, Nishimoto S, Liu I-LA, Harari A, et al. Incidence and prevalence of primary hyperparathyroidism in a racially mixed population. J Clin Endocrinol Metab. 2013;98(3):1122–9.
2. Klee GG, Kao PC, Heath H. Hypercalcemia. Endocrinol Metabol Clin North Am. 1988;17(3):28.
3. Lafferty FW. Differential diagnosis of hypercalcemia. J Bone Miner Res. 1991;6 Suppl 2:S51–9; discussion S61.
4. Wermers RAKS, Atkinson EJ, Achenbach SJ, Oberg AL, Grant CS, Melton LJ 3rd. Incidence of primary hyperparathyroidism in Rochester, Minnesota, 1993-2001: An update on the changing epidemiology of the disease. J Bone Miner Metab. 2016;21:171.
5. Wang S, McDonnell EH, Sedor FA, Toffaletti JG. pH effects on measurements of ionized calcium and ionized magnesium in blood. Arch Pathol Lab Med. 2002;126(8):947–50.
6. Pagana KD, Pagana TJ, Pagana TN. Mosby's diagnostic and laboratory test reference. 12th ed. St. Louis: Elsevier; 2015. p. 1–1094.
7. Walker MD, Silverberg SJ. Primary hyperparathyroidism. Nat Rev Endocrinol. 2018;14(2):115–25.
8. Conigrave AD. The calcium-sensing receptor and the parathyroid: past, present, future. Front Physiol. 2016;7:563.
9. Peng JB, Suzuki Y, Gyimesi G, Hediger MA. TRPV5 and TRPV6 calcium-selective channels. In: Kozak JA, Putney JW, Jr., editors. Calcium entry channels in non-excitable cells. Boca Raton: CRC Press/Taylor & Francis © 2017 by Taylor & Francis Group, LLC.; 2018. p. 241–74.
10. Glendenning P, Ratajczak T, Dick IM, Prince RL. Calcitriol upregulates expression and activity of the 1b isoform of the plasma membrane calcium pump in immortalized distal kidney tubular cells. Arch Biochem Biophys. 2000;380(1):126–32.

11. Thyagarajan B, Benn BS, Christakos S, Rohacs T. Phospholipase C-mediated regulation of transient receptor potential vanilloid 6 channels: implications in active intestinal Ca2+ transport. Mol Pharmacol. 2009;75(3):608–16.
12. Silva BC, Cusano NE, Bilezikian JP. Primary hyperparathyroidism. Best Pract Res Clin Endocrinol Metab. 2018;32(5):593–607.
13. Asonitis N, Angelousi A, Zafeiris C, Lambrou GI, Dontas I, Kassi E. Diagnosis, pathophysiology and management of hypercalcemia in malignancy: a review of the literature. Horm Metab Res. 2019;51(12):770–8.
14. Dent DM, Miller JL, Klaff L, Barron J. The incidence and causes of hypercalcaemia. Postgrad Med J. 1987;63(743):745–50.
15. Mitobe M, Kawamoto K, Suzuki T, Kiryu M, Nanba A, Suwabe T, et al. Anaplastic large cell lymphoma, with 1,25(OH)((2))D((3))-mediated hypercalcemia: a case report. J Clin Exp Hematop. 2019;59(1):22–8.
16. Catalano A, Chilà D, Bellone F, Nicocia G, Martino G, Loddo I, et al. Incidence of hypocalcemia and hypercalcemia in hospitalized patients: is it changing? J Clin Transl Endocrinol. 2018;13:9–13.
17. Stewart AF. Clinical practice. Hypercalcemia associated with cancer. N Engl J Med. 2005;352(4):373–9.
18. Ashrafi F, Iraj B, Nematollahi P, Darakhshandeh A. Pseudohypercalcemia in multiple myeloma: a case report. Int J Hematol Oncol Stem Cell Res. 2017;11(3):246–9.
19. Schwab JD, Strack MA, Hughes LD, Shaker JL. Pseudohypercalcemia in an elderly patient with multiple myeloma: report of a case and review of literature. Endocr Pract. 1995;1(6):390–2.
20. Jacobs TP, Bilezikian JP. Clinical review: rare causes of hypercalcemia. J Clin Endocrinol Metab. 2005;90(11):6316–22.
21. Hu ZD, Huang YL, Wang MY, Hu GJ, Han YQ. Predictive accuracy of serum total calcium for both critically high and critically low ionized calcium in critical illness. J Clin Lab Anal. 2018;32(9):e22589.
22. Gøransson LG, Skadberg Ø, Bergrem H. Albumin-corrected or ionized calcium in renal failure? What to measure? Nephrol Dial Transplant. 2005;20(10):2126–9.
23. Galor A, Leder HA, Thorne JE, Dunn JP. Transient band keratopathy associated with ocular inflammation and systemic hypercalcemia. Clin Ophthalmol. 2008;2(3):645–7.
24. Chorin E, Rosso R, Viskin S. Electrocardiographic manifestations of calcium abnormalities. Ann Noninvasive Electrocardiol. 2016;21(1):7–9.
25. Silverberg SJ, Lewiecki EM, Mosekilde L, Peacock M, Rubin MR. Presentation of asymptomatic primary hyperparathyroidism: proceedings of the third international workshop. J Clin Endocrinol Metab. 2009;94(2):351–65.
26. Lee JK, Chuang MJ, Lu CC, Hao LJ, Yang CY, Han TM, et al. Parathyroid hormone and parathyroid hormone related protein assays in the investigation of hypercalcemic patients in hospital in a Chinese population. J Endocrinol Investig. 1997;20(7):404–9.
27. Thakker RV. Genetics of parathyroid tumours. J Intern Med. 2016;280(6):574–83.
28. Pollak MR, Brown EM, Chou YH, Hebert SC, Marx SJ, Steinmann B, et al. Mutations in the human Ca(2+)-sensing receptor gene cause familial hypocalciuric hypercalcemia and neonatal severe hyperparathyroidism. Cell. 1993;75(7):1297–303.
29. Kamp K, Feelders RA, van Adrichem RC, de Rijke YB, van Nederveen FH, Kwekkeboom DJ, et al. Parathyroid hormone-related peptide (PTHrP) secretion by gastroenteropancreatic neuroendocrine tumors (GEP-NETs): clinical features, diagnosis, management, and follow-up. J Clin Endocrinol Metab. 2014;99(9):3060–9.
30. Mundy GR, Edwards JR. PTH-related peptide (PTHrP) in hypercalcemia. J Am Soc Nephrol JASN. 2008;19(4):672–5.
31. Simpson EL, Mundy GR, D'Souza SM, Ibbotson KJ, Bockman R, Jacobs JW. Absence of parathyroid hormone messenger RNA in nonparathyroid tumors associated with hypercalcemia. N Engl J Med. 1983;309(6):325–30.
32. Chukir T, Liu Y, Hoffman K, Bilezikian JP, Farooki A. Calcitriol elevation is associated with a higher risk of refractory hypercalcemia of malignancy in solid tumors. J Clin Endocrinol Metab. 2020;105(4):e1115–23.

33. Zagzag J, Hu MI, Fisher SB, Perrier ND. Hypercalcemia and cancer: differential diagnosis and treatment. CA Cancer J Clin. 2018;68(5):377–86.
34. Licata MJ, Janakiram M, Tan S, Fang Y, Shah UA, Verma AK, et al. Diagnostic challenges of adult T-cell leukemia/lymphoma in North America – a clinical, histological, and immunophenotypic correlation with a workflow proposal. Leuk Lymphoma. 2018;59(5):1188–94.
35. Shupp AB, Kolb AD, Mukhopadhyay D, Bussard KM. Cancer metastases to bone: concepts, mechanisms, and interactions with bone osteoblasts. Cancers (Basel). 2018;10(6):182.
36. Reddington JA, Mendez GA, Ching A, Kubicky CD, Klimo P Jr, Ragel BT. Imaging characteristic analysis of metastatic spine lesions from breast, prostate, lung, and renal cell carcinomas for surgical planning: osteolytic versus osteoblastic. Surg Neurol Int. 2016;7(Suppl 13):S361–S5.
37. Edwards CM, Zhuang J, Mundy GR. The pathogenesis of the bone disease of multiple myeloma. Bone. 2008;42(6):1007–13.
38. Oyajobi BO. Multiple myeloma/hypercalcemia. Arthritis Res Ther. 2007;9 Suppl 1(Suppl 1):S4.
39. Kyle RA, Gertz MA, Witzig TE, Lust JA, Lacy MQ, Dispenzieri A, et al. Review of 1027 patients with newly diagnosed multiple myeloma. Mayo Clin Proc. 2003;78(1):21–33.
40. Lowe H, Cusano NE, Binkley N, Blaner WS, Bilezikian JP. Vitamin D toxicity due to a commonly available "over the counter" remedy from the Dominican Republic. J Clin Endocrinol Metab. 2011;96(2):291–5.
41. Hathcock JN, Shao A, Vieth R, Heaney R. Risk assessment for vitamin D. Am J Clin Nutr. 2007;85(1):6–18.
42. Holick MF. Vitamin D deficiency. N Engl J Med. 2007;357(3):266–81.
43. Haddad JG, Chyu KJ. Competitive protein-binding radioassay for 25-hydroxycholecalciferol. J Clin Endocrinol Metab. 1971;33(6):992–5.
44. Lopez-Sublet M, Caratti di Lanzacco L, Danser AHJ, Lambert M, Elourimi G, Persu A. Focus on increased serum angiotensin-converting enzyme level: From granulomatous diseases to genetic mutations. Clinical biochemistry. 2018;59:1–8.
45. Vallet N, Ertault M, Delaye JB, Chalopin T, Villate A, Drieu La Rochelle L, et al. Hypercalcemia is associated with a poor prognosis in lymphoma a retrospective monocentric matched-control study and extensive review of published reported cases. Ann Hematol. 2020;99(2):229–39.
46. Kawahara C, Okada Y, Tanikawa T, Fukusima A, Misawa H, Tanaka Y. Severe hypercalcemia and hypernatremia associated with calcipotriol for treatment of psoriasis. J Bone Miner Metab. 2004;22(2):159–62.
47. Bourke JF, Mumford R, Whittaker P, Iqbal SJ, Le Van LW, Trevellyan A, et al. The effects of topical calcipotriol on systemic calcium homeostasis in patients with chronic plaque psoriasis. 1998/01/07 ed1997 Dec. 929–34 p.
48. Picolos MK, Lavis VR, Orlander PR. Milk-alkali syndrome is a major cause of hypercalcaemia among non-end-stage renal disease (non-ESRD) inpatients. Clin Endocrinol. 2005;63(5):566–76.
49. Patel AM, Goldfarb S. Got calcium? Welcome to the calcium-alkali syndrome. J Am Soc Nephrol JASN. 2010;21(9):1440–3.
50. Silverberg SJ, Walker MD, Bilezikian JP. Asymptomatic primary hyperparathyroidism. J Clin Densitom. 2013;16(1):14–21. https://doi.org/10.1016/j.jocd.2012.11.005.
51. Lee JY, Shoback DM. Familial hypocalciuric hypercalcemia and related disorders. Best Pract Res Clin Endocrinol Metab. 2018;32(5):609–19.
52. Buehlmeier J, Frings-Meuthen P, Mohorko N, Lau P, Mazzucco S, Ferretti JL, et al. Markers of bone metabolism during 14 days of bed rest in young and older men. J Musculoskelet Neuronal Interact. 2017;17(1):399–408.
53. Kanis JA, McCloskey EV. Bone turnover and biochemical markers in malignancy. Cancer. 1997;80(8 Suppl):1538–45.
54. Fohr B, Dunstan CR, Seibel MJ. Clinical review 165: markers of bone remodeling in metastatic bone disease. J Clin Endocrinol Metab. 2003;88(11):5059–75.
55. Jenkins JK, Best TR, Nicks SA, Murphy FY, Bussell KL, Vesely DL. Milk-alkali syndrome with a serum calcium level of 22 mg/dl and J waves on the ECG. South Med J. 1987;80(11):1444–9.

56. Felsenfeld AJ, Levine BS. Milk alkali syndrome and the dynamics of calcium homeostasis. Clin J Am Soc Nephrol. 2006;1(4):641–54.
57. Akmal M, Bishop JE, Telfer N, Norman AW, Massry SG. Hypocalcemia and hypercalcemia in patients with rhabdomyolysis with and without acute renal failure. J Clin Endocrinol Metab. 1986;63(1):137–42.
58. Jacobs TP, Kaufman M, Jones G, Kumar R, Schlingmann K-P, Shapses S, et al. A lifetime of hypercalcemia and hypercalciuria, finally explained. J Clin Endocrinol Metabol. 2014;99(3):708–12.
59. Carpenter TO. CYP24A1 loss of function: clinical phenotype of monoallelic and biallelic mutations. J Steroid Biochem Mol Biol. 2017;173:337–40.
60. Waghray A, Milas M, Nyalakonda K, Siperstein AE. Falsely low parathyroid hormone secondary to biotin interference: a case series. Endocr Pract. 2013;19(3):451–5.
61. Colon PJ, Greene DN. Biotin interference in clinical immunoassays. J Appl Lab Med. 2019;2(6):941–51.
62. Carter GD, Berry J, Cavalier E, Durazo-Arvizu R, Gunter E, Jones G, et al. Biotin supplementation causes erroneous elevations of results in some commercial serum 25-hydroxyvitamin d (25OHD) assays. J Steroid Biochem Mol Biol. 2020;200:105639.
63. Institute of Medicine Standing Committee on the Scientific Evaluation of Dietary Reference I, its Panel on Folate OBV, Choline. The National Academies Collection: Reports funded by National Institutes of Health. Dietary Reference Intakes for Thiamin, Riboflavin, Niacin, Vitamin B(6), Folate, Vitamin B(12), Pantothenic Acid, Biotin, and Choline. Washington (DC): National Academies Press (US) Copyright © 1998, National Academy of Sciences.; 1998.
64. Li D, Radulescu A, Shrestha RT, Root M, Karger AB, Killeen AA, et al. Association of Biotin Ingestion with Performance of hormone and nonhormone assays in healthy adults. JAMA. 2017;318(12):1150–60.
65. Li D, Ferguson A, Cervinski MA, Lynch KL, Kyle PB. AACC guidance document on biotin interference in laboratory tests. J Appl Lab Med. 2020;5(3):575–87.
66. Kummer S, Hermsen D, Distelmaier, F. Biotin Treatment Mimicking Graves' Disease. 2016; (375):704–6.
67. Laudes M, Frohnert J, Ivanova K, Wandinger K-P. PTH immunoassay interference due to human anti-mouse antibodies in a subject with obesity with normal parathyroid function. J Clin Endocrinol Metabol. 2019;104(12):5840–2.
68. Datta P. Chapter 6 – Immunoassay design and mechanisms of interferences. In: Dasgupta A, Sepulveda JL, editors. Accurate results in the clinical laboratory. San Diego: Elsevier; 2013. p. 63–73.
69. Lepage R, Roy L, Brossard JH, Rousseau L, Dorais C, Lazure C, et al. A non-(1-84) circulating parathyroid hormone (PTH) fragment interferes significantly with intact PTH commercial assay measurements in uremic samples. Clin Chem. 1998;44(4):805–9.
70. Silverberg SJ, Gao P, Brown I, LoGerfo P, Cantor TL, Bilezikian JP. Clinical utility of an immunoradiometric assay for parathyroid hormone (1-84) in primary hyperparathyroidism. J Clin Endocrinol Metab. 2003;88(10):4725–30.
71. Orloff JJ, Soifer NE, Fodero JP, Dann P, Burtis WJ. Accumulation of carboxy-terminal fragments of parathyroid hormone-related protein in renal failure. Kidney Int. 1993;43(6):1371–6.
72. Lum G. Falsely elevated parathyroid hormone-related protein (PTH-RP) in a patient with hypercalcemia and renal failure. Lab Med. 2011;42(12):726–8.
73. Khosla S, van Heerden JA, Gharib H, Jackson IT, Danks J, Hayman JA, et al. Parathyroid hormone-related protein and hypercalcemia secondary to massive mammary hyperplasia. N Engl J Med. 1990;322(16):1157.
74. Donovan PJ, Achong N, Griffin K, Galligan J, Pretorius CJ, McLeod DS. PTHrP-mediated hypercalcemia: causes and survival in 138 patients. J Clin Endocrinol Metab. 2015;100(5):2024–9.
75. Christensen S, Nissen P, Vestergaard P, Heickendorff L, Rejnmark L, Brixen K, Mosekilde L. Plasma 25-hydroxyvitamin D, 1,25-dihydroxyvitamin D, and parathyroid hormone in familial hypocalciuric hypercalcemia and primary hyperparathyroidism. Eur J Endocrinol. 2008;159(6):719–27.

Chapter 4
Diagnostic Approach and Treatment of the Pediatric Patient with Hypercalcemia

David R. Weber and Michael A. Levine

Introduction

Hypercalcemia is less common in children and adolescents than in adults. Nevertheless, there is a diverse and extensive catalog of genetic and acquired conditions that can cause hypercalcemia in the pediatric population. The clinical consequences of hypercalcemia are highly variable and range from an asymptomatic laboratory finding to a life-threatening medical emergency. In many cases, hypercalcemia presents as a diagnostic dilemma, as the pathophysiology underlying calcium metabolism is complex and the individual disorders causing hypercalcemia are rare. However, the correct diagnosis can usually be obtained using a mechanistic approach that systematically considers the diverse causes for dysregulated calcium homeostasis (Fig. 4.1). The objectives of this chapter are to review the epidemiology, pathophysiology, and clinical approach to childhood hypercalcemia. The chapter is organized according to the primary mechanism of hypercalcemia (Table 4.1), although an age-related approach can be useful as well (Fig. 4.2).

D. R. Weber · M. A. Levine (✉)
Division of Endocrinology and Diabetes and the Center for Bone Health, The Children's Hospital of Philadelphia, Philadelphia, PA, USA

Department of Pediatrics, University of Pennsylvania Perelman School of Medicine, Philadelphia, PA, USA
e-mail: WEBERD@chop.edu; levinem@chop.edu

© The Author(s), under exclusive license to Springer Nature Switzerland AG 2022
M. D. Walker (ed.), *Hypercalcemia*, Contemporary Endocrinology, https://doi.org/10.1007/978-3-030-93182-7_4

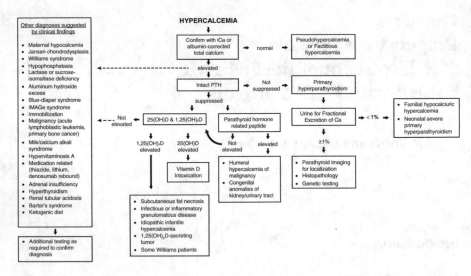

Fig. 4.1 Diagnostic algorithm for childhood hypercalcemia. The clinical approach begins by confirming the veracity of hypercalcemia either by correcting for albumin or ionized calcium. The differential diagnosis is then narrowed as PTH dependent or independent. The etiology of primary hyperparathyroidism should be determined as it will inform treatment. Further testing in PTH-independent cases will include assessment of vitamin D metabolites and PTHrP. In other cases, additional clinical findings will suggest the diagnosis (see text)

General Considerations

The physiologic mechanisms of calcium regulation are discussed in Chap. 1 and will not be covered here. It is necessary to emphasize several factors when assessing serum and urinary calcium concentrations in children, however. Total calcium is composed of both free (ionized, iCa) and substrate-bound calcium. Approximately 40% of total calcium is bound to protein, primarily albumin, with another 10% bound to small anions [1]. Total serum calcium must therefore be adjusted in the setting of hyperalbuminemia, by subtracting 0.8 mg/dL (0.2 mmol/L) for each 1 g/dL increase in albumin over 4 g/dL. Calcium binding to albumin is decreased in the setting of acidemia, resulting in a relatively greater fraction of iCa. Improper specimen collection, handling, or prolonged transport time can result in a downward drift in pH and rise in iCa. Interpretation of iCa is most accurate when the specimen can be analyzed immediately and when the blood pH at the time of sample collection is known. Additionally, it is important to use age-appropriate reference ranges when interpreting serum and urine calcium concentrations. The upper limit of normal for serum calcium is highest in infancy and declines through childhood. For example, the upper limit for total calcium was determined to fall from 11.1 mg/dL (2.8 mmol/L) for infants <90 days old to 10.2 mg/dL (2.6 mmol/L) for children ≥12 years of age in a large single-center study [2]. Likewise, the upper limit for the random urinary calcium/creatinine (Uca/Ucr) ratio declines from ~0.9 mg/mg (2.4 mmol/mmol) in

Table 4.1 Hypercalcemic disorders of childhood – categorized by primary physiologic mechanism

Disorders of parathyroid hormone excess/action
 Inactivating mutations in *CASR*, *GNA11*, and *AP2S1*
  Familial hypocalciuric hypercalcemia
  Neonatal severe primary hyperparathyroidism
 Primary hyperparathyroidism
  Single adenoma
  Multi-gland disease
 Parathyroid carcinoma
 Tertiary hyperparathyroidism
 Parathyroid hormone related peptide (PTHrP) excess
  Malignancy
  Congenital anomalies of kidney and urinary tract
 Jansen's metaphyseal chondrodysplasia (activating mutation in *PTH1R*)
Disorders of excess vitamin D action or sensitivity
 Hypervitaminosis D (vitamin D intoxication)
 Granulomatosis
  Subcutaneous fat necrosis
  Infectious (tuberculosis, etc.)
  Inflammatory (sarcoidosis, etc.)
  Genetic (Blau syndrome)
 Idiopathic infantile hypercalcemia (inactivating mutations in *CYP24A1 or SLC34A1*)
Disorders of excess gastrointestinal absorption (not vitamin D-mediated)
 Milk (calcium) alkali syndrome
 Congenital lactase deficiency
 Congenital sucrase-isomaltase deficiency
Disorders of excess bone mineral resorption/diminished bone mineral deposition
 Malignancy
  Acute lymphoblastic leukemia, lymphoma, primary bone cancer, and metastatic
 Immobilization
 Hyperthyroidism
 Hypervitaminosis A
 Rebound hypercalcemia following denosumab withdrawal
 Hypophosphatasia
Disorders of excess renal calcium reabsorption
 Thiazide diuretics
 Barters syndrome
 Adrenal insufficiency
Unknown/multifactorial mechanism
 Ketogenic diet
 Williams syndrome
 Renal tubular acidosis
 Blue diaper syndrome
 Extreme low birth weight in prematurity

[1]Germline mutations in *MEN1* (multiple endocrine neoplasia 1), *RET* (multiple endocrine neoplasia 2A), *CDKN1B* (multiple endocrine neoplasia 4), *CDC73* (hyperparathyroidism-jaw tumor syndrome and familial isolated hyperparathyroidism), or GCM2 (familial isolated hyperparathyroidism) underlie a significant proportion of primary hyperparathyroidism in children. Risk of germline mutation is greater in younger children and with multigland disease.

newborns to ~0.2 mg/mg (0.6 mmol/mmol) after age 6–8 years [3]. Older children should excrete no more than 4 mg/kg of calcium per day.

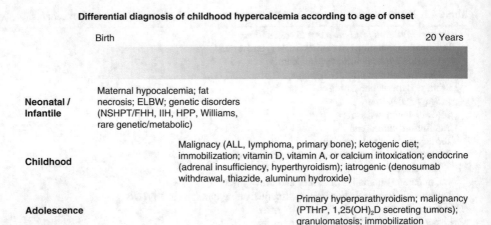

Fig. 4.2 Hypercalcemia disorders of childhood by typical age of onset. The age of presentation of hypercalcemia will help narrow the differential diagnosis. Maternal and perinatal factors and genetic disorders are more likely to underlying neonatal/infantile onset disease. Acquired forms of hypercalcemia begin to arise during childhood and persist through adolescence. The differential diagnosis of adolescent hypercalcemia begins to mimic that of adults, with primary hyperparathyroidism due to solitary adenoma becoming more likely

Factitious hypercalcemia can be the result of acute increases in the serum albumin level due to dehydration or prolonged application of a tourniquet during phlebotomy. Pseudohypercalcemia may occur in patients with thrombocytosis as a result of platelet lysis in the collecting tube.

Hypercalcemic Disorders of Childhood

Parathyroid Hormone (PTH) Excess

Primary hyperparathyroidism (PHPT) is far less prevalent in children compared with adults. The incidence during childhood is commonly cited as 2–5 cases per 100,000 children; [4] however, accurate population-level data are lacking. Single center reports have found that the incidence of PHPT increases with age and may be slightly higher in females [5–9]. Blood and urine calcium levels at diagnosis are generally higher in children than adults [10]. Additionally, most children with PHPT are symptomatic at presentation, which is in contrast to adults who commonly present with asymptomatic hypercalcemia that is discovered by routine biochemical assessments [11, 12]. The well-described mnemonic of "stones, bones, abdominal groans, thrones, and psychiatric overtones" to emphasize the common presenting symptoms of hyperparathyroidism generally applies to children. This phrase describes the effects of PTH excess including nephrocalcinosis, nephrolithiasis, and hematuria (stones); low bone density, fracture, and osteitis fibrosa cystica (bones);

abdominal pain due to gastritis or pancreatitis (groans); bowel and bladder symptoms including constipation and polyuria (thrones); and changes in mental status, behavior, or cognitive function (psychiatric overtones). In infants and young children, the signs/symptoms of hypercalcemia may be vague and include lethargy, feeding intolerance, dehydration, and failure to thrive.

The diagnosis of PHPT is based on biochemical findings of an elevated or inappropriately normal PTH concentration in the setting of hypercalcemia. It is also important to determine vitamin D status, as coexisting vitamin D deficiency can moderate hypercalcemia and/or hypercalciuria. Moreover, it is important to distinguish patients with PHPT from those with a primary deficiency in vitamin D; these patients will have secondary (i.e., adaptive) hyperparathyroidism, in which elevations in PTH are accompanied by serum calcium levels that are within the mid to lower reference range, low urinary calcium excretion, and serum concentrations of 25-OH-vitamin D levels that are below 20 ng/mL (< 50 nmol/L).

Once the diagnosis of PHPT is confirmed, further evaluation is required to determine the etiology, as this informs the treatment approach. It is critically important to distinguish *familial hypocalciuric hypercalcemia (FHH)* from other forms of PHPT, as the management differs markedly. A detailed discussion of the etiology of FHH can be found in Chaps. 7 and 8. Briefly, FHH is typically a benign condition that is usually due to a heterozygous inactivating mutation in the calcium-sensing receptor gene (*CASR,* OMIM 601199). The calcium sensing receptor (CASR) is a G-protein coupled receptor that is highly expressed in the chief cells of the parathyroid glands and the proximal and distal tubules of the kidney, skeleton, gastrointestinal tract, and elsewhere [13]. In the parathyroid cell, binding of extracellular iCa to the CASR activates a signaling pathway that leads to decreased secretion and synthesis of PTH. In the renal tubules, activation of the CASR reduces urinary calcium reabsorption and together with excess PTH reduces the fractional excretion of calcium (FeCa).

The biochemical hallmark of FHH is hypocalciuria due to an inappropriately low FeCa. The FeCA can be determined using either a random urine or a 24-hour collection [(urine calcium concentration X serum creatinine concentration)/(serum calcium concentration X urine creatinine concentration)] and is typically less than 1%. Patients with FHH usually have mild hypercalcemia (serum calcium typically <12 mg/dL [3 mmol/L]) and normal to mildly elevated PTH [14]. Other factors supporting the diagnosis of FHH include a family history of hypercalcemia following an autosomal dominant inheritance pattern, normal or elevated serum magnesium (typically decreased in other forms of PHPT), normal serum 1,25(OH)$_2$D (typically elevated in other forms of PHPT), and normal bone mineral density (may be diminished in other forms of PHPT) [15]. Genetic testing should be considered to confirm the diagnosis, as there is overlap in the biochemical findings of FHH and other forms of PHPT. Not all patients with FHH have FeCa <1% and hypocalciuria may occur in other forms of PHPT with coexistent vitamin D deficiency. Heterozygous mutations in *GNA11* (OMIM 139313) and *AP2S1* (OMIM 602242) cause *FHH2* and *FHH3*, respectively. These latter genes encode proteins required for CASR function, and therefore, FHH2 and FHH3 have similar features to FHH1.

Accordingly, all three genes should be analyzed when FHH is suspected. Once confirmed, patients with FHH can usually be managed conservatively, as they typically do not develop significant sequelae and surgical intervention is rarely effective. In rare cases of symptomatic FHH, a therapeutic trial with a calcimimetic can be considered (see below). The genetics and clinical features of FHH are further discussed further in Chaps. 7 and 8.

In contrast to FHH, *neonatal severe primary hyperparathyroidism (NSHPT)* is a potentially life-threatening condition characterized by marked hypercalcemia (serum calcium often >17.5 mg/dL [4.5 mmol/L]) that presents in infancy [16]. Most cases of NSPHT are due to biallelic inactivating mutations in *CASR* or other genes that cause FHH2 and FHH3, but some heterozygous *CASR* mutations have been described in which the mutant CASR has features of a dominant negative protein that impairs function of the CASR produced by the wild type allele [17]. In addition, NSPHT is more likely to occur in newborns who carry a single mutant CASR allele when the mother is unaffected (i.e., the mutation is de novo or paternally inherited) due to exposure of the fetus to normal maternal calcium levels during pregnancy.

Affected newborns require urgent intervention to lower calcium and PTH. Aggressive administration of normal saline is used to restore intravascular volume but is of limited benefit in lowering serum calcium, with or without loop diuretics, due to the loss of CASR in the kidney. Calcitonin and/or bisphosphonates are often necessary to reduce serum calcium levels [18] and have the additional benefit of decreasing PTH-mediated bone resorption. The very high levels of PTH cause severe skeletal demineralization, leading to weakness and deformity of the chest cage that can cause respiratory insufficiency or failure. PTH excess also causes hypophosphatemia due to reduced renal tubular reabsorption of phosphorus (TRP). Hypophosphatemia can cause muscle weakness and aggravate hypercalcemia, and many infants will require phosphate supplementation. Subtotal parathyroidectomy may provide short-term improvement but is typically not effective in achieving long-term control of hypercalcemia. Total parathyroidectomy has been traditionally advocated once the patient has been stabilized [19]. This is a challenging procedure in infants and results in permanent hypoparathyroidism. Emerging data suggest that NSHPT can improve over time in some patients [17], spurring interest in the use of cinacalcet, an orally administered calcimimetic, to delay or prevent the need for parathyroidectomy. There have been several reports describing the successful use of cinacalcet as first- or second-line therapy in newborns [20–23]. The dosing regimen to achieve control of hypercalcemia varied from ~20 to 200 mg/m^2/day [22], or from ~0.4 to 2 mg/kg/day [18], typically divided into two daily doses. It is prudent to initiate therapy at a low dose and titrate upward to achieve target serum calcium levels at or slightly above the upper limit of the reference range, with careful monitoring for hypocalcemia. A successful response to cinacalcet requires functional CASR protein on the surface of the parathyroid cells; biallelic mutations that result in absent or dysfunctional protein or that inhibit membrane trafficking may explain cases where cinacalcet was ineffective [24].

The conventional treatment of PHPT not due to FHH/NSHP in children is surgical removal of the abnormal parathyroid gland(s). Data from pediatric case series' have shown that between 65% and 91% of PHPT cases were attributable to a solitary adenoma [5, 9, 12, 25]. Parathyroid adenomas are generally the result of a sporadic, somatic mutation arising in a single parathyroid cell, although they can occur secondary to germline mutations in *MEN1* (OMIM 131100; multiple endocrine neoplasia 1), *RET* (OMIM 164761; multiple endocrine neoplasia 2A), *CDKN1B* (OMIM 600778; multiple endocrine neoplasia 4), *CDC73* [OMIM 607393; hyperparathyroidism jaw-tumor syndrome (HPT-JTS) and familial isolated hyperparathyroidism], or *GCM2* (OMIM 603716; familial isolated hyperparathyroidism) [26]. It is therefore important to consider genetic conditions in which multiple parathyroid glands will be involved prior to undertaking surgery (see Chap. 7). The approach taken by the authors is to evaluate first degree relatives for hypercalcemia and/or other features of MEN syndromes and in many cases to perform genetic testing.

In most cases, parathyroid imaging should be performed prior to surgery. The objective is not to confirm the diagnosis of PHPT but rather to assist in surgical planning. Similar to adult practice at many institutions, minimally invasive parathyroidectomy (MIP) is the preferred surgical approach for solitary parathyroid adenoma in children. Preoperative localization complements a comprehensive surgical plan for successful MIP that includes a highly experienced surgeon and the ability to perform near-real time intraoperative PTH measurement. Ultrasound examination of the neck and radionucleotide scanning with technetium-^{99}m sestamibi (MIBI), with or without single-photon emission computerized tomography, are the most commonly used imaging techniques in children. The sensitivity and specificity of these tests, either in isolation or in combination, to identify an abnormal parathyroid gland vary considerably, and centers should individualize their approach based upon local expertise. Four-dimensional CT is increasingly used in adults [27]. However, there are concerns about this technique in children because of the greater radiation exposure to thyroid [28].

Multi-gland parathyroid hyperplasia underlies ~20–25% of pediatric PHPT. Multi-gland disease is more common in younger children and suggests the presence of a germline mutation in one of the genes listed above [12]. *Ectopic parathyroid adenomas* have been reported in children at all levels of thymic descent from the angle of mandible to the mediastinum, providing additional justification for referring patients to highly experienced operators who are familiar with the sites in which ectopic parathyroid glands occur [25, 29, 30]. Enlarged parathyroid glands in patients with multi-gland disease are usually not detected by ultrasound or MIBI scans, and often ectopic adenomas will escape detection by these techniques as well. When parathyroid imaging does not suggest the presence of a single adenoma, a surgical approach that includes bilateral parathyroid exploration, with potential extension to other cervical sites and the thymus, may be necessary, with biochemical cure confirmed by intraoperative PTH [25]. With the exception of NSHPT, subtotal parathyroidectomy (removing 3 ½ of 4 glands) or total parathyroidectomy with autotransplantation of a portion of the most normal-appearing gland into the sternocleidomastoid or brachioradialis muscle is the preferred approach for multi-gland disease [31]. Parathyroidectomy, whether for single adenoma or multi-gland disease, is highly effective in children, with cure rates >90% [32, 33].

Genetic testing of the aforementioned genes should be considered in all children diagnosed with PHPT [26]. The likelihood that PHPT is due to an underlying germ-line mutation is greater in younger patients compared with older adults [34]. The true prevalence of pathogenic mutations in children with PHPT is unknown but has been reported to range from 10% to 52% [25, 35]. PHPT can be the initial manifestation of MEN1, providing justification for genetic testing, as a diagnosis would require additional screening for pancreatic and pituitary tumors. Likewise, a diagnosis of HPT-JTS requires regular monitoring for the development of parathyroid carcinoma, ossifying fibromas of the jaw, renal cysts, adenomas and carcinomas, and endometrial hyperplasia, uterine leiomyomas, and adenofibromas (females). Multi-gene sequencing and copy-number-variant panels are increasingly available at commercial laboratories and can be performed in the absence of a phenotype suggestive of a specific disorder. See Chap. 7 for a detailed discussion of inherited forms and the genetics causes of PHPT.

Parathyroid carcinoma is extremely rare in childhood [36]. Clinical features suggestive of parathyroid carcinoma include markedly elevated serum calcium, palpable mass, and adenoma size >3 cm [36]. The diagnosis is confirmed by histopathology [37], and the treatment includes *en bloc* resection of the tumor along with adjacent involved structures [38]. Parathyroid carcinoma has been reported in association with somatic and germline mutations in *CDC73* [39, 40]and less commonly in *MEN1* [41].

Secondary hyperparathyroidism, in which PTH levels are appropriately elevated due to vitamin D deficiency, renal disease with impaired 1-alpha-hydroxylase (CYP27B1) activity, and/or insufficient calcium absorption, usually does not cause hypercalcemia. Several caveats apply, however. First, patients with vitamin D deficiency may experience transient hypercalcemia if they are treated with high doses of vitamin D (e.g., stoss therapy), as elevated serum PTH levels stimulate rapid and excessive conversion of rising levels of 25(OH)D to 1,25(OH)$_2$D. Second, infants exposed to *maternal hypocalcemia in utero* may develop secondary hyperparathyroidism that results in transient hypercalcemia, skeletal demineralization, and fracture [42]. Transient neonatal hyperparathyroidism can also occur in infants who carry biallelic mutations in *TRPV6,* due to impaired maternal–fetal calcium transport in the placenta, but hypercalcemia has not yet been reported [43]. Third, in some cases of chronic kidney disease, *tertiary hyperparathyroidism* may develop, which is characterized by parathyroid gland hyperplasia and autonomous PTH secretion. The development of hypercalcemia with tertiary hyperparathyroidism generally requires parathyroidectomy [44].

Other Forms of PTH1R Activation

Hypercalcemia due to excess production of *parathyroid hormone-related peptide (PTHrP)* is exceedingly uncommon in childhood. PTHrP shares homology with PTH and binds to the type 1 PTH receptor (PTH1R). At high concentrations, PTHrP may induce hypercalcemia through increased osteoclast mediated bone resorption and increased renal calcium reabsorption [45, 46]; increased synthesis of $1,25(OH)_2D$ is characteristically absent. A variety of malignancies have been reported to secrete PTHrP and must be considered with a finding of elevated PTHrP [47]. PTHrP is also expressed in the urinary tract, and hypercalcemia in association with elevated PTHrP levels in patients with congenital anomalies of the kidney and urinary tract has been reported [48]. Carboxy-terminal fragments of PTHrP accumulate in renal insufficiency; therefore, confirmation of elevated PTHrP should be performed using an assay targeted to the amino-terminal of PTHrP in patients with kidney disease [49].

Jansen-type metaphyseal chondrodysplasia is a rare disorder caused by monoallelic activating mutations in *PTH1R* (OMIM 168468). The biochemical findings mimic those of PHPT, with the exception of PTH, which is suppressed [50]. Other features include craniofacial dysmorphism, short limbs, bowed legs, undermineralized bones, and metaphyseal irregularities [51]. Bisphosphonates have been used to manage hypercalcemia and hypercalciuria [52].

Excessive Vitamin D Action

Excessive vitamin D action can be the result of either vitamin D intoxication or endogenous defects in vitamin D metabolism. Ingestion of excessive quantities of vitamin D supplements may cause hypercalcemia from excess gastrointestinal calcium absorption and increased bone resorption. Hypercalcemia generally does not develop until serum 25(OH)D levels rise above at least 90 ng/mL (220 nmol/L) [53] and is usually accompanied by hyperphosphatemia and hypercalciuria. PTH is suppressed, and serum concentrations of $1,25(OH)_2D$ are typically not elevated when measured using assays that are unaffected by high levels of 25(OH)D [54].

Endogenous forms of vitamin D-mediated hypercalcemia occur because of overproduction or underdegradation of $1,25(OH)_2D$. *Subcutaneous fat necrosis* can occur in infants with traumatic births or who have been treated with therapeutic hypothermia for hypoxic ischemic encephalopathy. Subcutaneous fat necrosis is a noninfectious panniculitis that manifests the properties of a granulomatous disease with local macrophage activation in response to necrotic fat. Activated macrophages express CYP27B1, and in some cases, the local production of $1,25(OH)_2D$ is sufficient to induce hypercalcemia and hypercalciuria [55]. Classically, violaceous skin lesions are described. However, in practice, the skin findings may be subtle or even resolved prior to presentation. Other forms of *granulomatous disease-mediated hypercalcemia* in children are uncommon but include infection (tuberculosis, *Pneumocystis jirovecii*) and genetic or inflammatory granulomatosis such as Blau syndrome and sarcoid [56–59]. Ectopic $1,25(OH)_2D$ production by malignant tumors has also been described [60].

The treatment of hypervitaminosis D consists of eliminating exogenous vitamin D supply and reducing dietary calcium intake. Infants may respond to a low calcium, vitamin D-free formula such as Calcilo XD. Additional measures may be necessary in cases of symptomatic or severe hypercalcemia (initial corrected calcium >14 mg/dL [3.5 mmol/L]), including hyperhydration with normal saline. Treatment with high-dose glucocorticoids has no role in cases of exogenous vitamin D intoxication. In children, the benefit of glucocorticoid therapy in granulomatous disorders is uncertain and outweighed by the risk of steroid exposure [61]. By contrast, calcitonin and intravenous bisphosphonates (often a single dose) are efficacious and have excellent safety profiles [62–64].

Idiopathic infantile hypercalcemia (IIH) is most commonly caused by biallelic inactivating mutations in *CYP24A1* (OMIM 126065) leading to reduced function of the 24-hydroxylase enzyme that is chiefly responsible for vitamin D inactivation [65]. Patients with this condition typically present during infancy with hypercalcemia, hypercalciuria, and suppressed PTH with inappropriately elevated $1,25(OH)_2D$. There are reports describing the successful medical management of IIH with ketoconazole [66] and fluconazole; [67] inhibitors of the CYP27B1 enzyme responsible for $1,25(OH)_2D$ synthesis; and rifampin, an inducer of the CYP3A4 enzyme, which provides an alternative pathway for vitamin D catabolism [68]. Intravenous bisphosphonates can also provide transient improvement [69]. Patients with IIH due to inactivating mutations in *SLC34A1* (encoding renal sodium-phosphate cotransporter 2A (NaPi-IIa) may be treated with oral phosphate [70].

Other Disorders of Excess Gastrointestinal Calcium Absorption

Hypercalcemia in an infant with failure to thrive and watery diarrhea should prompt consideration of metabolic diseases including *congenital lactase deficiency* and *sucrase-isomaltase deficiency* [71]. It is hypothesized that non-hydrolyzed lactose stimulates calcium absorption [72]. Hypercalcemia resolves with institution of a lactose free diet. Hypercalcemia due to excess calcium ingestion can occur as a part of the *milk (or calcium) – alkali syndrome* – in which the accompanying alkalosis (typically from calcium carbonate ingestion) reduces urinary calcium excretion [73].

Non-PTH, PTHrP, or Vitamin D-Mediated Excess Bone Mineral Resorption

Children have high bone turnover and are at risk of hypercalcemia secondary to pathologies that either increase bone mineral resorption or diminish bone mineral deposition. Osteolysis is the most common mechanism of *hypercalcemia of malignancy (HCM)* in children. The prevalence of hypercalcemia in pediatric cancer is low, reported to be 0.2–0.8% [74]. However, hypercalcemia can be the presenting sign of acute lymphoblastic leukemia and may occur before deficits in peripheral blood counts or peripheral blasts are detectable [75]. Other childhood malignancies associated with hypercalcemia include lymphoma, brain tumors, and primary bone cancers [74]. A finding of hypercalcemia with suppressed PTH, hypercalciuria, and the absence of elevated vitamin D suggests the possibility of HCM. Additional testing including radiographs (for lytic lesions), technetium bone scan (for focal areas of increased bone metabolism), bone marrow aspirate, and/or bone biopsy may be required to confirm the diagnosis.

Rapidly growing children and adolescents who acutely lose weight-bearing ability due to trauma or other etiology are at risk of *hypercalcemia of immobility*. This condition is thought to be the result of "uncoupling" of bone turnover, whereby osteoblast-mediated bone formation declines with the loss of mechanosensation, while osteoclastic-mediated bone resorption continues or even increases [76]. Hypercalciuria typically precedes the development of hypercalcemia. *Rebound hypercalcemia* following discontinuation of denosumab, an anti-RANKL osteoporosis drug occasionally used in children, has been described [77]. The mechanism is thought to be due to a robust activation of quiescent osteoclasts as the concentration of anti-RANKL wanes. Other processes that increase bone resorption including *hyperthyroidism* [78] and *hypervitaminosis A* [79, 80] may also cause hypercalcemia. Hypercalcemia due to increased bone resorption of any etiology typically responds well to antiresorptive therapy with calcitonin and/or bisphosphonates [81–83].

Diminished Bone Mineral Deposition

Loss of function mutations in *ALPL* (OMIM 171760) causes *hypophosphatasia (HPP)*. Reduced activity of alkaline phosphatase leads to an accumulation of extracellular inorganic pyrophosphate, which in turn diminishes the deposition of calcium and phosphorus into bone [84]. HPP should be suspected when hypercalcemia is accompanied by low serum ALP and radiographic findings of rickets. Enzyme replacement with asfotase alpha is used for severe forms of HPP; [85] mild hypercalcemia in the setting of less severe disease can be managed with dietary calcium restriction. *Adynamic bone disease* secondary to CKD is an uncommon cause of hypercalcemia in children [86].

Diminished Renal Excretion of Calcium

Congenital and acquired conditions that increase renal tubular calcium reabsorption may cause hypercalcemia and include *Bartter's syndrome* due to *SLC12A1* (OMIM: 600839, which also manifests with PTH excess) [87] and *thiazide diuretic* use. Conditions that acutely reduce glomerular filtration rate including *adrenal insufficiency* may also reduce urinary calcium excretion and cause hypercalcemia [88].

Pathophysiology Unknown

Hypercalcemia occurs in some children treated with a *ketogenic diet* [89]. The mechanism is hypothesized to be multifactorial and related to impaired bone mineral deposition and insufficient renal calcium excretion [90]. *Williams syndrome*, a disorder due to 7q11.23 chromosomal deletion that is characterized by facial dysmorphisms, cardiovascular disease, and intellectual disability, is accompanied by mild hypercalcemia in about 20% of cases [91]. Onset is typically before 3 years of age and can usually be managed with vitamin D and calcium restriction. Hypercalcemia is common in *extremely low birth weight infants* and may be associated with delayed or insufficient provision of phosphorus in total parental nutrition and inadequate renal calcium excretion [92]. *Renal tubular acidosis* is occasionally associated with hypercalcemia [93]. Other rare forms of hypercalcemia are listed in Fig. 4.1.

Diagnostic and Treatment Approach

As outlined above, establishing the underlying cause of the hypercalcemia is critical to developing a definitive management plan. The key aspects of the history, physical exam, and biochemical testing protocol are provided in Table 4.2. On the other hand, immediate intervention to treat symptomatic hypercalcemia is based on standard principles in which treatment is guided by the degree of hypercalcemia.

In cases of symptomatic or severe hypercalcemia [albumin-corrected calcium >14 mg/dL (3.5 mmol/L)], medical stabilization is often required in parallel with the diagnostic work-up. The goals of treatment are to lower serum calcium by (1) promoting renal calcium excretion, (2) limiting gastrointestinal calcium absorption, and (3) decreasing calcium resorption from bone. All calcium and vitamin D supplements should be discontinued at presentation. Intravenous rehydration with normal saline is provided to restore intravascular volume and thereby lower serum calcium concentration via dilution; increased renal perfusion and glomerular filtration rate will also promote calciuresis. The benefit of loop diuretics to induce calciuresis beyond what is achieved through normal saline hydration is uncertain. Their

Table 4.2 Key aspects of the history, physical, biochemical, and imaging evaluation of the hypercalcemic child

---

History[1]

  Birth history: maternal hypocalcemia, birth trauma
  Medications: calcium, vitamin D, vitamin A, thiazide diuretics, antacids, and lithium
  Dietary history: infant formula, dairy/calcium rich foods, and ketogenic diet
  Activity: ambulatory status – especially recent change
  Family History: hypercalcemia, hypercalciuria, and kidney stones

---

Review of systems

  Constitutional: fatigue, nausea, anorexia, and failure to thrive
  Gastrointestinal: diarrhea, constipation, change in stooling pattern, and pain
  Urinary: polyuria, dysuria, hematuria, and crystalluria
  Nervous system: change in mental status andconfusion
  Musculoskeletal: bone pain
  Skin: bruises, rash, and lesion
  Hematology: bleeding

Physical exam

  General: overall appearance
  HEENT: dry mucus membranes, sunken fontanel, and dysmorphisms
  Neck: central or lateral mass
  Nervous system: confusion and lethargy
  Musculoskeletal: focal skeletal tenderness
  Extremities: cool and slow capillary refills
  Skin: lesions, hyperpigmentation, and bruising

Laboratory evaluation

<u>*Standard*</u>

  Blood: comprehensive metabolic panel (with focus on calcium, albumin, alkaline phosphatase, bicarbonate, and potassium), phosphorus, magnesium, intact parathyroid hormone, 25-OH vitamin D, $1,25(OH)_2$ vitamin D, and ionized calcium (if proper specimen handling can be obtained)
  Urine: random fasting urine for calcium, creatinine, and phosphorus (to calculate urine calcium/creatinine ratio; tubular resorption of phosphate)

<u>*As suggested by history/exam/initial laboratory findings*</u>

  Blood: endocrine hormones (thyroid function tests, adrenocorticotropic hormone, and cortisol); complete blood count; parathyroid hormone-related peptide; markers of bone formation (bone specific alkaline phosphatase); and bone resorption [collagen type I c-telopeptide (Beta CTX)]
  Urine: 24-hour urine calcium, creatinine; 4–6 hour fasting urine for phosphorus, creatinine (with midway blood draw for phosphorus, creatinine for tubular maximum reabsorption rate of phosphate to glomerular filtration rate)

Imaging evaluation

  Neck/parathyroid ultrasound; parathyroid MIBI scan – if primary hyperparathyroidism confirmed biochemically
  Skeletal survey – if malignancy or skeletal dysplasia suspected
  Technetium bone scan – if malignancy or other bone destructive process suspected

---

Other Evaluation

  Bone marrow aspirate or bone biopsy – if malignancy suspected or unknown bone lesion identified
  Bone densitometry by dual energy x-ray absorptiometry (to monitor bone mass in cases of immobilization, ketogenic diet, primary hyperparathyroidism, etc.)

---

[1]Not all aspects are relevant to every child; history, exam, and testing will be guided by factors including patient age and clinical presentation

use should absolutely be avoided in the initial phase of fluid resuscitation, as they counteract the benefits of volume expansion and may exacerbate kidney injury. Phosphate supplementation should be considered if hypophosphatemia is present (common in PTH mediated hypercalcemia). Repletion of serum phosphate facilitates calcium deposition into bone and allows FGF-23 secretion to rise, which has an inhibitory effect on $1,25(OH)_2D$ synthesis.

Pharmacotherapy to inhibit osteoclastic resorption and thereby reduce mobilization of calcium (and phosphorus) from bone should be considered for hypercalcemia refractory to hyperhydration. With few exceptions (e.g., calcium gluttony, adynamic bone disease, and HPP) excessive osteoclastic bone resorption is an important driver of hypercalcemia in children. Calcitonin (salmon) may be administered subcutaneously at a starting dose of 1–4 international units/kg every 6–12 hours. The calcium-lowering effect of calcitonin is modest (1–2 mg/dL). Although the benefit of calcitonin may be limited due to tachyphylaxis, this loss of effectiveness appears to be more common in adults than in children, who may show a response for longer periods of time. The principal advantages of calcitonin are its rapid onset of effect, a relative lack of toxicity, reversibility, and dosing flexibility. Moreover, a response to calcitonin confirms the role of osteoclastic bone resorption in the pathophysiology of hypercalcemia and provides reassurance that other antiresorptive therapies will be effective.

Pamidronate and zoledronic acid are the most widely used intravenous bisphosphonates and are both highly efficacious for treatment of hypercalcemia. A single dose of pamidronate at 0.25 mg/kg may be effective, although follow-up doses of 0.5 mg/kg on 1–2 subsequent days may be required [94]. Zoledronic acid is more potent and typically administered as a single dose of 0.025–0.05 mg/kg up to 4 mg, the usual adult dose for hypercalcemia [95]. Both of these bisphosphonates have been associated with nephrotoxicity, and they should be used with caution (e.g., at reduced dosage and infused over longer time period) in patients with renal insufficiency. Careful monitoring for post-infusion hypocalcemia and acute phase reaction (fever, myalgia, and gastrointestinal upset) is required [96]. Zoledronic acid has longer duration of effect than pamidronate. However, the duration of the calcium lowering effect is highly variable, and redosing of either formulation may be required in the ensuing weeks to months. Denosumab (anti-RANKL) is a pharmacologically appealing alternative to bisphosphonates in that it is less persistent in the body and not nephrotoxic. However, its use in pediatrics has been extremely limited [97], and the appropriate dose to treat hypercalcemia but avoid hypocalcemia is not known. Dialysis can be considered if other interventions fail.

Conclusion

In conclusion, a thoughtful and stepwise approach to the hypercalcemic child is necessary to establish the underlying cause. It is useful to recall key aspects of calcium physiology including the potential sources of calcium excess (increased gastrointestinal absorption, increased bone resorption or diminished bone deposition, and increased renal reabsorption or diminished renal excretion) and the actions of calciometabolic hormones (PTH and vitamin D) when formulating a differential diagnosis and interpreting laboratory findings. Urgent medical stabilization is required for symptomatic or severe hypercalcemia and typically includes hydration and anti-bone-resorptive therapy. It is critical to establish a definitive diagnosis, when possible, as this will inform the definitive or long-term treatment approach.

Funding   This work was funded in part by grants from the National Institutes of Health (R01 DK112955) to MAL.

References

1. Bushinsky DA, Monk RD. Electrolyte quintet: Calcium. Lancet. 1998;352(9124):306–11.
2. Roizen JD, Shah V, Levine MA, Carlow DC. Determination of reference intervals for serum total calcium in the vitamin D-replete pediatric population. J Clin Endocrinol Metab. 2013;98(12):E1946–50.
3. Sargent JD, Stukel TA, Kresel J, Klein RZ. Normal values for random urinary calcium to creatinine ratios in infancy. J Pediatr. 1993;123(3):393–7.
4. Roizen J, Levine MA. Primary hyperparathyroidism in children and adolescents. J Chin Med Assoc. 2012;75(9):425–34.
5. Kollars J, Zarroug AE, van Heerden J, et al. Primary hyperparathyroidism in pediatric patients. Pediatrics. 2005;115(4):974–80.
6. Durkin ET, Nichol PF, Lund DP, Chen H, Sippel RS. What is the optimal treatment for children with primary hyperparathyroidism? J Pediatr Surg. 2010;45(6):1142–6.
7. Chesney RW. Primary hyperparathyroidism in pediatric patients: clear-cut differences from adult patients. Pediatrics. 2005;115(4):1073.
8. Wang W, Kong J, Nie M, et al. Primary hyperparathyroidism in Chinese children and adolescents: a single-centre experience at Peking Union Medical College Hospital. Clin Endocrinol. 2017;87(6):865–73.
9. Sharanappa V, Mishra A, Bhatia V, et al. Pediatric primary hyperparathyroidism: experience in a tertiary care referral center in a developing country over Three Decades. World J Surg. 2021;45(2):488–95.
10. Roizen J, Levine MA. A meta-analysis comparing the biochemistry of primary hyperparathyroidism in youths to the biochemistry of primary hyperparathyroidism in adults. J Clin Endocrinol Metab. 2014;99(12):4555–64.
11. Hsu SC, Levine MA. Primary hyperparathyroidism in children and adolescents: the Johns Hopkins Children's Center experience 1984-2001. J Bone Miner Res. 2002;17(Suppl 2):N44–50.
12. Zivaljevic V, Jovanovic M, Diklic A, Zdravkovic V, Djordjevic M, Paunovic I. Differences in primary hyperparathyroidism characteristics between children and adolescents. J Pediatr Surg. 2020;55(8):1660–2.
13. Brown EM, MacLeod RJ. Extracellular calcium sensing and extracellular calcium signaling. Physiol Rev. 2001;81(1):239–97.
14. Christensen SE, Nissen PH, Vestergaard P, Heickendorff L, Brixen K, Mosekilde L. Discriminative power of three indices of renal calcium excretion for the distinction between familial hypocalciuric hypercalcaemia and primary hyperparathyroidism: a follow-up study on methods. Clin Endocrinol. 2008;69(5):713–20.

15. Lee JY, Shoback DM. Familial hypocalciuric hypercalcemia and related disorders. Best Pract Res Clin Endocrinol Metab. 2018;32(5):609–19.
16. Alagaratnam S, Brain C, Spoudeas H, et al. Surgical treatment of children with hyperparathyroidism: single centre experience. J Pediatr Surg. 2014;49(11):1539–43.
17. Marx SJ, Sinaii N. Neonatal severe hyperparathyroidism: novel insights from calcium, PTH, and the CASR gene. J Clin Endocrinol Metab. 2020;105(4):1061–78.
18. Mayr B, Schnabel D, Dörr HG, Schöfl C. Genetics in endocrinology: gain and loss of function mutations of the calcium-sensing receptor and associated proteins: current treatment concepts. Eur J Endocrinol. 2016;174(5):R189–208.
19. Savas-Erdeve S, Sagsak E, Keskin M, et al. Treatment experience and long-term follow-up data in two severe neonatal hyperparathyroidism cases. J Pediatr Endocrinol Metab. 2016;29(9):1103–10.
20. Reh CM, Hendy GN, Cole DE, Jeandron DD. Neonatal hyperparathyroidism with a heterozygous calcium-sensing receptor (CASR) R185Q mutation: clinical benefit from cinacalcet. J Clin Endocrinol Metab. 2011;96(4):E707–12.
21. Fisher MM, Cabrera SM, Imel EA. Successful treatment of neonatal severe hyperparathyroidism with cinacalcet in two patients. Endocrinol Diabetes Metab Case Rep. 2015;2015:150040.
22. Gulcan-Kersin S, Kirkgoz T, Eltan M, et al. Cinacalcet as a first-line treatment in neonatal severe hyperparathyroidism secondary to calcium sensing receptor (CaSR) mutation. Horm Res Paediatr. 2020;93(5):313–21.
23. Gannon AW, Monk HM, Levine MA. Cinacalcet monotherapy in neonatal severe hyperparathyroidism: a case study and review. J Clin Endocrinol Metab. 2014;99(1):7–11.
24. Atay Z, Bereket A, Haliloglu B, et al. Novel homozygous inactivating mutation of the calcium-sensing receptor gene (CASR) in neonatal severe hyperparathyroidism-lack of effect of cinacalcet. Bone. 2014;64:102–7.
25. Rampp RD, Mancilla EE, Adzick NS, et al. Single gland, ectopic location: adenomas are common causes of primary hyperparathyroidism in children and adolescents. World J Surg. 2020;44(5):1518–25.
26. Marini F, Cianferotti L, Giusti F, Brandi ML. Molecular genetics in primary hyperparathyroidism: the role of genetic tests in differential diagnosis, disease prevention strategy, and therapeutic planning. A 2017 update. Clin Cases Miner Bone Metab. 2017;14(1):60–70.
27. Yeh R, Tay YD, Tabacco G, et al. Diagnostic performance of 4D CT and Sestamibi SPECT/CT in localizing parathyroid adenomas in primary hyperparathyroidism. Radiology. 2019;291(2):469–76.
28. Mahajan A, Starker LF, Ghita M, Udelsman R, Brink JA, Carling T. Parathyroid four-dimensional computed tomography: evaluation of radiation dose exposure during preoperative localization of parathyroid tumors in primary hyperparathyroidism. World J Surg. 2012;36(6):1335–9.
29. Kordahi AM, Newfield RS, Bickler SW, et al. Undescended retropharyngeal parathyroid adenoma with adjacent thymic tissue in a 13-year-old boy with primary hyperparathyroidism. Oxf Med Case Reports. 2019;2019(12):519–23.
30. Liu X, Sun L, Shao M, et al. Primary hyperparathyroidism due to ectopic parathyroid adenoma in an adolescent: a case report and review of the literature. Endocrine. 2019;64(1):38–42.
31. Burke JF, Chen H, Gosain A. Parathyroid conditions in childhood. Semin Pediatr Surg. 2014;23(2):66–70.
32. Jamshidi R, Egan JC. Pediatric parathyroid disease. Semin Pediatr Surg. 2020;29(3):150923.
33. Li CC, Yang C, Wang S, Zhang J, Kong XR, Ouyang J. A 10-year retrospective study of primary hyperparathyroidism in children. Exp Clin Endocrinol Diabetes. 2012;120(4):229–33.
34. Starker LF, Akerström T, Long WD, et al. Frequent germ-line mutations of the MEN1, CASR, and HRPT2/CDC73 genes in young patients with clinically non-familial primary hyperparathyroidism. Horm Cancer. 2012;3(1–2):44–51.
35. El Allali Y, Hermetet C, Bacchetta J, et al. Presenting features and molecular genetics of primary hyperparathyroidism in the paediatric population. Eur J Endocrinol. 2020.

36. Dutta A, Pal R, Jain N, et al. Pediatric parathyroid carcinoma: a case report and review of the literature. J Endocr Soc. 2019;3(12):2224–35.
37. Howell VM, Gill A, Clarkson A, et al. Accuracy of combined protein gene product 9.5 and parafibromin markers for immunohistochemical diagnosis of parathyroid carcinoma. J Clin Endocrinol Metab. 2009;94(2):434–41.
38. Rodrigo JP, Hernandez-Prera JC, Randolph GW, et al. Parathyroid cancer: an update. Cancer Treat Rev. 2020;86:102012.
39. Korpi-Hyövälti E, Cranston T, Ryhänen E, et al. CDC73 intragenic deletion in familial primary hyperparathyroidism associated with parathyroid carcinoma. J Clin Endocrinol Metab. 2014;99(9):3044–8.
40. Shattuck TM, Välimäki S, Obara T, et al. Somatic and germ-line mutations of the HRPT2 gene in sporadic parathyroid carcinoma. N Engl J Med. 2003;349(18):1722–9.
41. Cinque L, Sparaneo A, Salcuni AS, et al. MEN1 gene mutation with parathyroid carcinoma: first report of a familial case. Endocr Connect. 2017;6(8):886–91.
42. Alikasifoglu A, Gonc EN, Yalcin E, Dogru D, Yordam N. Neonatal hyperparathyroidism due to maternal hypoparathyroidism and vitamin D deficiency: a cause of multiple bone fractures. Clin Pediatr (Phila). 2005;44(3):267–9.
43. Yamashita S, Mizumoto H, Sawada H, Suzuki Y, Hata D. TRPV6 gene mutation in a Dizygous twin with transient neonatal hyperparathyroidism. J Endocr Soc. 2019;3(3):602–6.
44. Patel A, Lee CY, Sloan DA, Randle RW. Parathyroidectomy for tertiary hyperparathyroidism: a multi-institutional analysis of outcomes. J Surg Res. 2021;258:430–4.
45. Lai NK, Martinez D. Physiological roles of parathyroid hormone-related protein. Acta Biomed. 2019;90(4):510–6.
46. Mirrakhimov AE. Hypercalcemia of malignancy: an update on pathogenesis and management. N Am J Med Sci. 2015;7(11):483–93.
47. Stokes VJ, Nielsen MF, Hannan FM, Thakker RV. Hypercalcemic disorders in children. J Bone Miner Res. 2017;32(11):2157–70.
48. Kodous N, Filler G, Sharma AP, Van Hooren TA. PTHrP-related Hypercalcaemia in infancy and congenital anomalies of the kidney and urinary tract (CAKUT). Can J Kidney Health Dis. 2015;2:21.
49. Orloff JJ, Soifer NE, Fodero JP, Dann P, Burtis WJ. Accumulation of carboxy-terminal fragments of parathyroid hormone-related protein in renal failure. Kidney Int. 1993;43(6):1371–6.
50. Saito H, Noda H, Gatault P, et al. Progression of mineral ion abnormalities in patients with Jansen metaphyseal chondrodysplasia. J Clin Endocrinol Metab. 2018;103(7):2660–9.
51. Nampoothiri S, Fernández-Rebollo E, Yesodharan D, et al. Jansen metaphyseal chondrodysplasia due to heterozygous H223R-PTH1R mutations with or without overt hypercalcemia. J Clin Endocrinol Metab. 2016;101(11):4283–9.
52. Sharwood E, Harris M. Bisphosphonate Treatment of Hypercalcemia in a Child with Jansen'S Metaphyseal Chondrodysplasia. ESPE Abstracts. 86(P2):155.
53. Vieth R. Vitamin D supplementation, 25-hydroxyvitamin D concentrations, and safety. Am J Clin Nutr. 1999;69(5):842–56.
54. Hawkes CP, Schnellbacher S, Singh RJ, Levine MA. 25-Hydroxyvitamin D can interfere with a common assay for 1,25-Dihydroxyvitamin D in vitamin D intoxication. J Clin Endocrinol Metab. 2015;100(8):2883–9.
55. Bikle DD, Patzek S, Wang Y. Physiologic and pathophysiologic roles of extra renal CYP27b1: case report and review. Bone Rep. 2018;8:255–67.
56. Kilinc S, Bostan O, Erol M, Erturk S, Dilek D, Yigit O. Successful management with bisphosphonate treatment in a child with tuberculosis-associated hypercalcemia. North Clin Istanb. 2020;7(4):411–4.
57. VanSickle JS, Srivastava T, Alon US. Life-Threatening Hypercalcemia During Prodrome of Pneumocystis jiroveci Pneumonia in an Immunocompetent Infant. Glob Pediatr Health. 2017;4:2333794x17705955.

58. Baughman RP, Janovcik J, Ray M, Sweiss N, Lower EE. Calcium and vitamin D metabolism in sarcoidosis. Sarcoidosis Vasc Diffuse Lung Dis. 2013;30(2):113–20.
59. Whyte MP, Lim E, McAlister WH, et al. Unique variant of NOD2 pediatric granulomatous arthritis with severe 1,25-Dihydroxyvitamin D-mediated hypercalcemia and generalized Osteosclerosis. J Bone Miner Res. 2018;33(11):2071–80.
60. Colak U, Mutlu GY, Sozmen BO, Yucel EB, Kayserili H, Hatun S. Zoledronate-responsive calcitriol-mediated hypercalcemia in a 5-year-old case with squamous cell carcinoma on the background of xeroderma pigmentosum. J Pediatr Endocrinol Metab. 2019;32(12):1403–6.
61. Demir K, Döneray H, Kara C, et al. Comparison of treatment regimens in Management of Severe Hypercalcemia due to vitamin D intoxication in children. J Clin Res Pediatr Endocrinol. 2019;11(2):140–8.
62. Chesover AD, Harrington J, Mahmud FH. Pamidronate as first-line treatment of hypercalcemia in neonatal subcutaneous fat necrosis: a case series. Paediatr Child Health. 2021;26(1):e52–6.
63. Militello MA, Re MP, Vitaliti G, Finazzo F, Manzoni P, Vitaliti SM. Use of zoledronic acid in a neonate with subcutaneous fat necrosis complicated with severe, refractory hypercalcemia. Am J Perinatol. 2019;36(S 02):S134–8.
64. Barrueto F Jr, Wang-Flores HH, Howland MA, Hoffman RS, Nelson LS. Acute vitamin D intoxication in a child. Pediatrics. 2005;116(3):e453–6.
65. Dauber A, Nguyen TT, Sochett E, et al. Genetic defect in CYP24A1, the vitamin D 24-hydroxylase gene, in a patient with severe infantile hypercalcemia. J Clin Endocrinol Metab. 2012;97(2):E268–74.
66. Nguyen M, Boutignon H, Mallet E, et al. Infantile hypercalcemia and hypercalciuria: new insights into a vitamin D-dependent mechanism and response to ketoconazole treatment. J Pediatr. 2010;157(2):296–302.
67. Sayers J, Hynes AM, Srivastava S, et al. Successful treatment of hypercalcaemia associated with a CYP24A1 mutation with fluconazole. Clin Kidney J. 2015;8(4):453–5.
68. Hawkes CP, Li D, Hakonarson H, Meyers KE, Thummel KE, Levine MA. CYP3A4 induction by rifampin: an alternative pathway for vitamin D inactivation in patients with CYP24A1 mutations. J Clin Endocrinol Metab. 2017;102(5):1440–6.
69. Skalova S, Cerna L, Bayer M, Kutilek S, Konrad M, Schlingmann KP. Intravenous pamidronate in the treatment of severe idiopathic infantile hypercalcemia. Iran J Kidney Dis. 2013;7(2):160–4.
70. Schlingmann KP, Ruminska J, Kaufmann M, et al. Autosomal-recessive mutations in SLC34A1 encoding sodium-phosphate cotransporter 2A cause idiopathic infantile hypercalcemia. J Am Soc Nephrol. 2016;27(2):604–14.
71. Belmont JW, Reid B, Taylor W, et al. Congenital sucrase-isomaltase deficiency presenting with failure to thrive, hypercalcemia, and nephrocalcinosis. BMC Pediatr. 2002;2:4.
72. Saarela T, Similä S, Koivisto M. Hypercalcemia and nephrocalcinosis in patients with congenital lactase deficiency. J Pediatr. 1995;127(6):920–3.
73. Henry RK, Gafni RI. Hypercalcemia due to milk-alkali syndrome and fracture-induced immobilization in an adolescent boy with hypoparathyroidism. Horm Res Paediatr. 2016;86(3):201–5.
74. Jick S, Li L, Gastanaga VM, Liede A, Hernandez RK. Prevalence of hypercalcemia of malignancy among pediatric cancer patients in the UK clinical practice research datalink database. Clin Epidemiol. 2017;9:339–43.
75. Hoyoux C, Lombet J, Nicolescu CR. Malignancy-induced hypercalcemia-diagnostic challenges. Front Pediatr. 2017;5:233.
76. Walls TJ, Ashworth B, Saunders M. Immobilisation hypercalcaemia complicating polyneuropathy in adolescent boys. J Neurol Neurosurg Psychiatry. 1984;47(11):1232–5.
77. Boyce AM, Chong WH, Yao J, et al. Denosumab treatment for fibrous dysplasia. J Bone Miner Res. 2012;27(7):1462–70.
78. Hui WH, Lee CY. Hypercalcaemia and hypertransaminasaemia in a child with hyperthyroidism. J Paediatr Child Health. 2004;40(11):646–8.

79. Lorenzo M, Nadeau M, Harrington J, Gill PJ. Refractory hypercalcemia owing to vitamin A toxicity in a 4-year-old boy. CMAJ. 2020;192(25):E671–e675.
80. O'Neal S, Foster TP, Bhatt A, Lossius MN, Dayton K. Hypercalcemia from hypervitaminosis A in a child with autism. J Pediatr Endocrinol Metab. 2020.
81. Sydlik C, Dürr HR, Pozza SB, Weißenbacher C, Roeb J, Schmidt H. Hypercalcaemia after treatment with denosumab in children: bisphosphonates as an option for therapy and prevention? World J Pediatr. 2020;16(5):520–7.
82. Mathur M, Sykes JA, Saxena VR, Rao SP, Goldman GM. Treatment of acute lymphoblastic leukemia-induced extreme hypercalcemia with pamidronate and calcitonin. Pediatr Crit Care Med. 2003;4(2):252–5.
83. Allgrove J. Use of bisphosphonates in children and adolescents. J Pediatr Endocrinol Metab. 2002;15(Suppl 3):921–8.
84. Whyte MP. Hypophosphatasia: an overview for 2017. Bone. 2017;102:15–25.
85. Whyte MP, Simmons JH, Moseley S, et al. Asfotase alfa for infants and young children with hypophosphatasia: 7 year outcomes of a single-arm, open-label, phase 2 extension trial. Lancet Diabetes Endocrinol. 2019;7(2):93–105.
86. Wesseling K, Bakkaloglu S, Salusky I. Chronic kidney disease mineral and bone disorder in children. Pediatr Nephrol. 2008;23(2):195–207.
87. Wongsaengsak S, Vidmar AP, Addala A, et al. A novel SLC12A1 gene mutation associated with hyperparathyroidism, hypercalcemia, nephrogenic diabetes insipidus, and nephrocalcinosis in four patients. Bone. 2017;97:121–5.
88. Schoelwer MJ, Viswanathan V, Wilson A, Nailescu C, Imel EA. Infants with congenital adrenal hyperplasia are at risk for hypercalcemia, hypercalciuria, and nephrocalcinosis. J Endocr Soc. 2017;1(9):1160–7.
89. Hawkes CP, Roy SM, Dekelbab B, et al. Hypercalcemia in children using the ketogenic diet: a multicenter study. J Clin Endocrinol Metab. 2021;106(2):e485–95.
90. Hawkes CP, Levine MA. Ketotic hypercalcemia: a case series and description of a novel entity. J Clin Endocrinol Metab. 2014;99(5):1531–6.
91. Kim YM, Cho JH, Kang E, et al. Endocrine dysfunctions in children with Williams-Beuren syndrome. Ann Pediatr Endocrinol Metab. 2016;21(1):15–20.
92. Hair AB, Chetta KE, Bruno AM, Hawthorne KM, Abrams SA. Delayed introduction of parenteral phosphorus is associated with hypercalcemia in extremely preterm infants. J Nutr. 2016;146(6):1212–6.
93. Ehlayel AM, Copelovitch L. Uncommon cribfellows: an infant with hypercalcemia, nephrocalcinosis, and acidosis: answers. Pediatr Nephrol. 2018;33(10):1697–9.
94. Auron A, Tal L, Srivastava T, Alon US. Reversal of hypercalcemic acute kidney injury by treatment with intravenous bisphosphonates. Pediatr Nephrol. 2009;24(3):613–7.
95. Bowden SA, Mahan JD. Zoledronic acid in pediatric metabolic bone disorders. Transl Pediatr. 2017;6(4):256–68.
96. George S, Weber DR, Kaplan P, Hummel K, Monk HM, Levine MA. Short-term safety of zoledronic acid in young patients with bone disorders: an extensive institutional experience. J Clin Endocrinol Metab. 2015;100(11):4163–71.
97. Mamedova E, Kolodkina A, Vasilyev EV, Petrov V, Belaya Z, Tiulpakov A. Successful use of denosumab for life-threatening hypercalcemia in a pediatric patient with primary hyperparathyroidism. Horm Res Paediatr. 2020;93(4):272–8.

Chapter 5
General Management and Treatment of Acute and Chronic Hypercalcemia in Adults

Elizabeth Shane

Introduction

The normal physiology of calcium metabolism, the pathophysiology, causes and clinical manifestations of hypercalcemia, and the diagnostic approach to the patient with hypercalcemia have been covered in earlier chapters. This chapter will focus on the treatment of hypercalcemia, particularly hypercalcemia of malignancy, and will limit discussions of its pathophysiology, and its signs and symptoms, to their strategic relationship to therapy.

Pathophysiology, Metabolic Effects, and Clinical Manifestations of Hypercalcemia

A detailed discussion of the pathophysiology, metabolic effects, and clinical manifestations of hypercalcemia is presented in Chap. 2. The diagnostic approach to the adult patient with hypercalcemia is covered in detail in Chap. 3. For completeness, several points of particular therapeutic relevance will be reemphasized in this chapter.

In addition to its established importance in skeletal development and maintenance, extracellular calcium concentrations also play key roles in other metabolic processes, including excitation-contraction coupling, cellular membrane stability and permeability, and transmembrane signaling [1]. Because of these important metabolic functions, serum calcium is tightly regulated by the movement of ionized calcium between the skeleton, intestines, kidney, and by the binding of ionized

E. Shane (✉)
Division of Endocrinology, Columbia University Irving Medical Center, New York, NY, USA
e-mail: es54@cumc.columbia.edu

© The Author(s), under exclusive license to Springer Nature Switzerland AG 2022
M. D. Walker (ed.), *Hypercalcemia*, Contemporary Endocrinology,
https://doi.org/10.1007/978-3-030-93182-7_5

calcium to serum proteins [1]. Hypercalcemia develops when there are abnormalities in the movement of ionized calcium between the extracellular fluid (ECF) and one of these compartments or when there is abnormal binding of calcium to serum proteins [1, 2].

Because calcium in serum is bound to proteins, principally albumin, total serum calcium concentrations in patients with low or high serum albumin levels may not accurately reflect the ionized calcium concentration [1]. In patients with hypoalbuminemia, total serum calcium concentration may be normal when serum ionized calcium is elevated, and the measured serum calcium concentration should be corrected for albumin concentration, as described in Chap. 3. Conversely, patients with hyperalbuminemia due to severe volume depletion and rarely those with multiple myeloma and a calcium-binding paraprotein may have increased protein binding of calcium. This can cause an elevation in the serum total calcium concentration while the serum ionized calcium concentration remains normal – pseudohypercalcemia or factitious hypercalcemia. Algorithms to adjust for hyperalbuminemia are less well-validated than those for hypoalbuminemia. In complex situations, serum ionized calcium can be measured accurately in most laboratories [1].

Elevation of ionized calcium causes hyperpolarization of neuromuscular cell membranes, which causes them to become refractory to stimulation [1]. This hyperpolarization can result in neuropsychiatric disturbances, gastrointestinal abnormalities, musculoskeletal symptoms, and cardiovascular disease. In addition, hypercalcemia impairs renal function through several mechanisms of therapeutic relevance. Hypercalcemia causes afferent arteriolar vasoconstriction and activation of the calcium receptor in the distal nephron, which reduces the glomerular filtration rate (GFR). It can also cause a form of nephrogenic diabetes insipidus with associated polydipsia and polyuria. As a result, the ECF volume is reduced and the GFR further lowered, which has the effect of increasing further serum ionized calcium concentrations.

General Considerations in the Treatment of Hypercalcemia

The most common causes of hypercalcemia are primary hyperparathyroidism (Chap. 6) [3–5] and malignancy (Chaps. 9, 10, and 11) [6–8]. Hypercalcemia may be associated with a spectrum of clinical manifestations (Chap. 2) [2]. Patients with mild hypercalcemia (<12 mg/dl) commonly manifest few or no symptoms. In contrast, severe hypercalcemia (>13–15 mg/dl) is usually symptomatic. Whether a patient develops symptoms may also depend on how rapidly hypercalcemia develops. If the increase in serum calcium occurs very gradually, there may be fewer associated symptoms than might otherwise be expected, even though the serum calcium concentration may be very high (>15 mg/dL). Conversely, if the rise in serum calcium is very rapid, symptoms may occur at lower levels than might be expected (<12 mg/dL). Older age and the presence of other comorbidities, such as diabetes, renal insufficiency, and heart disease, may be associated with more severe manifestations.

Indications for Treatment

The degree of hypercalcemia, along with the rate of rise of the serum calcium, and the presence or absence of symptoms usually determines both whether urgent therapy is necessary and the approach to such therapy [7]. Of particular clinical importance in therapeutic decision-making are the neurological signs and symptoms, which can range in severity from mild confusion to severe obtundation and coma (Chap. 2). Similarly, the cardiological manifestations of hypercalcemia, which may include brady and tachyarrhythmias, electrocardiogram abnormalities such as shortening of the QTc interval, prolonged PR interval, widened QRS complex are very important considerations in the decision to initiate therapy.

Patients with chronic asymptomatic or mildly symptomatic hypercalcemia (albumin-corrected total calcium <12 mg/dL) do not require immediate treatment. They do require evaluation to determine the etiology of the hypercalcemia, if unknown. Medications that may cause or exacerbate hypercalcemia (high dose calcium or vitamin D, thiazide diuretics, and lithium) should be discontinued if possible, and prolonged bed rest should be avoided. Oral hydration (six to eight glasses of water daily) should be recommended. Additional therapy should be specific to the cause of the hypercalcemia.

Individuals with chronic moderate hypercalcemia (albumin-corrected total calcium between 12 and 14 mg/dL) may not require urgent therapy. If they have no symptoms or mild symptoms such as constipation, they may be managed as described above for mild hypercalcemia. In contrast, if they are experiencing marked fatigue or lethargy, nausea, and mental status changes (stupor) or have electrocardiogram abnormalities, an approach similar to that described below for severe hypercalcemia is warranted. Severe hypercalcemia, defined as an albumin-corrected total calcium >14 mg/dL, is considered a medical emergency and requires treatment, regardless of symptoms.

The therapeutic goals are twofold. First and foremost, it is important to lower the serum calcium concentration. Second, it is important to treat the underlying cause of the hypercalcemia if it is possible to do so, and if not, to target as specifically as possible, the pathophysiology of hypercalcemia in that patient. In general, effective therapies reduce serum calcium by one of three main mechanisms (Table 5.1): increasing ECF volume and urinary calcium excretion, inhibiting bone resorption, or decreasing intestinal calcium absorption.

Table 5.1 Therapy of acute severe hypercalcemia[a]

Intervention	Mechanism of action	Onset	Duration
Saline hydration	Replenishes intravascular volume.	Within hours	During therapy
Salmon calcitonin	Inhibits bone resorption by directly and reversibly inhibiting osteoclast activity. Increases urinary calcium excretion.	4–6 hours	48 hours
Bisphosphonates	Inhibit bone resorption by interfering with osteoclast recruitment and function.	24–72 hours	2–4 weeks
Denosumab	Inhibits bone resorption by preventing RANKL-mediated osteoclast maturation, function and survival.	4–10 days	4–15 weeks
Loop diuretics	Inhibit calcium reabsorption in the distal nephron, increase urinary calcium excretion.	Within hours	During therapy
Glucocorticoids	Decrease 1,25(OH)2D synthesis by activated mononuclear cells in granulomatous diseases and certain lymphoproliferative diseases. Inhibit intestinal calcium absorption.		
Calcimimetics	Reduces PTH secretion by acting as CaSR agonist.	2–3 days	During therapy
Dialysis	Promotes removal of ionized calcium from extracellular fluid.	Hours	During therapy

RANKL receptor activator of nuclear factor kappa-B ligand
PTH parathyroid hormone
CaSR calcium-sensing receptor
[a]Adapted from Shane E, Berenson JR, Treatment of hypercalcemia. UpToDate

Therapy of Severe Hypercalcemia

Fundamental Approach

The initial approach to treatment includes intravenous hydration with isotonic saline, calcitonin, and potent antiresorptive agents like bisphosphonates or denosumab (Table 5.1). Concurrent administration of saline and calcitonin substantially lowers serum calcium concentrations within 12–48 hours. The bisphosphonate effect will become apparent by the second to fourth day and will last several days to weeks, thereby maintaining serum calcium in the normal range or substantially reduced compared to pretreatment levels. Denosumab is an alternative option for patients who are refractory to bisphosphonates or have renal dysfunction that precludes bisphosphonate use. The maximum effect of bisphosphonates occurs two to four days after initiation and of denosumab four to seven days after initiation. To emphasize, because their onset of action is slower than saline and calcitonin, it is important to initiate bisphosphonates or denosumab concurrently with fluids and calcitonin.

Intravenous Hydration with Isotonic Saline

Virtually, all patients with severe hypercalcemia are very hypovolemic due to hypercalcemia-induced urinary salt wasting and, in some cases, vomiting. Hypovolemia further reduces renal clearance of calcium and worsens hypercalcemia. Therefore, ECF repletion with isotonic saline is the cornerstone of therapy. The initial rate of administration should be 200–300 mL/hour for 3–4 hours, after which the rate may be adjusted to maintain urine output at 100–150 mL/hour. Higher initial rates may be considered if the patient is hypotensive. Conversely, lower initial rates should be considered when fluid overload is a concern, such as in older patients and those with underlying congestive heart failure or known chronic kidney disease. In such individuals, careful monitoring is crucial, and judicious use of loop diuretics may be required. In the past, it was a standard practice to add loop diuretics once fluid repletion had been achieved with the goal of further increasing urinary calcium excretion. However, in the absence of renal failure or heart failure, loop diuretic therapy is no longer recommended, because of potential fluid and electrolyte complications (hypokalemia, hypomagnesemia, and volume depletion) and because of the availability of drugs that inhibit bone resorption [9].

Salmon Calcitonin

Intravenous saline rarely normalizes serum calcium concentrations in patients with moderate or severe hypercalcemia [10]. In addition, excessive bone resorption is the central cause of hypercalcemia in the majority of patients. Therefore, salmon calcitonin, which has a rapid onset of action to increase renal calcium excretion and to decrease osteoclast-mediated bone resorption [11], should be initiated at the same time as intravenous saline. The recommended dose of calcitonin is 4 international units/kg subcutaneously or intramuscularly every 12 hours for 48 hours. However, if necessary, the dose may be increased up to 6–8 international units/kg every six hours. Although calcitonin is a relatively weak antiresorptive agent, it rapidly lowers serum calcium by 1–2 mg/dL (0.3–0.5 mmol/L) by four to six hours after initiation (Table 5.1) [12]. Because tachyphylaxis develops rapidly to calcitonin therapy, perhaps due to receptor downregulation, it should be discontinued after 48 hours. Calcitonin is very safe, although it may cause nausea. Nasal calcitonin is not effective for treatment of hypercalcemia [13].

Intravenous Bisphosphonates

The majority of patients treated for severe hypercalcemia, particularly malignant hypercalcemia, respond only partially and temporarily to isotonic saline and calcitonin. Therefore, concurrent intravenous bisphosphonate therapy should be initiated at the same time [2, 6–8, 14–16]. Bisphosphonates are nonhydrolyzable analogs of inorganic pyrophosphate that adsorb to the surface of bone hydroxyapatite and inhibit calcium release by interfering with osteoclast-mediated bone resorption. Bisphosphonates are more effective than saline and calcitonin for moderate or severe hypercalcemia [2, 7, 8, 11, 14, 17–21].

Zoledronic acid (4 mg intravenously over 15 minutes) is the preferred intravenous bisphosphonate for severe hypercalcemia. *Pamidronate (60–90 mg over 2 hours)* is an alternative option if zoledronic acid is not available. Zoledronic acid is preferred over pamidronate because it is more effective at lowering serum calcium in patients with malignant hypercalcemia (~87% vs 70%), it controls serum calcium for longer (32–43 versus 18 days) [19], and it can be administered in 15 minutes versus the 2 hours required for pamidronate. If pamidronate is chosen, infusion times of 2–4 hours are safe and maintain normocalcemia for two or more weeks. Although the 90 mg dose is maximally hypocalcemic, some adjust the dose to the degree of hypercalcemia: 60 mg if the serum calcium concentration is up to 13.5 mg/dL (3 to 3.4 mmol/L) and 90 mg for higher levels [18, 22]. Pamidronate should not be repeated sooner than a minimum of seven days. The most common side effect is fever. *Ibandronate* may also be used to treat hypercalcemia of malignancy. Doses of 2, 4, and 6 mg infused over 2 hours are safe and well tolerated; the 4 and 6 mg doses are more effective and comparable in efficacy to pamidronate [23, 24]. Oral bisphosphonates are not used to treat severe or acute hypercalcemia, and the use of etidronate has been abandoned.

Intravenous bisphosphonates are generally well tolerated. Occasionally, flu-like symptoms (fever, arthralgias, myalgia, fatigue, and bone pain), ocular inflammation (uveitis), hypocalcemia, and hypophosphatemia may occur. Intravenous bisphosphonates may also cause impaired renal function. In patients with impaired renal function at baseline, avoiding intravenous bisphosphonates altogether may not be necessary, since the renal failure may in fact be due to acute hypercalcemia. However, in such cases, it is especially important to ensure adequate hydration with saline. One can also use a lower dose and/or slower infusion rate (4 mg zoledronic acid over 30–60 minutes or 30–45 mg pamidronate over four hours) to minimize risk. Finally, one can substitute denosumab for intravenous bisphosphonates.

Denosumab

Denosumab, a human monoclonal antibody to receptor activator of NF kappa-B ligand (RANKL) that inhibits osteoclast activity and bone resorption, is approved by the FDA for treatment of osteoporosis and prevention of skeletal-related events in patients with certain cancers. Denosumab is not renally cleared; therefore, there is no restriction to its use in patients with chronic kidney disease, for whom bisphosphonates are used with caution or contraindicated. Denosumab has been studied in patients with hypercalcemia of malignancy, particularly in those resistant to bisphosphonates [2, 7, 8, 11, 15, 25–28]. In one series, 33 patients with hypercalcemia of malignancy with persistently elevated serum calcium levels after bisphosphonate treatment received denosumab 120 mg subcutaneously weekly for four weeks and then monthly thereafter. Within ten days, 64% had serum calcium levels <11.5 mg/dL [29]. In 2014, denosumab (60 mg subcutaneously) was approved for hypercalcemia refractory to bisphosphonates, with repeat dosing based on response. Hypocalcemia may occur following denosumab administration particularly in patients with renal dysfunction or vitamin D deficiency. Thus, it may be wise to start with a lower dose of 30 mg, with a second dose administered if the goal calcium is not achieved within approximately one week. It is also prudent to measure serum 25-hydroxyvitamin D (25-OHD) levels. While awaiting the results of the serum 25-OHD level, one could consider repleting with one or two days of vitamin D, 50,000 international units daily. If the patient is vitamin D deficient, it may help prevent hypocalcemia, and if they are vitamin D replete, the supplementation can be stopped.

Glucocorticoids

Glucocorticoids inhibit gastrointestinal calcium absorption. They are the preferred treatment for hypercalcemia due to excessive intestinal calcium absorption [30]. Increased absorption of dietary calcium is primarily, although not completely, responsible for the hypercalcemia associated with the excess administration or ingestion of vitamin D, milk-alkali syndrome, and with the endogenous overproduction of calcitriol (1,25-dihydroxyvitamin D), the most active metabolite of vitamin D. Increased calcitriol production can occur in patients with chronic granulomatous diseases (e.g., sarcoidosis) and in patients with lymphoma. In such patients, glucocorticoids (prednisone 20–40 mg/day) will usually reduce serum calcium concentrations within two to five days by decreasing calcitriol production by the activated mononuclear cells in the lung and lymph nodes. However, long-term therapy is often required to maintain normocalcemia.

Ketoconazole is an imidazole antifungal that inhibits macrophage 1 alpha-hydroxylation of 25-hydroxyvitamin D3. Ketoconazole reduces granulomatous production of $1,25(OH)_2D_3$ associated with diseases such as sarcoidosis [31] and tuberculosis [31–35], and in granulomas secondary to silicone and mineral oil injections [36–38]. It is also effective in lowering serum and urine calcium in patients with paraneoplastic hypercalcemia and inactivating mutations of CYP24A1 [30, 39–41]. In such disorders, ketoconazole may permit the maintenance dose of glucocorticoids to be reduced or discontinued. Thus, ketoconazole may be considered as an alternative or adjunctive glucocorticoid-sparing therapy for $1,25(OH)_2D_3$-dependent hypercalcemia. Additional measures include a low dietary calcium intake, low vitamin D intake, limiting sun exposure, and encouraging adequate hydration. Medications that induce hypercalcemia should be discontinued.

Renal Replacement Therapy

Occasionally, more aggressive measures are necessary in patients with very severe, symptomatic hypercalcemia. Hemodialysis with a low or zero calcium dialysate and peritoneal dialysis (though it is slower) are both effective therapies for hypercalcemia [6–8, 11, 16]. Dialysis may be indicated in patients with severe malignancy-associated hypercalcemia and renal insufficiency or heart failure, in whom hydration cannot be safely administered [42]. Hemodialysis should be considered in addition to the above treatments, in hemodynamically stable patients with serum calcium concentrations above 18–20 mg/dL (4.5–5 mmol/L) and neurologic symptoms or in those with severe hypercalcemia complicated by end-stage renal failure. In hypercalcemic patients with concomitant hypophosphatemia, hemodialysis with a dialysis solution enriched with phosphorus (final phosphorous concentration of 4 mg/dL) [43] may be necessary.

Calcimimetics

The CaSR is the regulator of PTH synthesis and secretion; it is expressed in parathyroid cells, the nephron, and other tissues. Cinacalcet increases the sensitivity of the CaSR to extracellular calcium, thus decreasing PTH secretion and serum calcium concentrations. Cinacalcet is approved for use in patients with chronic kidney disease and secondary hyperparathyroidism and for patients with severe primary hyperparathyroidism who cannot undergo parathyroidectomy [4, 44]. It can also be used to treat severe hypercalcemia from tertiary hyperparathyroidism or due to parathyroid carcinoma [45]. Calcimimetic agents reduce serum calcium concentration in patients with severe hypercalcemia due to parathyroid carcinoma and in hemodialysis patients with an elevated calcium-phosphorous product and secondary or tertiary hyperparathyroidism. A few case reports exist in which patients with hypercalcemia of malignancy refractory to usual therapy have responded to the addition of cinacalcet [11, 46, 47].

Prevention of Hypercalcemia Recurrence

After acute hypercalcemia has resolved, follow-up therapy may be necessary to prevent recurrence. In patients with malignancy, tumor progression may often result in recurrent and/or progressive hypercalcemia. Therefore, it is important to treat the underlying cancer if possible. Patients with cancer metastatic to the skeleton typically receive zoledronic acid or denosumab every three to four weeks as part of their treatment to prevent skeletal complications; such regimens typically prevent hypercalcemia. Additional measures include a low dietary calcium intake, low vitamin D intake, limiting sun exposure, and encouraging adequate hydration. Medications that induce hypercalcemia should be discontinued.

Disease-Specific Approaches to Management of Hypercalcemia

The general approaches to management described above apply to all patients with severe hypercalcemia. Below is a brief overview of treatment considerations specific to certain causes of hypercalcemia that are covered in more detail in other chapters.

Primary hyperparathyroidism, the most common cause of mild hypercalcemia in the outpatient setting (Chap. 6), may occasionally present with or be complicated by severe hypercalcemia particularly in patients who are otherwise seriously ill or bedridden. In patients with mild hypercalcemia, treatment typically focuses on parathyroidectomy to correct the underlying cause of the hyperparathyroidism. Patients who do not meet surgical guidelines should be monitored for complications of primary hyperparathyroidism (Chap. 6). Acute severe hypercalcemia in a patient with primary hyperparathyroidism (parathyroid crisis) should be managed as described above with saline hydration and antiresorptive drugs (calcitonin, IV bisphosphonates, or denosumab). *Parathyroid carcinoma* is a rare cause of hyperparathyroidism. Patients typically present with marked hypercalcemia, markedly elevated parathyroid hormone concentrations, and a neck mass. The primary treatment of parathyroid carcinoma is surgery. When the tumor can no longer be managed surgically because of local invasion or distant metastases, control of hypercalcemia with medical therapy becomes the therapeutic goal. While this goal can often be achieved with bisphosphonates or denosumab, calcimimetic agents may play a more central role. Severe hypercalcemia is unusual with familial hypocalciuric hypercalcemia (Chap. 8).

Lymphoma, sarcoidosis, and other granulomatous causes of hypercalcemia have enhanced intestinal calcium absorption due to increased endogenous calcitriol production. The major modalities of therapy are a low calcium diet, glucocorticoids, ketoconazole, and treatment of the underlying disease (Chap. 11). Additional measures include a low dietary calcium intake, low vitamin D intake, limiting sun exposure, and encouraging adequate hydration. Medications that induce hypercalcemia should be discontinued.

Vitamin D intoxication may also cause hypercalcemia. This can occur due to excessive intake of parent vitamin D in the form of supplements or to calcitriol therapy for hypoparathyroidism or for hyperparathyroidism secondary to renal failure. Hypercalcemia due to calcitriol therapy is generally short-lived because of the relatively short biologic half-life of calcitriol. Thus, stopping the calcitriol, increasing salt and fluid intake, and hydrating with intravenous saline if necessary may be all that is required. Hypercalcemia due to excess intake of parent vitamin D or calcidiol may take longer to resolve because this form of vitamin D is stored in adipose tissue. Thus, more aggressive therapy with saline hydration, parenteral antiresorptive therapy (zoledronic acid or denosumab), and glucocorticoids to decrease intestinal calcium absorption may be necessary.

Summary

Mild hypercalcemia (calcium <12 mg/dL) is usually asymptomatic or mildly symptomatic, and immediate intervention to lower serum calcium is not necessary. The main goal is to determine the etiology of the hypercalcemia and to treat accordingly. Such patients should be advised to avoid dehydration, dietary calcium intakes above 1000 mg/day, and prolonged bed rest, all of which can exacerbate hypercalcemia. If possible, thiazide diuretics, lithium, and vitamin D supplements should be discontinued. Chronic moderate hypercalcemia (calcium between 12 and 14 mg/dL) that is asymptomatic or only mildly symptomatic may not require immediate intervention to lower serum calcium. If, however, such a patient has gastrointestinal symptoms (e.g., nausea) and/or abnormal mental status, the therapeutic approach should be similar to patients with severe hypercalcemia.

Severe hypercalcemia (calcium >14 mg/dL) requires hydration with isotonic saline at an initial rate of 200–300 mL/hour that is then adjusted to maintain the urine output at 100–150 mL/hour. Loop diuretics should be avoided unless the patient has renal insufficiency or heart failure and is thus at risk of fluid overload. To achieve rapid lowering of serum calcium, salmon calcitonin should be started concurrently with hydration, (4 international units/kg subcutaneously or intramuscularly every 12 hours for 48 hours). Calcitonin should be discontinued after 48 hours because of tachyphylaxis. To achieve longer-term control of severe hypercalcemia, particularly when due to excessive bone resorption, intravenous zoledronic acid (4 mg over 30 minutes) or pamidronate (60–90 mg over 2 hours) should be initiated. Denosumab can be used instead for patients with hypercalcemia refractory to bisphosphonates or in whom bisphosphonates are contraindicated due to severe renal impairment. However, careful monitoring of serum calcium levels is necessary in these patients because there is a higher risk of hypocalcemia with denosumab than with bisphosphonates. Moreover, in many cases, the renal impairment, especially if it is acute in onset and accompanied the development of hypercalcemia, may be reversed with IV bisphosphonates. Glucocorticoids are effective in treating hypercalcemia due to some lymphomas, sarcoid, or other granulomatous diseases. Dialysis is generally reserved for those with severe hypercalcemia.

References

1. Vautour L, Goltzman D. Regulation of calcium homeostasis. In: Primer on the metabolic bone diseases and disorders of mineral metabolism; 2018. p. 163–72.
2. Minisola S, Pepe J, Piemonte S, Cipriani C. The diagnosis and management of hypercalcaemia. BMJ. 2015;350:h2723.
3. Bilezikian JP. Approach to parathyroid disorders. In: Primer on the metabolic bone diseases and disorders of mineral metabolism; 2018. p. 611–8.
4. Silverberg SJ, Bandeira F, Liu J, Marcocci C, Walker MD. Primary hyperparathyroidism. In: Primer on the metabolic bone diseases and disorders of mineral metabolism. Malden: Wiley-Blackwell; 2018. p. 619–28.
5. Walker MD, Silverberg SJ. Primary hyperparathyroidism. Nat Rev Endocrinol. 2018;14:115–25.
6. Ahmad S, Kuraganti G, Steenkamp D. Hypercalcemic crisis: a clinical review. Am J Med. 2015;128:239–45.
7. Horwitz MJ. Non-parathyroid hypercalcemia. In: Primer on the Metabolic Bone Diseases and Disorders of Mineral Metabolism; 2018. p. 639–45.
8. Zagzag J, Hu MI, Fisher SB, Perrier ND. Hypercalcemia and cancer: differential diagnosis and treatment. CA Cancer J Clin. 2018;68:377–86.
9. LeGrand SB, Leskuski D, Zama I. Narrative review: furosemide for hypercalcemia: an unproven yet common practice. Ann Intern Med. 2008;149:259–63.
10. Hosking DJ, Cowley A, Bucknall CA. Rehydration in the treatment of severe hypercalcaemia. Q J Med. 1981;50:473–81.
11. Sternlicht H, Glezerman IG. Hypercalcemia of malignancy and new treatment options. Ther Clin Risk Manag. 2015;11:1779–88.
12. Wisneski LA. Salmon calcitonin in the acute management of hypercalcemia. Calcif Tissue Int. 1990;46(Suppl):S26–30.
13. Dumon JC, Magritte A, Body JJ. Nasal human calcitonin for tumor-induced hypercalcemia. Calcif Tissue Int. 1992;51:18–9.
14. Berenson JR. Treatment of hypercalcemia of malignancy with bisphosphonates. Semin Oncol. 2002;29:12–8.
15. Goltzman D. Nonparathyroid Hypercalcemia. Front Horm Res. 2019;51:77–90.
16. Maier JD, Levine SN. Hypercalcemia in the intensive care unit: a review of pathophysiology, diagnosis, and modern therapy. J Intensive Care Med. 2015;30:235–52.
17. Body JJ, Bartl R, Burckhardt P, et al. Current use of bisphosphonates in oncology. International Bone and Cancer Study Group. J Clin Oncol. 1998;16:3890–9.
18. Gucalp R, Theriault R, Gill I, et al. Treatment of cancer-associated hypercalcemia. Double-blind comparison of rapid and slow intravenous infusion regimens of pamidronate disodium and saline alone. Arch Intern Med. 1994;154:1935–44.
19. Major P, Lortholary A, Hon J, et al. Zoledronic acid is superior to pamidronate in the treatment of hypercalcemia of malignancy: a pooled analysis of two randomized, controlled clinical trials. J Clin Oncol. 2001;19:558–67.
20. Major PP, Coleman RE. Zoledronic acid in the treatment of hypercalcemia of malignancy: results of the international clinical development program. Semin Oncol. 2001;28:17–24.
21. Stewart AF. Clinical practice. Hypercalcemia associated with cancer. N Engl J Med. 2005;352:373–9.

22. Nussbaum SR, Younger J, Vandepol CJ, et al. Single-dose intravenous therapy with pamidronate for the treatment of hypercalcemia of malignancy: comparison of 30-, 60-, and 90-mg dosages. Am J Med. 1993;95:297–304.
23. Pecherstorfer M, Ludwig H, Schlosser K, Buck S, Huss HJ, Body JJ. Administration of the bisphosphonate ibandronate (BM 21.0955) by intravenous bolus injection. J Bone Miner Res. 1996;11:587–93.
24. Pecherstorfer M, Herrmann Z, Body JJ, et al. Randomized phase II trial comparing different doses of the bisphosphonate ibandronate in the treatment of hypercalcemia of malignancy. J Clin Oncol. 1996;14:268–76.
25. Thosani S, Hu MI. Denosumab: a new agent in the management of hypercalcemia of malignancy. Future Oncol. 2015;11:2865–71.
26. Hu MI, Glezerman IG, Leboulleux S, et al. Denosumab for treatment of hypercalcemia of malignancy. J Clin Endocrinol Metab. 2014;99:3144–52.
27. Dietzek A, Connelly K, Cotugno M, Bartel S, McDonnell AM. Denosumab in hypercalcemia of malignancy: a case series. J Oncol Pharm Pract. 2015;21:143–7.
28. Cicci JD, Buie L, Bates J, van Deventer H. Denosumab for the management of hypercalcemia of malignancy in patients with multiple myeloma and renal dysfunction. Clin Lymphoma Myeloma Leuk. 2014;14:e207–11.
29. Adhikaree J, Newby Y, Sundar S. Denosumab should be the treatment of choice for bisphosphonate refractory hypercalcaemia of malignancy. BMJ Case Rep. 2014;2014:bcr2013202861.
30. Tebben PJ, Singh RJ, Kumar R. Vitamin D-mediated hypercalcemia: mechanisms, diagnosis, and treatment. Endocr Rev. 2016;37:521–47.
31. Conron M, Beynon HL. Ketoconazole for the treatment of refractory hypercalcemic sarcoidosis. Sarcoidosis Vasc Diffuse Lung Dis. 2000;17:277–80.
32. Adams JS, Sharma OP, Diz MM, Endres DB. Ketoconazole decreases the serum 1,25-dihydroxyvitamin D and calcium concentration in sarcoidosis-associated hypercalcemia. J Clin Endocrinol Metab. 1990;70:1090–5.
33. Hilderson I, Van Laecke S, Wauters A, Donck J. Treatment of renal sarcoidosis: is there a guideline? Overview of the different treatment options. Nephrol Dial Transplant. 2014;29:1841–7.
34. Saggese G, Bertelloni S, Baroncelli GI, Di Nero G. Ketoconazole decreases the serum ionized calcium and 1,25-dihydroxyvitamin D levels in tuberculosis-associated hypercalcemia. Am J Dis Child. 1993;147:270–3.
35. Sharma OP. Hypercalcemia in granulomatous disorders: a clinical review. Curr Opin Pulm Med. 2000;6:442–7.
36. Eldrup E, Theilade S, Lorenzen M, et al. Hypercalcemia after cosmetic oil injections: unraveling etiology, pathogenesis, and severity. J Bone Miner Res. 2021;36:322–33.
37. Negri AL, Rosa Diez G, Del Valle E, et al. Hypercalcemia secondary to granulomatous disease caused by the injection of methacrylate: a case series. Clin Cases Miner Bone Metab. 2014;11:44–8.
38. Shirvani A, Palermo NE, Holick MF. Man of steel syndrome: silicone and mineral oil injections with associated hypercalcemia, hypophosphatemia, and proximal muscle weakness. JBMR Plus. 2019;3:e10208.
39. Carpenter TO. Take another CYP: confirming a novel mechanism for "idiopathic" hypercalcemia. J Clin Endocrinol Metab. 2012;97:768–71.
40. Jacobs TP, Kaufman M, Jones G, et al. A lifetime of hypercalcemia and hypercalciuria, finally explained. J Clin Endocrinol Metab. 2014;99:708–12.
41. Sayers J, Hynes AM, Srivastava S, et al. Successful treatment of hypercalcaemia associated with a CYP24A1 mutation with fluconazole. Clin Kidney J. 2015;8:453–5.
42. Koo WS, Jeon DS, Ahn SJ, Kim YS, Yoon YS, Bang BK. Calcium-free hemodialysis for the management of hypercalcemia. Nephron. 1996;72:424–8.
43. Leehey DJ, Ing TS. Correction of hypercalcemia and hypophosphatemia by hemodialysis using a conventional, calcium-containing dialysis solution enriched with phosphorus. Am J Kidney Dis. 1997;29:288–90.

44. Silva BC, Cusano NE, Bilezikian JP. Primary hyperparathyroidism. Best Pract Res Clin Endocrinol Metab. 2018;32:593–607.
45. Silverberg SJ, Rubin MR, Faiman C, et al. Cinacalcet hydrochloride reduces the serum calcium concentration in inoperable parathyroid carcinoma. J Clin Endocrinol Metab. 2007;92:3803–8.
46. Asonitis N, Kassi E, Kokkinos M, Giovanopoulos I, Petychaki F, Gogas H. Hypercalcemia of malignancy treated with cinacalcet. Endocrinol Diabetes Metab Case Rep. 2017;2017:17-0118.
47. Takeuchi Y, Takahashi S, Miura D, et al. Cinacalcet hydrochloride relieves hypercalcemia in Japanese patients with parathyroid cancer and intractable primary hyperparathyroidism. J Bone Miner Metab. 2017;35:616–22.

Chapter 6
Primary Hyperparathyroidism

John P. Bilezikian

Introduction

In primary hyperparathyroidism (PHPT), the serum calcium and the parathyroid hormone level are classically above normal. These patients will sometimes show levels of PTH that are in the normal range, but given the exquisite physiological relationship between calcium and PTH, normal levels of PTH are distinctly abnormal in the context of hypercalcemia. The disease has undergone a clinical evolution from one in which the skeleton and kidney were invariably involved and the serum calcium was typically more than 1 mg/dL above normal [1–3] to one in which patients are now discovered incidentally in the context of routine biochemical screening [4–8]. A further clinical evolution, due undoubtedly to our proactive approach to the evaluation of patients with low bone density, is the phenotype now known as normocalcemic PHPT [9]. These patients typically have consistently normal adjusted total and ionized serum calcium levels but persistently elevated levels of PTH in the absence of secondary causes.

Risk Factors, Pathology, and Anatomical Location

Most patients with PHPT have the sporadic form in which there is no family history nor any known predisposing elements such as external neck radiation, lithium, or hydrochlorothiazide use [10–12]. Less certain risk factors include prolonged low calcium intake and higher body weight [13, 14]. The single, benign parathyroid

J. P. Bilezikian (✉)
Division of Endocrinology, Department of Medicine, Vagelos College of Physicians and Surgeons, Columbia University, New York, NY, USA
e-mail: JPB2@cumc.columbia.edu

© The Author(s), under exclusive license to Springer Nature Switzerland AG 2022
M. D. Walker (ed.), *Hypercalcemia*, Contemporary Endocrinology,
https://doi.org/10.1007/978-3-030-93182-7_6

adenoma occurs in about 80% of patients [15]. Less commonly, in about 15% of patients, four-gland parathyroid hyperplasia is seen [16]. Multiple parathyroid adenomas are rarely encountered, in less than 5% [17]. Parathyroid carcinoma is exceedingly rare with most series reporting an incidence of well under <1% [18]. Even more rare are patients who have parathyromatosis in which benign but overactive parathyroid tissue is seeded throughout the neck and, sometimes, in the mediastinum [19]. Hyperfunctioning parathyroid tissue is found in typical anatomical locations, namely, at the four poles of the thyroid gland, but they can be found literally anywhere in the neck, retroesophageal space, or mediastinum [20–23].

Epidemiology

The incidence of PHPT has changed over the past half-century, primarily as a function of technology and practice [24, 25]. The multichannel autoanalyzer in the early 1970s marked the demarcation between a rare, symptomatic disease to a common, asymptomatic disease. The incidence rose from 7.8 cases per 100,000 to 51.1 cases per 100,000. After this wave and an expected decline in incidence to 27 per 100,000, another increase in the United States has been reported [24, 26–28]. Again, one can attribute this second peak to a more proactive approach to screening for general health in the population. In particular, attention to a complete skeletal evaluation among those referred for osteoporosis or low bone density has been responsible also for the more recently recognized normocalcemic variant of PHPT [29]. In most series, the incidence of NPHPT ranges from 0.2% to 0.4% [30–32]. PHPT is more likely to be seen in the early postmenopausal years among women who predominate by a ratio of 3–4:1.

Diagnosis and Differential Diagnosis

Other chapters in this book cover the differential diagnosis of hypercalcemia and will, therefore, not be covered in detail here. The diagnosis is quite readily made in individuals whose serum calcium and PTH levels are as noted above. The other most common cause of hypercalcemia, namely that due to malignancy is differentiated readily by suppressed levels of PTH. Moreover, such individuals are typically symptomatic of a malignancy in other ways. The true ectopic production of PTH from a malignant tumor is exceedingly rare [33]. Familial hypocalciuric hypercalcemia (FHH) is usually not a diagnostic dilemma because these individuals have a family history, are typically much younger, and have exceedingly low urinary excretion of calcium [34–36].

Normocalcemic primary hyperparathyroidism (NPHPT), as noted above, is the third generational phenotype of this disease. While there is considerable uncertainty about diagnostic criteria [31, 37], because secondary causes for the elevated PTH levels in normocalcemic individuals have not always been ruled out definitely in publications, it is nevertheless a recognized entity. In the recent publication by Schini et al., [31] the adjusted serum calcium in NPHPT was 10.2 ± 0.2 mg/dL, lower than the PHPT group in which the adjusted serum calcium was 11.0 ± 0.4. Both groups had similarly elevated levels of PTH (107 vs 102 pg/mL). Part of the natural history of NPHPT in some, but not all patients, is progression to overt hypercalcemia or intermittently elevated levels [29, 31, 38, 39].

Other biochemical features of PHPT in comparison with NPHPT are illustrated in Table 6.1. A tendency for the serum phosphorus concentration to be in the low normal range is more likely than frank hypophosphatemia. The average urinary calcium excretion tends to be in the upper range of normal but hypercalciuria is not uncommon. Serum 25-hydroxyvitamin D levels tend to be in the lower end of the normal range. They are higher in more recent series because many patients are receiving supplemental vitamin D whereas in the past they were not [40, 41]. 1,25-dihydroxyvitamin D levels are elevated in about 1/3 of patients [42].

Pathophysiology of Hypercalcemia in PHPT

The pathophysiology of the hypercalcemia of PHPT is due to the effects of PTH on its target organs, the kidney and the skeleton. The physiological actions of PTH are to conserve calcium filtered at the glomerulus, thus contributing to hypercalcemia by virtue of the greater amount of calcium filtered. Skeletal resorption of calcium which exceeds calcium accretion is another pathophysiological feature of the hypercalcemia. In some situations, particularly, in those with elevated levels of 1,25-dihydroxyvitamin D and high dietary calcium, the gastrointestinal tract can participate in these pathophysiological mechanisms [43].

Table 6.1 A comparison of biochemical indices in those with normocalcemic and with hypercalcemic primary hyperparathyroidism

Index	Controls($n = 300$)	NPHPT($n = 11$)	PHPT($n = 17$)
% Women	71%	92%	88%
PTH (pg/mL)[a]	42.5 (40.8, 44.2)	107 (86.9124)	102 (89,112)
Cal (adj) mg/dL[a]	9.48 (± 0.32)	10.2 (± 0.2)	11.0 (± 0.44)
P (mg/dL)[a]	3.36 (± 0.5)	3.12 (± 0.42)	2.67 (±0.48)
25-OH D (ng/mL)	31.6 (±13)	25.1 (±9)	28.6 (±12)
Urinary Calcium (mg/24 hr)		170	300

[a]$P < 0.001$ controls vs two PHPT groups. There were no significant differences in any of the indices between the two PHPT groups
Adapted from Ref. [31]

Clinical Presentation: Asymptomatic Versus Symptomatic PHPT

In countries where biochemical screening is a standard of care, most patients with PHPT will not have experienced overt, classical signs or symptoms of the disease, apart from the hypercalcemia. The terminology used widely to describe these individuals is "asymptomatic PHPT." They constitute, by far, the majority of patients with this disease in the developed world. It is important to distinguish this terminology from involvement of target organs that may become apparent *after* patients are evaluated. For example, discovery of low bone density by dual energy absorptiometry (DXA) or a kidney stone by ultrasound does not redefine these patients as symptomatic, but rather, the terminology is modified to indicate that they have target organ involvement. The term symptomatic PHPT is reserved for those individuals who are truly symptomatic. This could take the form of symptomatic hypercalcemia, a clinical event such as a fracture or a kidney stone, or very rarely, a proximal myopathy. The vague, nonspecific descriptors of weakness, easy fatigability, depression, and intellectual weariness do not enter into this discussion of symptomatic PHPT because they lack specificity (see below) [44]. The physical examination is generally unremarkable. If a mass is felt in the neck, it is likely to be a thyroid nodule or, if the clinical setting is suggestive, a parathyroid malignancy.

This chapter will not discuss concomitant diseases that have historically or more recently been linked to PHPT such as peptic ulcer disease, gout, pseudogout, or celiac disease [45–50]. In the asymptomatic form of the disease, they all lack a clear etiological relationship [51]. This chapter also does not consider specific presentations of PHPT beyond the traditional ones, acute primary hyperparathyroidism, PHPT in pregnancy, parathyroid cancer, or parathyromatosis. These variants are also covered elsewhere [52]. Genetic forms of PHPT are covered elsewhere in this book.

Target Organs: Skeleton

Classical radiographic features of PHPT, although rare in asymptomatic disease, are seen more often in symptomatic patients [53, 54]. With the introduction of DXA in the 1980s, it became possible to determine whether, to what extent, and with what selectivity the skeleton is involved in asymptomatic patients. The application of other imaging modalities, such as bone histomorphometry, new imaging technologies, and bone turnover markers all have given a more complete understanding of how this target organ is affected in this disease.

Bone Mineral Densitometry and Other Imaging Modalities

Bone density is an indispensable tool for the noninvasive evaluation of the skeleton in any disorder associated with low bone mass, such as osteoporosis. In osteoporosis, many centers measure only the lumbar spine and the hip regions. In PHPT, however, it is essential to measure also the distal third radius site because of the known proclivity of PTH to be catabolic at the cortical compartment of bone. The distal 1/3 radius is primarily cortical bone and thus can show changes when the lumbar spine (more trabecular bone) and the hip regions (more even admixtures of cortical and trabecular bone) may not. A typical pattern, first shown by Silverberg et al., [55] is for the distal third radius to be preferentially involved, with relative preservation of trabecular bone (lumbar spine) and an intermediate measurement at the hip regions [55–58]. However, this pattern is the typical presentation, not the only one. About 15% of patients with PHPT will have reduced bone density of the lumbar spine [59]. In fact, any pattern of bone density can be seen in PHPT [60]. This impression, namely, that in PHPT, the cortical compartment of bone is compromised, has been confirmed by histomorphometric analysis of bone biopsies [61–63].

The classical approaches to evaluating the skeleton in PHPT by BMD and by bone biopsies have been augmented by newer noninvasive skeletal imaging technologies, such as the trabecular bone score (TBS) and high-resolution peripheral quantitative tomography. By these two approaches, it has been shown clearly that not only the cortical compartment of bone is compromised in PHPT but also the trabecular compartment is at risk [64–67]. This is a high bone turnover state as shown by dynamic bone histomorphometry and by bone turnover markers [68–72]. The combination of both cortical and trabecular bone involvement along with the high turnover state characteristic of many patients with asymptomatic PHPT leads to certain expectations about fracture risk.

Fractures

Although in symptomatic primary hyperparathyroidism, fractures are experienced, the possibility of increased fracture incidence in asymptomatic PHPT has been more difficult to ascertain. Based upon BMD, one might expect that fracture risk would be increased at cortical sites but not necessarily at trabecular sites. However, studies by Kholsa et al. [73] first raised the possibility that fracture incidence might be increased uniformly at both nonverbetral and vertebral sites. Of interest, trabecular regions were specifically demonstrated to be at risk [73–77]. Ejlsmark-Svensson et al. have documented, in a meta-analysis, an increase in "any fracture," forearm

Table 6.2 Fracture risk in primary hyperparathyroidism

Site	Odds Ratio	95% CI
Any	2.01	1.61–2.50*
Forearm	2.36	1.64–3.38*
Vertebral	3.00	1.41–6.37*
Hip	1.27	0.97–1.66

Adapted from Ref. [78]

and vertebral fracture in PHPT [78] (Table 6.2). A significant increase in hip fracture could not be demonstrated.

Target Organs: The Kidney

The pathogenesis of kidney stones and calcifications in PHPT can be explained readily by the pathophysiology of renal handling as described above [79–82]. In addition, local urinary factors that contribute to stone risk, such as a reduction in inhibitor activity or an increase in stone-promoting factors, may be important [82, 83]. Hypomagnesuria has recently been associated with kidney stones in PHPT [84].

Given that the pathophysiology of kidney stones formation in PHPT is multifactorial and not completely understood, it is nevertheless clear that their incidence is increased. Most series still place the percentage of kidney stones in PHPT to be 15–20% [85]. If one screens for prevalence among those with asymptomatic PHPT, these percentages are in fact much higher [86–90]. Other renal manifestations of PHPT include hypercalciuria, nephrocalcinosis, and renal impairment [87, 91–95].

Nonclassical Organ Involvement

Space does not permit a discussion of PHPT as it may be relevant to non-classical targets such as the cardiovascular system but a recent study about the putative neurocognitive aspects of PHPT is noteworthy. The possibility of specific neuropsychologic abnormities to account for subjective complaints of patients with PHPT has been a vexing challenge for many years [44, 96]. They do not appear to be associated with a well-documented and reversible neuromuscular disease [97–100]. In asymptomatic PHPT such abnormalities are not demonstrable [101].

Three RCTs that investigated the reversibility of reduced quality of life (QOL) and psychiatric symptoms were neither conclusive nor consistent [102–104]. Even more sophisticated testing of cognition, cerebrovascular function, and functional magnetic resonance imaging has not yielded insight into a putative link between CNS function and PHPT [105–116].

The most recent attempt to demonstrate an effect of parathyroidectomy on quality of life in PHPT was published by Pretorius et al. [117]. In their ten-year prospective clinical trial, 192 subjects with asymptomatic PHPT were randomized 1:1 to parathyroid surgery or to observation. Two quality of life metrics were used. Those who underwent parathyroidectomy achieved biochemical cure. In the group that was observed without surgery, hypercalcemia and elevated levels of PTH persisted. With the exception of only 1 metric of the SF-36 scale (vitality), there were no significant differences between the two groups when both quality of life metrics were monitored during and at the ten-year time point. It is apparent from this well-designed prospective study that parathyroid surgery does not improve quality of life in PHPT. Another clear result of this study is the observation that no surgery does not worsen quality of life [118].

Evaluation

After the diagnosis of PHPT is secured biochemically, other laboratory measurements should include the serum phosphorus, alkaline phosphatase activity, 25-hydroxyvitamin D, and creatinine. An index of urinary calcium excretion should be obtained either as a 2-hour morning or a full 24-hour urine collection. Despite being more cumbersome, most experts prefer the 24-hour urinary calcium excretion to account for diurnal variability. Bone turnover markers such as the serum osteocalcin and CTX give information about the activity of bone turnover. All patients should have bone densitometry by DXA at the lumbar spine, hip, and distal 1/3 radius. In view of the increased vertebral fracture risk in PHPT, despite bone density values that may not be low, additional spine imaging by vertebral X-rays or vertebral fracture assessment is recommended. The TBS score can be helpful to assess skeletal quality [119]. In view of an appreciable incidence of silent kidney stones and/or nephrocalcinosis, renal ultrasound, CT, or abdominal x-ray is recommended [89].

Natural History: Observational Experience

One of the conundrums that has led to uncertainty to recommend parathyroidectomy more uniformly in this disease is related to the natural history of the disease. Among the noteworthy studies for their duration to address this point are those published by Silverberg, Rubin, and their colleagues [94, 120]. Their observations over a period of 15 years among those who did or did not have surgery constitute the longest natural-history study of this disorder [120].

After Surgery

Successful parathyroidectomy cures the disease with persistent normalization of the serum calcium and PTH levels in virtually all patients. After surgery, BMD increases at all sites. While the increase is approximately 10% at the lumbar spine, hip and distal forearm regions, there is a difference in the rate at which bone mineral accrues. The lumbar spine shows the fastest gains; the distal 1/3 radius shows the slowest gains. This is to be expected since the two sites are so different in their intrinsic skeletal metabolism. The lumbar spine with much more rapid bone turnover than the 1/3 radius gains bone mineral within the first few years after surgery while the distal 1/3 radius takes longer [94, 120]. While this study included those who did or did not meet surgical guidelines, the similar gains between these two groups helps to confirm that skeletal improvements can be expected on all patients who undergo parathyroidectomy, irrespective of meeting accepted surgical guidelines.

Without Surgery

This study included a large number of subjects who were observed without parathyroid surgery. Except for the serum calcium that tended to rise minimally after year 12, all other indices such as the PTH, 25-hydroxyvitamin D, and urinary calcium excretion did not change over the entire 15-year period [120]. Long-term stability was also observed by the measurement of lumbar spine BMD. The hip and forearm regions, however, began to decline after year 8 with the distal radius showing substantial reductions after year 10. A loss of 10% or more was seen in a majority of the subjects after 15 years of observation. Taking into account accepted guidelines for surgery (Table 6.3), approximately 1/3 of subjects met at least one guideline for surgery after 15 years. Another way to consider this is that a majority of subjects followed for 15 years did not meet a guideline for surgery even after that period of time.

Table 6.3 Indications for surgery in asymptomatic primary hyperparathyroidism

Recommended index	4th Int'l Workshop (Bilezikian et al. [89])
Serum calcium (above normal)	> 1 mg/dL
Skeletal	DXA: T-Score < −2.5 at any site; Vert Fx by X-ray or VFA
Renal	Creatinine clearance <60 cc/min Stone by X-ray, CT, or ultrasound Urinary calcium: >400 mg/d plus other urinary biochemical indices of increased stone risk
Age	< 50

Adapted from Ref. [89]

Natural History: Randomized Controlled Trials

The aforementioned experience has been confirmed by more rigorous prospective natural history, but they have been much shorter. In the studies of Rao et al. [121], Bollerslev et al. [102], and Ambrogini et al. [104] short-term gains in bone density were seen uniformly.

Who Should Be Recommended to Have Parathyroid Surgery? Guidelines for Surgical Intervention

Five International Workshops on the management of asymptomatic PHPT have been held since 1991, with the most recent one in 2021 [89, 122–125]. The reason for periodic reassessment of guidelines for surgery relates to the natural history studies summarized above. While parathyroid surgery is the only way to cure this disease, its natural history is rather benign in the majority of patients. On the other hand, patients can experience kidney stones, lose bone mass, and fractures over time. These possible sequelae might be of greater concern if the initial evaluation were to show nephrocalcinosis, a silent kidney stone, marked hypercalciuria, low bone density, or a silent vertebral fracture. As the guidelines from 2021 have not been published yet, the guidelines from the 2013 conference are still current at this time. There has never been any dispute that symptomatic PHPT is a call for surgical intervention. For asymptomatic PHPT, the following guidelines based upon the best available evidence were established (see Table 6.3):

1. Serum calcium >1 mg/dL above the upper limit of normal
2. Renal issues: reduction in creatinine clearance to <60 mL/min; urinary calcium excretion >400 mg/24 h with increased stone risk; or the presence of nephroli-thiasis or nephrocalcinosis on renal imaging
3. Skeletal issues: T-score < −2.5 at any site; vertebral compression fracture by vertebral imaging
4. Age: < 50 years

These guidelines were established as individual criteria, which mean that any endpoint would be consistent with a recommendation for surgery. It is noteworthy, and explained above, that neurocognitive, cardiovascular, and other nonclassical features of PHPT are not included among the guidelines for surgery. Most experts do not recommend surgery in PHPT if patients demonstrate these nonclassical features because of the uncertainty linking them etiologically and little evidence that surgery has any effects on them.

Surgery

It is important to note that surgery in PHPT can be conducted with the concurrence of the patient and the physician, even though surgical guidelines may not be met. On the other hand, patients who meet one or more surgical guidelines may opt not to have parathyroid surgery. Furthermore, intercurrent medical conditions can be a contraindication to surgery. The patient may have had previous, unsuccessful parathyroid surgery. The decision for or against surgery is not necessarily a simple matter of deciding whether or not guidelines are met.

Preoperative Localization of Hyperfunctioning Parathyroid Tissue

In the old days, before imaging of hyperfunctioning parathyroid tissue became a standard of care, the expert parathyroid surgeon was successful as often as those today who have the advantage of preoperative parathyroid imaging. In both cases, success rates of 95% have been reported. Preoperative parathyroid imaging, however, has become an essential guide. One reason for this is the anatomic variability of parathyroid tissue. The offending gland can be found in many places, apart from their typical sites at the four poles of the thyroid. In addition, a patient who has undergone previous anterior neck surgery is likely to have distorted anatomical landmarks, making it more difficult to identify parathyroid tissue. With the advent of minimally invasive parathyroid surgery, preoperative localization has become even more important. A key point to bear in mind is that parathyroid imaging is not used to diagnose the disease. It should be reserved for those who are going to undergo parathyroid surgery. If there are no plans for the patient to have parathyroid surgery, there is no justification for parathyroid imaging.

Most parathyroid imaging is noninvasive. The various approaches include technetium (Tc)-99 m sestamibi scintigraphy, ultrasound, computed tomography (CT) scanning, magnetic resonance imaging (MRI), and positron emission tomography (PET) scanning. Each has strengths and weaknesses. To a certain extent, it depends upon the capacities of the center and its experience [126–128]. Four-dimensional (4D) CT has emerged as a promising method and was shown in a recent study, to be superior to sestamibi SPECT/CT [129]. Invasive imaging consists of parathyroid fine-needle aspiration (FNA) [130] or arteriography with selective venous sampling for PTH [131]. FNA carries with it the theoretical risk of autoseeding of parathyroid tissue. Selective venous sampling is reserved for the most difficult clinical situations, such as those in whom other localization maneuvers have failed and/or those who have had previous unsuccessful parathyroid surgery. This approach requires an experienced interventional radiologist.

Parathyroidectomy

One of the first dictums in parathyroid surgery is that it should be done by someone who is experienced and acknowledged to be an expert. Standard approaches include the four-gland exploration that can be done under general or regional anesthesia. Another approach that has gained popularity is the unilateral minimally invasive parathyroidectomy (MIP) in which only the offending gland, previously visualized by preoperative localization, is removed. The intraoperative PTH level is expected to fall by >50% into the normal range by 10 minutes after removal of the adenoma. This approach has comparable success rates to the standard operation [132] but has the advantage in being faster and less invasive [133, 134]. Successful preoperative localization is essential for this procedure [135]. MIP is reported to have a success rate of 95% to 98% [136, 137]. In a recent meta-analysis that included >12,000 patients, there was no difference between MIP and the more conventional procedure in terms of success rate, recurrent or persistent PHPT, failure, or the need for repeat surgery [138]. Variations on the MIP approach include endoscopy and perioperative sestamibi scanning [139, 140].

Successful surgery is associated with not only rapid normalization of the PTH level but also correction of the hypercalcemia. Typically, patients with asymptomatic PHPT do not experience postoperative hypocalcemia, a situation that is still possible in those with symptomatic disease. In addition to normalization of the serum calcium and PTH, postoperative reduction in urinary calcium by as much as 50% is also expected [94, 141]. BMD also improves.

Table 6.4 Guidelines for the management of asymptomatic primary hyperparathyroidism in those who are not going to have parathyroid surgery

Measurement	Frequency
Serum calcium	Annually
Twenty-four-hour urinary calcium	Not recommended unless clinically indicated
Creatinine clearance	Not recommended unless clinically indicated
Serum creatinine	Annually
Bone density	Annually or biannually
Abdominal x-ray	Not recommended unless clinically indicated

Adapted from Ref. [89]

In the context of symptomatic disease, the improvement in BMD can truly be dramatic as shown by Kulak et al. [53] with 2.6- to 4.3-fold gain in BMD 3–4 years after surgery.

Nonsurgical Management

In patients who do not meet guidelines for surgery or in those who do but are not going to have parathyroid surgery, monitoring guidelines have been useful [89] (Table 6.4). This includes annual measurements of the serum calcium concentration, a calculated or estimated creatinine clearance, and regular monitoring of BMD.

General Measures

General approaches that are advised for all patients include maintaining good hydration and avoiding medications that can lead to dehydration such as diuretics. Prolonged immobilization is also to be avoided, if at all possible. Dietary management includes nutritional amounts of calcium. This advice has seemed counterintuitive to patients because they assume that calcium in the diet will worsen their hypercalcemia. Clinicians need to instruct patients that this is almost never the case. Rather, restricted calcium diets can lead to increases in PTH and worsen the disease [142–144]. There is some evidence that dietary calcium, when increased, can reduce PTH levels in PHPT [145]. The only exception to this general rule is to recognize that a high level of 1,25-dihydroxyvitamin D could lead to enhanced absorption to high dietary calcium and lead to increased urinary calcium excretion [43]. Nutritional amounts of calcium are best provided through the diet, but calcium supplements are not contraindicated in PHPT if dietary calcium cannot meet nutritional guidelines of approximately 1000 mg/day [146]. Vitamin D adequacy is also an important general guideline in PHPT. While guidelines endorse a 25-hydroxyvitamin D level in the range of 21–30 ng/ml using daily vitamin D doses of 600–1000 IU, [147] levels up to 38 ng/ml were shown to lower PTH, increase lumbar spine BMD, and to maintain baseline levels of serum and urinary calcium [148].

Pharmacological Approaches to PHPT

Pharmacological measures are available in PHPT. However, those patients for whom these approaches are considered are virtually always candidates for parathyroid surgery. They typically meet a guideline such as a serum calcium >1 mg/dL above the upper limit of normal or reduced BMD to < −2.5. It is a given, then, that these agents are considered only when candidates for parathyroidectomy are not going to have surgery for reasons already stated.

Estrogens and selective estrogen receptor modulators like raloxifene have been associated with reductions in the serum calcium [149–151]. Estrogen and medroxyprogesterone (5 mg daily) were shown in one RCT to increase BMD at all skeletal sites. These approaches are not generally favored by clinicians or patients because of general concerns about estrogen as well as the extremely limited data with raloxifene.

Antiresorptives such as the bisphosphonates and denosumab may have a role because they appear to improve bone density. Among the bisphosphonates that have been studied, the most extensive and positive experience has been with alendronate [152–155]. With much more limited experience, denosumab also appears to increase BMD in postmenopausal women with PHPT [156, 157]. Despite the improvement in BMD, these antiresorptives do not reliably reduce the serum calcium concentration.

A more specific approach to the medical management of PHPT is to inhibit PTH secretion. To this point, the calcimimetic, cinacalcet, has been studied extensively. It reduces the serum calcium often to normal [158, 159]. PTH levels fall by an average of 35–50%. Even after 5 years of therapy, however, average BMD does not improve [160]. Cinacalcet can be particularly effective in those with intractable PHPT [159] or in inoperable parathyroid carcinoma [161].

When it is considered important to take measures to reduce the serum calcium and to increase BMD, combination use of cinacalcet and a bisphosphonate has been used [162]. More recently combination therapy with denosumab and cinacalcet has been reported [163]. With combination therapy but not with either agent alone, the serum calcium became normal in two-thirds of the patients. Bone density was higher with combination than denosumab alone: 5.4% vs 4.1% at the lumbar spine. Similarly, at the femoral neck, combination therapy gave somewhat higher gains than denosumab

Case

A 52-year-old healthy woman was found to have mild hypercalcemia (serum calcium 10.5 mg/dL; reference range 8.5–10.2 mg/dL) on routine blood work performed in the course of laboratory testing done at the time of her annual physical examination. Repeat testing confirmed the hypercalcemia with a value of 10.6 mg/dL. The parathyroid hormone level was 77 pg/mL (normal 15–65 pg/mL) and albumin was 4.0 g/dL. The ionized calcium was also mildly elevated at 5.7 mg/dL (Normal, < 5.5 mg/dL). Renal function was normal. She had menopause three years prior. She had no other medical history except for osteopenia at the lumbar spine and hip when bone mineral density was measured by dual x-ray absorptiometry. She had no history of nephrolithiasis or fracture. There was no family history of hypercalcemia. Review of systems was negative for constitutional or gastrointestinal symptoms. Her physical examination was normal. Review of her prior serum calcium levels revealed one prior elevated serum calcium 2 years ago.

Her physician referred her to an endocrinologist. Serum calcium and PTH were repeated along with a 25-hydroxyvitamin D, a 24-hour urine collection for calcium and serum phosphate: serum calcium 10.7 mg/dL, PTH

64 pg/mL, 25-hydroxyvitamin D 25 ng/ml, urine calcium 322 mg/24 hours (normal, < 250 mg/24 hours), and phosphorus of 2.7 mg/dL (normal 2.5–4.5). A dual x-ray absorptiometry scan of the 1/3-radius was obtained indicating a T-score of −2.6. She was referred to an experienced parathyroid surgeon. A 4D-CT indicated an enlarged parathyroid gland in the left superior position of the thyroid. She underwent minimally invasive parathyroid surgery with identification and removal of a 0.5 x 0.5 x 0.5 cm parathyroid adenoma in the location identified by 4D-CT. The serum PTH level fell intraoperatively from 147→ 69→ 24 pg/mL from baseline, before the surgery, to 5 and 10 minutes, respectively, after the excision of the adenoma. Postoperatively her serum calcium and PTH levels normalized. Pathology was consistent with a 0.5 gram parathyroid adenoma. One-year post parathyroidectomy, her bone mineral density at the lumbar spine had improved by 7%, and there were nonsignificant "trends" toward improvement at the other skeletal sites. Three years post-parathyroidectomy, she had significant improvements in bone mineral density at all skeletal sites compared with her baseline scan pre-parathyroidectomy and her 1/3-forearm was now in the osteopenic range.

This case illustrates the clinical features of asymptomatic PHPT. The patient's demographics match that of the most commonly affected population, post-menopausal women. As is most often the case today in the United States, this patient presented with asymptomatic PHPT and incidentally identified, mildly elevated calcium levels (within 1 mg/dL of the upper limit of normal). The patient's other biochemistries were characteristic of those seen in asymptomatic PHPT. Her PTH level was mildly elevated on one occasion (within two times the upper limit of normal) and "inappropriately normal" on the second measurement, both of which are consistent with a diagnosis of PHPT. Further diagnostic testing revealed "subclinical" end-organ evidence of bone loss with a reduction in bone mineral density at all sites and preferential loss at the 1/3-radius. Hypercalciuria was also present. The patient met criteria for recommending parathyroidectomy based on her T-score < −2.5. This case further highlights the value of preoperative imaging, which can be highly predictive of the location of the enlarged parathyroid gland. This patient was cured after surgery and she had a single adenoma as the cause of her PHPT, which is most often the case. This patient had a robust increase in bone density at the lumbar spine, a site rich in trabecular bone, in the first year following parathyroidectomy with gains at other sites that contain a greater proportion of cortical bone in subsequent years. This pattern is typical of the differential rates of bone mass accrual at skeletal sites that have varying amounts of trabecular versus cortical bone.

alone, 4.5% vs. 3.8%. With denosumab alone or combined with cinacalcet, the PTH rose by 40% above baseline and then fell but remained 13% higher.

Summary

This chapter has summarized the historical and current evidence for the presentation and management of PHPT. This disorder continues to present challenges in evaluation and management, but over the past 50 years, our new knowledge has provided reasonable, evidence-based guidelines as to its evaluation and management.

Acknowledgments This work was supported in part by National Institutes of Health grants NIDDK 32333.

References

1. Albright F, Bauer W, Claflin D, Cockrill JR. Studies in parathyroid physiology III. The effect of phosphate ingestion in clinical hyperparathyroidism. J Clin Invest. 1932;11:411–35.
2. Albright F, Aub J, Bauer W. Hyperparathyroidism: common and polymorphic condition as illustrated by seventeen proven cases in one clinic. JAMA. 1934;102:1276.
3. Bauer W, Federman DD. Hyperparathyroidism epitomized: the case of captain Charles E. Martell. Metabolism. 1962;11:21–9.
4. Silverberg SJ, Bilezikian JP. Clinical presentation of primary hyperparathyroidism. In: Bilezikian JP, Marcus R, Levine M, editors. The parathyroids. 2nd ed. San Diego: Academic Press; 2001. p. 349–60.
5. Heath H 3rd, Hodgson SF, Kennedy MA. Primary hyperparathyroidism. Incidence, morbidity, and potential economic impact in a community. N Engl J Med. 1980;302:189–93.
6. Mundy GR, Cove DH, Fisken R. Primary hyperparathyroidism: changes in the pattern of clinical presentation. Lancet. 1980;1:1317–20.
7. Scholz DA, Purnell DC. Asymptomatic primary hyperparathyroidism. 10-year prospective study. Mayo Clin Proc. 1981;56:473–8.
8. Silverberg SJ, Bilezikian JP. The diagnosis and management of asymptomatic primary hyperparathyroidism. Nat Clin Pract Endocrinol Metab. 2006;2:494–503.
9. Pawlowska M, Cusano NE. An overview of normocalcemic primary hyperparathyroidism. Curr Opin Endocrinol Diabetes Obes. 2015;22:413–21.
10. Bendz H, Sjodin I, Toss G, Berglund K. Hyperparathyroidism and long-term lithium therapy--a cross-sectional study and the effect of lithium withdrawal. J Intern Med. 1996;240:357–65.
11. Rao SD, Frame B, Miller MJ, Kleerekoper M, Block MA, Parfitt AM. Hyperparathyroidism following head and neck irradiation. Arch Intern Med. 1980;140:205–7.
12. Nordenstrom J, Strigard K, Perbeck L, Willems J, Bagedahl-Strindlund M, Linder J. Hyperparathyroidism associated with treatment of manic-depressive disorders by lithium. Eur J Surg. 1992;158:207–11.
13. Vaidya A, Curhan GC, Paik JM, Wang M, Taylor EN. Body size and the risk of primary hyperparathyroidism in women: a cohort study. J Bone Miner Res. 2017;32:1900–6.
14. Paik JM, Curhan GC, Taylor EN. Calcium intake and risk of primary hyperparathyroidism in women: prospective cohort study. BMJ. 2012;345:e6390.

15. Golden SH, Robinson KA, Saldanha I, Anton B, Ladenson PW. Clinical review: prevalence and incidence of endocrine and metabolic disorders in the United States: a comprehensive review. J Clin Endocrinol Metab. 2009;94:1853–78.
16. Barczynski M, Branstrom R, Dionigi G, Mihai R. Sporadic multiple parathyroid gland disease--a consensus report of the European Society of Endocrine Surgeons (ESES). Langenbeck's Arch Surg. 2015;400:887–905.
17. Attie JN, Bock G, Auguste LJ. Multiple parathyroid adenomas: report of thirty-three cases. Surgery. 1990;108:1014–9; discussion 9-20.
18. Bilezikian JP, Bandeira L, Khan A, Cusano NE. Hyperparathyroidism. Lancet. 2018;391:168–78.
19. Jain M, Krasne DL, Singer FR, Giuliano AE. Recurrent primary hyperparathyroidism due to type 1 parathyromatosis. Endocrine. 2017;55:643–50.
20. Nudelman IL, Deutsch AA, Reiss R. Primary hyperparathyroidism due to mediastinal parathyroid adenoma. Int Surg. 1987;72:104–8.
21. Sloane JA, Moody HC. Parathyroid adenoma in submucosa of esophagus. Arch Pathol Lab Med. 1978;102:242–3.
22. Joseph MP, Nadol JB, Pilch BZ, Goodman ML. Ectopic parathyroid tissue in the hypopharyngeal mucosa (pyriform sinus). Head Neck Surg. 1982;5:70–4.
23. Gilmour JR. Some developmental abnormalities of the thymus and parathyroids. J Pathol Bacteriol. 1941;52:213–8.
24. Wermers RA, Khosla S, Atkinson EJ, Hodgson SF, O'Fallon WM, Melton LJ 3rd. The rise and fall of primary hyperparathyroidism: a population-based study in Rochester, Minnesota, 1965-1992. Ann Intern Med. 1997;126:433–40.
25. Melton LJ 3rd. The epidemiology of primary hyperparathyroidism in North America. J Bone Miner Res. 2002;17(Suppl 2):N12–7.
26. Wermers RA, Khosla S, Atkinson EJ, et al. Incidence of primary hyperparathyroidism in Rochester, Minnesota, 1993-2001: an update on the changing epidemiology of the disease. J Bone Miner Res. 2006;21:171–7.
27. Griebeler ML, Kearns AE, Ryu E, Hathcock MA, Melton LJ 3rd, Wermers RA. Secular trends in the incidence of primary hyperparathyroidism over five decades (1965-2010). Bone. 2015;73:1–7.
28. Yeh MW, Ituarte PH, Zhou HC, et al. Incidence and prevalence of primary hyperparathyroidism in a racially mixed population. J Clin Endocrinol Metab. 2013;98:1122–9.
29. Lowe H, McMahon DJ, Rubin MR, Bilezikian JP, Silverberg SJ. Normocalcemic primary hyperparathyroidism: further characterization of a new clinical phenotype. J Clin Endocrinol Metab. 2007;92:3001–5.
30. Cusano NE, Maalouf NM, Wang PY, et al. Normocalcemic hyperparathyroidism and hypoparathyroidism in two community-based nonreferral populations. J Clin Endocrinol Metab. 2013;98:2734–41.
31. Schini M, Jacques RM, Oakes E, Peel NFA, Walsh JS. Eastell R. Normocalcemic Hyperparathyroidism: Study of its Prevalence and Natural History. J Clin Endocrinol Metab; 2020. p. 105.
32. Vignali E, Cetani F, Chiavistelli S, et al. Normocalcemia primary hyperparathyroidism: a survey in a small village of southern Italy. Endocr Connect. 2015;4:172–8.
33. Jacobs TP, Bilezikian JP. Clinical review: rare causes of hypercalcemia. J Clin Endocrinol Metab. 2005;90:6316–22.
34. Eastell R, Arnold A, Brandi ML, et al. Diagnosis of asymptomatic primary hyperparathyroidism: proceedings of the third international workshop. J Clin Endocrinol Metab. 2009;94:340–50.
35. Nesbit MA, Hannan FM, Howles SA, et al. Mutations affecting G-protein subunit alpha11 in hypercalcemia and hypocalcemia. N Engl J Med. 2013;368:2476–86.
36. Nesbit MA, Hannan FM, Howles SA, et al. Mutations in AP2S1 cause familial hypocalciuric hypercalcemia type 3. Nat Genet. 2013;45:93–7.

37. Zavatta G, Clarke BL. Normocalcemic hyperparathyroidism: a heterogenous disorder often misdiagnosed. JBMR Plus. 2020;4:e10391.
38. Hagag P, Revet-Zak I, Hod N, Horne T, Rapoport MJ, Weiss M. Diagnosis of normocalcemic hyperparathyroidism by oral calcium loading test. J Endocrinol Investig. 2003;26:327–32.
39. Silverberg SJ, Bilezikian JP. "incipient" primary hyperparathyroidism: a "forme fruste" of an old disease. J Clin Endocrinol Metab. 2003;88:5348–52.
40. Silverberg SJ, Shane E, Dempster DW, Bilezikian JP. The effects of vitamin D insufficiency in patients with primary hyper-parathyroidism. Am J Med. 1999;107:561–7.
41. Walker MD, Cong E, Lee JA, Kepley A, Zhang C, McMahon DJ, Bilezikian JP, Silverberg SJ. Low vitamin D levels have become less common in primary hyperparathyroidism. Osteoporos Int. 2015;26:2837–43.
42. Vieth R, Bayley TA, Walfish PG, Rosen IB, Pollard A. Relevance of vitamin D metabolite concentrations in supporting the diagnosis of primary hyperparathyroidism. Surgery. 1991;110:1043–6; discussion 6-7.
43. Locker FG, Silverberg SJ, Bilezikian JP. Optimal dietary calcium intake in primary hyperparathyroidism. Am J Med. 1997;102:543–50.
44. Silverberg SJ. Non-classical target organs in primary hyperparathyroidism. J Bone Miner Res. 2002;17(Suppl 2):N117–25.
45. Ringe JD. Reversible hypertension in primary hyperparathyroidism--pre- and posteroperative blood pressure in 75 cases. Klin Wochenschr. 1984;62:465–9.
46. Broulik PD, Horky K, Pacovsky V. Blood pressure in patients with primary hyperparathyroidism before and after parathyroidectomy. Exp Clin Endocrinol. 1985;86:346–52.
47. Rapado A. Arterial hypertension and primary hyperparathyroidism. Incidence and follow-up after parathyroidectomy. Am J Nephrol. 1986;6(Suppl 1):49–50.
48. Bilezikian JP, Connor TB, Aptekar R, et al. Pseudogout after parathyroidectomy. Lancet. 1973;1:445–6.
49. Geelhoed GW, Kelly TR. Pseudogout as a clue and complication in primary hyperparathyroidism. Surgery. 1989;106:1036–41, discussion 41-2.
50. Ludvigsson JF, Kampe O, Lebwohl B, Green PH, Silverberg SJ, Ekbom A. Primary hyperparathyroidism and celiac disease: a population-based cohort study. J Clin Endocrinol Metab. 2012;97:897–904.
51. Bilezikian JP. Primary hyperparathyroidism. In Oxford textbook of endocrinology and diabetes, 3rd. Wass, J, Arlt W, and Semple R, eds, (in press), 2021.
52. Silverberg SJ, Bilezikian JP. Primary hyperparathyroidism. In: Jameson JL, LJ DG, editors. Endocrinology. 7th ed. Saunders: Elsevier; 2015. p. 1105–24.
53. Kulak CA, Bandeira C, Voss D, et al. Marked improvement in bone mass after parathyroidectomy in osteitis fibrosa cystica. J Clin Endocrinol Metab. 1998;83:732–5. 266. Tritos NA, Hartzband P. Rapid improvement of osteoporosis following
54. Misiorowski W, Czajka-Oraniec I, Kochman M, Zgliczynski W, Bilezikian JP. Osteitis fibrosa cystica-a forgotten radiological feature of primary hyperparathyroidism. Endocrine. 2017;58:380–5.
55. Silverberg SJ, Shane E, de la Cruz L, et al. Skeletal disease in primary hyperparathyroidism. J Bone Miner Res. 1989;4:283–91.
56. Bilezikian JP, Silverberg SJ, Shane E, Parisien M, Dempster DW. Characterization and evaluation of asymptomatic primary hyperparathyroidism. J Bone Miner Res. 1991;6(Suppl 2):S85–9. discussion S121-4
57. Dempster DW, Cosman F, Parisien M, Shen V, Lindsay R. Anabolic actions of parathyroid hormone on bone. Endocr Rev. 1993;14:690–709.
58. Bilezikian JP, Rubin MR, Finkelstein JS. Parathyroid hormone as an anabolic therapy for women and men. J Endocrinol Investig. 2005;28:41–9.
59. Silverberg SJ, Locker FG, Bilezikian JP. Vertebral osteopenia: a new indication for surgery in primary hyperparathyroidism. J Clin Endocrinol Metab. 1996;81:4007–12.
60. Bilezikian JP. Primary hyperparathyroidism. J Clin Endocrinol Metab. 2018;103:3993–4004.

61. Parisien M, Silverberg SJ, Shane E, et al. The histomorphometry of bone in primary hyperparathyroidism: preservation of cancellous bone structure. J Clin Endocrinol Metab. 1990;70:930–8.
62. Parfitt AM. Accelerated cortical bone loss: primary and secondary hyperparathyroidism. In: Uhthoff H, Stahl E, editors. Current concepts in bone fragility. New York: Mary Ann Liebert. p. 7–14.
63. van Doorn L, Lips P, Netelenbos JC, Hackeng WH. Bone histomorphometry and serum concentrations of intact parathyroid hormone (PTH(1-84)) in patients with primary hyperparathyroidism. Bone Miner. 1993;23:233–42.
64. Silva BC, Boutroy S, Zhang C, et al. Trabecular bone score (TBS)--a novel method to evaluate bone microarchitectural texture in patients with primary hyperparathyroidism. J Clin Endocrinol Metab. 2013;98:1963–70.
65. Stein EM, Silva BC, Boutroy S, et al. Primary hyperparathyroidism is associated with abnormal cortical and trabecular microstructure and reduced bone stiffness in postmenopausal women. J Bone Miner Res. 2013;28:1029–40.
66. Hansen S, Hauge EM, Rasmussen L, Jensen JE, Brixen K. Parathyroidectomy improves bone geometry and microarchitecture in female patients with primary hyperparathyroidism. A 1-year prospective controlled study using high resolution peripheral quantitative computed tomography. J Bone Miner Res. 2012.
67. Vu TD, Wang XF, Wang Q, et al. New insights into the effects of primary hyperparathyroidism on the cortical and trabecular compartments of bone. Bone. 2013;55:57–63.
68. Silverberg SJ, Gartenberg F, Jacobs TP, et al. Longitudinal measurements of bone density and biochemical indices in untreated primary hyperparathyroidism. J Clin Endocrinol Metab. 1995;80:723–8.
69. van Lierop AH, Witteveen JE, Hamdy NA, Papapoulos SE. Patients with primary hyperparathyroidism have lower circulating sclerostin levels than euparathyroid controls. Eur J Endocrinol. 2010;163:833–7.
70. Costa AG, Cremers S, Rubin MR, et al. Circulating sclerostin in disorders of parathyroid gland function. J Clin Endocrinol Metab. 2011;96:3804–10.
71. Seibel MJ, Gartenberg F, Silverberg SJ, Ratcliffe A, Robins SP, Bilezikian JP. Urinary hydroxypyridinium cross-links of collagen in primary hyperparathyroidism. J Clin Endocrinol Metab. 1992;74:481–6.
72. Dempster DW, Parisien M, Silverberg SJ, et al. On the mechanism of cancellous bone preservation in postmenopausal women with mild primary hyperparathyroidism. J Clin Endocrinol Metab. 1999;84:1562–6.
73. Khosla S, Melton LJ 3rd, Wermers RA, Crowson CS, O'Fallon W, Riggs B. Primary hyperparathyroidism and the risk of fracture: a population-based study. J Bone Miner Res. 1999;14:1700–7.
74. Vignali E, Viccica G, Diacinti D, et al. Morphometric vertebral fractures in postmenopausal women with primary hyperparathyroidism. J Clin Endocrinol Metab. 2009;94:2306–12.
75. De Geronimo S, Romagnoli E, Diacinti D, D'Erasmo E, Minisola S. The risk of fractures in postmenopausal women with primary hyperparathyroidism. Eur J Endocrinol. 2006;155:415–20.
76. Dauphine RT, Riggs BL, Scholz DA. Back pain and vertebral crush fractures: an unemphasized mode of presentation for primary hyperparathyroidism. Ann Intern Med. 1975;83:365–7.
77. Liu M, Williams J, Kuo J, Lee JA, Silverberg SJ, Walker MD. Risk factors for vertebral fracture in primary hyperparathyroidism. Endocrine. 2019;66:682–90.
78. Ejlsmark-Svensson H, rolighed L, Harslof T, Rejnmark L. Risk of fractures in PHPT: a systeamtic review and meta-analysis. Osteoporosis Int. 2021.
79. Pak CY, Oata M, Lawrence EC, Snyder W. The hypercalciurias. Causes, parathyroid functions, and diagnostic criteria. J Clin Invest. 1974;54:387–400.
80. Kaplan RA, Haussler MR, Deftos LJ, Bone H, Pak CY. The role of 1 alpha, 25-dihydroxyvitamin D in the mediation of intestinal hyperabsorption of calcium in primary hyperparathyroidism and absorptive hypercalciuria. J Clin Invest. 1977;59:756–60.

81. Broadus AE, Horst RL, Lang R, Littledike ET, Rasmussen H. The importance of circulating 1,25-dihydroxyvitamin D in the pathogenesis of hypercalciuria and renal-stone formation in primary hyperparathyroidism. N Engl J Med. 1980;302:421–6.

82. Pak CY, Nicar MJ, Peterson R, Zerwekh JE, Snyder W. A lack of unique pathophysiologic background for nephrolithiasis of primary hyperparathyroidism. J Clin Endocrinol Metab. 1981;53:536–42.

83. Pak CY. Effect of parathyroidectomy on crystallization of calcium salts in urine of patients with primary hyperparathyroidism. Investig Urol. 1979;17:146–8.

84. Saponaro F, Marcocci C, Apicella M, et al. Hypomagnesuria is Associated With Nephrolithiasis in Patients With Asymptomatic Primary Hyperparathyroidism. J Clin Endocrinol Metab. 2020;105:e-2789–95.

85. Peacock M. Primary hyperparathyroidism and the kidney. In: Bilezikian JP, editor. The parathyroids: basic and clinical concepts. San Diego: Elsevier, Academic Press; 2015. p. 455–68.

86. Cipriani C, Biamonte F, Costa AG, et al. Prevalence of kidney stones and vertebral fractures in primary hyperparathyroidism using imaging technology. J Clin Endocrinol Metab. 2015;100:1309–15.

87. Rejnmark L, Vestergaard P, Mosekilde L. Nephrolithiasis and renal calcifications in primary hyperparathyroidism. J Clin Endocrinol Metab. 2011;96:2377–85.

88. Cassibba S, Pellegrino M, Gianotti L, et al. Silent renal stones in primary hyperparathyroidism: prevalence and clinical features. Endocr Pract. 2014;20:1137–42.

89. Bilezikian JP, Brandi ML, Eastell R, et al. Guidelines for the management of asymptomatic primary hyperparathyroidism: summary statement from the Fourth International Workshop. J Clin Endocrinol Metab. 2014;99:3561–9.

90. Tay YD, Liu M, Bandeira L, et al. Occult urolithiasis in asymptomatic primary hyperparathyroidism. Endocr Res. 2018;43:106–15.

91. Tassone F, Gianotti L, Emmolo I, Ghio M, Borretta G. Glomerular filtration rate and parathyroid hormone secretion in primary hyperparathyroidism. J Clin Endocrinol Metab. 2009;94:4458–61.

92. Walker MD, Nickolas T, Kepley A, et al. Predictors of renal function in primary hyperparathyroidism. J Clin Endocrinol Metab. 2014;99:1885–92.

93. Walker MD, Dempster DW, McMahon DJ, et al. Effect of renal function on skeletal health in primary hyperparathyroidism. J Clin Endocrinol Metab. 2012;97:1501–7.

94. Silverberg SJ, Shane E, Jacobs TP, Siris E, Bilezikian JP. A 10-year prospective study of primary hyperparathyroidism with or without parathyroid surgery. N Engl J Med. 1999;341:1249–55.

95. Rao DS, Wilson RJ, Kleerekoper M, Parfitt AM. Lack of biochemical progression or continuation of accelerated bone loss in mild asymptomatic primary hyperparathyroidism: evidence for biphasic disease course. J Clin Endocrinol Metab. 1988;67:1294–8.

96. Cope O. The study of hyperparathyroidism at the Massachusetts General Hospital. N Engl J Med. 1966;274:1174–82.

97. Vicale CT. Diagnostic features of muscular syndrome resulting from hyperparathyroidism, osteomalacia owing to renal tubular acidosis and perhaps related disorders of calcium metabolism. Trans Am Neurol Assoc. 1949;74:143–7.

98. Patten BM, Bilezikian JP, Mallette LE, Prince A, Engel WK, Aurbach GD. Neuromuscular disease in primary hyperparathyroidism. Ann Intern Med. 1974;80:182–93.

99. Frame B, Heinze EG Jr, Block MA, Manson GA. Myopathy in primary hyperparathyroidism. Observations in three patients. Ann Intern Med. 1968;68:1022–7.

100. Rollinson RD, Gilligan BS. Primary hyperparathyroidism presenting as a proximal myopathy. Aust NZ J Med. 1977;7:420–1.

101. Turken SA, Cafferty M, Silverberg SJ, et al. Neuromuscular involvement in mild, asymptomatic primary hyperparathyroidism. Am J Med. 1989;87:553–7.

102. Bollerslev J, Jansson S, Mollerup CL, et al. Medical observation, compared with parathyroidectomy, for asymptomatic primary hyperparathyroidism: a prospective, randomized trial. J Clin Endocrinol Metab. 2007;92:1687–92.

103. Talpos GB, Bone HG 3rd, Kleerekoper M, et al. Randomized trial of parathyroidectomy in mild asymptomatic primary hyperparathyroidism: patient description and effects on the SF-36 health survey. Surgery. 2000;128:1013–20;discussion 20–1.
104. Ambrogini E, Cetani F, Cianferotti L, et al. Surgery or surveillance for mild asymptomatic primary hyperparathyroidism: a prospective, randomized clinical trial. J Clin Endocrinol Metab. 2007;92:3114–21.
105. Perrier ND, Balachandran D, Wefel JS, et al. Prospective, randomized, controlled trial of parathyroidectomy versus observation in patients with "asymptomatic" primary hyperparathyroidism. Surgery. 2009;146:1116–22.
106. Walker MD, McMahon DJ, Inabnet WB, et al. Neuropsychological features in primary hyperparathyroidism: a prospective study. J Clin Endocrinol Metab. 2009;94:1951–8.
107. Roman SA, Sosa JA, Mayes L, et al. Parathyroidectomy improves neurocognitive deficits in patients with primary hyperparathyroidism. Surgery. 2005;138:1121–8; discussion 8-9.
108. Benge JF, Perrier ND, Massman PJ, Meyers CA, Kayl AE, Wefel JS. Cognitive and affective sequelae of primary hyperparathyroidism and early response to parathyroidectomy. J Int Neuropsychol Soc. 2009;15:1002–11.
109. Chiang CY, Andrewes DG, Anderson D, Devere M, Schweitzer I, Zajac JD. A controlled, prospective study of neuropsychological outcomes post parathyroidectomy in primary hyperparathyroid patients. Clin Endocrinol. 2005;62:99–104.
110. Numann PJ, Torppa AJ, Blumetti AE. Neuropsychologic deficits associated with primary hyperparathyroidism. Surgery. 1984;96:1119–23.
111. Babinska D, Barczynski M, Stefaniak T, et al. Evaluation of selected cognitive functions before and after surgery for primary hyperparathyroidism. Langenbeck's Arch Surg. 2012;397:825–31.
112. Lourida I, Thompson-Coon J, Dickens CM, et al. Parathyroid hormone, cognitive function and dementia: a systematic review. PLoS One. 2015;10:e0127574.
113. Dotzenrath CM, Kaetsch AK, Pfingsten H, et al. Neuropsychiatric and cognitive changes after surgery for primary hyperparathyroidism. World J Surg. 2006;30:680–5.
114. Goyal A, Chumber S, Tandon N, Lal R, Srivastava A, Gupta S. Neuropsychiatric manifestations in patients of primary hyperparathyroidism and outcome following surgery. Indian J Med Sci. 2001;55:677–86.
115. Liu M, Sum M, Cong E, et al. Cognition and cerebrovascular function in primary hyperparathyroidism before and after parathyroidectomy. J Endocrinol Investig. 2020;43:369–79.
116. Gazes Y, Liu M, Sum M, et al. Functional magnetic resonance imaging in primary hyperparathyroidism. Eur J Endocrinol. 2020;183:21–30.
117. Pretorius M, Lundstam K, Hellstrom M, et al. Effect of parathyroidectomy on quality of life: 10 years data from a prospective randomized controlled trial on primary hyperparathyroidism. J Bone Miner Res. 2020;36:3–11.
118. Walker MD, Silverberg SJ. Quality of life in primary hyperparathyroidism revisited: keep calm and carry on? J Bone Miner Res. 2020;36:1–2.
119. Silva BC, Boutroy S, Zhang C, et al. Trabecular bone score-TBS-a novel method to evaluate bone microarchitectural texture in patients with primary hyperparathyroidism. J Clin Endocrinol Metab. 2013;2013(98):1963–70.
120. Rubin MR, Bilezikian JP, McMahon DJ, et al. The natural history of primary hyperparathyroidism with or without parathyroid surgery after 15 years. J Clin Endocrinol Metab. 2008;93:3462–70.
121. Rao DS, Phillips ER, Divine GW, Talpos GB. Randomized controlled clinical trial of surgery versus no surgery in patients with mild asymptomatic primary hyperparathyroidism. J Clin Endocrinol Metab. 2004;89:5415–22.
122. Bilezikian JP, Potts JT Jr, Fuleihan Gel H, et al. Summary statement from a workshop on asymptomatic primary hyperparathyroidism: a perspective for the 21st century. J Clin Endocrinol Metab. 2002;87:5353–61.
123. Khan AA, Bilezikian JP, Potts JT Jr. The diagnosis and management of asymptomatic primary hyperparathyroidism revisited. J Clin Endocrinol Metab. 2009;94:333–4.

124. Bilezikian JP, Khan AA, Potts JT Jr. Guidelines for the management of asymptomatic primary hyperparathyroidism: summary statement from the third international workshop. J Clin Endocrinol Metab. 2009;94:335–9.
125. Silverberg SJ, Clarke BL, Peacock M, et al. Current issues in the presentation of asymptomatic primary hyperparathyroidism: proceedings of the fourth international workshop. J Clin Endocrinol Metab. 2014;99:3580–94.
126. Civelek AC, Ozalp E, Donovan P, Udelsman R. Prospective evaluation of delayed technetium-99m sestamibi SPECT scintigraphy for preoperative localization of primary hyperparathyroidism. Surgery. 2002;131:149–57.
127. Van Husen R, Kim LT. Accuracy of surgeon-performed ultrasound in parathyroid localization. World J Surg. 2004;28:1122–6.
128. Mortenson MM, Evans DB, Lee JE, et al. Parathyroid exploration in the reoperative neck: improved preoperative localization with 4D-computed tomography. J Am Coll Surg. 2008;206:888–95; discussion 95-6.
129. Yeh R, Tay YD, Tabacco G, et al. Diagnostic performance of 4D CT and Sestamibi SPECT/CT in localizing parathyroid adenomas in primary hyperparathyroidism. Radiology. 2019;291:469–76.
130. Maser C, Donovan P, Santos F, et al. Sonographically guided fine needle aspiration with rapid parathyroid hormone assay. Ann Surg Oncol. 2006;13:1690–5.
131. Udelsman R, Donovan PI. Remedial parathyroid surgery: changing trends in 130 consecutive cases. Ann Surg. 2006;244:471–9.
132. Clark OH. How should patients with primary hyperparathyroidism be treated? J Clin Endocrinol Metab. 2003;88:3011–4.
133. Udelsman R. Six hundred fifty-six consecutive explorations for primary hyperparathyroidism. Ann Surg. 2002;235:665–70; discussion 70-2.
134. Irvin GL 3rd, Solorzano CC, Carneiro DM. Quick intraoperative parathyroid hormone assay: surgical adjunct to allow limited parathyroidectomy, improve success rate, and predict outcome. World J Surg. 2004;28:1287–92.
135. Udelsman R, Donovan PI, Sokoll LJ. One hundred consecutive minimally invasive parathyroid explorations. Ann Surg. 2000;232:331–9.
136. Westerdahl J, Bergenfelz A. Unilateral versus bilateral neck exploration for primary hyperparathyroidism: five-year follow-up of a randomized controlled trial. Ann Surg. 2007;246:976–80; discussion 80-1.
137. Russell CF, Dolan SJ, Laird JD. Randomized clinical trial comparing scan-directed unilateral versus bilateral cervical exploration for primary hyperparathyroidism due to solitary adenoma. Br J Surg. 2006;93:418–21.
138. Jinih M, O'Connell E, O'Leary DP, Liew A, Redmond HP. Focused versus bilateral parathyroid exploration for primary hyperparathyroidism: a systematic review and meta-analysis. Ann Surg Oncol. 2017;24:1924–34.
139. Miccoli P, Berti P, Materazzi G, Ambrosini CE, Fregoli L, Donatini G. Endoscopic bilateral neck exploration versus quick intraoperative parathormone assay (qPTHa) during endoscopic parathyroidectomy: a prospective randomized trial. Surg Endosc. 2008;22:398–400.
140. Henry JF, Sebag F, Tamagnini P, Forman C, Silaghi H. Endoscopic parathyroid surgery: results of 365 consecutive procedures. World J Surg. 2004;28:1219–23.
141. Silverberg SJ, Gartenberg F, Jacobs TP, et al. Increased bone mineral density after parathyroidectomy in primary hyperparathyroidism. J Clin Endocrinol Metab. 1995;80:729–34. Parathyroidectomy in a premenopausal woman with acute primary hyperparathyroidism. Arch Intern Med 1999;159:1495–8.
142. Dawson-Hughes B, Stern DT, Shipp CC, Rasmussen HM. Effect of lowering dietary calcium intake on fractional whole body calcium retention. J Clin Endocrinol Metab. 1988;67:62–8.
143. Barger-Lux MJ, Heaney RP. Effects of calcium restriction on metabolic characteristics of premenopausal women. J Clin Endocrinol Metab. 1993;76:103–7.
144. Calvo MS, Kumar R, Heath H. Persistently elevated parathyroid hormone secretion and action in young women after four weeks of ingesting high phosphorus, low calcium diets. J Clin Endocrinol Metab. 1990;70:1334–40.

145. Insogna KL, Mitnick ME, Stewart AF, Burtis WJ, Mallette LE, Broadus AE. Sensitivity of the parathyroid hormone-1,25-dihydroxyvitamin D axis to variations in calcium intake in patients with primary hyperparathyroidism. N Engl J Med. 1985;313:1126–30.
146. Jorde R, Szumlas K, Haug E, Sundsfjord J. The effects of calcium supplementation to patients with primary hyperparathyroidism and a low calcium intake. Eur J Nutr. 2002;41:258–63.
147. Marcocci C, Bollerslev J, Khan AA, Shoback DM. Medical management of primary hyperparathyroidism: proceedings of the fourth international workshop on the Management of Asymptomatic Primary Hyperparathyroidism. J Clin Endocrinol Metab. 2014;99:3607–18.
148. Rolighed L, Rejnmark L, Sikjaer T, et al. Vitamin D treatment in primary hyperparathyroidism: a randomized placebo controlled trial. J Clin Endocrinol Metab. 2014;99:1072–80.
149. Gallagher JC, Nordin BE. Treatment with with oestrogens of primary hyperparathyroidism in post-menopausal women. Lancet. 1972;1:503–7.
150. Marcus R, Madvig P, Crim M, Pont A, Kosek J. Conjugated estrogens in the treatment of postmenopausal women with hyperparathyroidism. Ann Intern Med. 1984;100:633–40.
151. Rubin MR, Lee KH, McMahon DJ, Silverberg SJ. Raloxifene lowers serum calcium and markers of bone turnover in postmenopausal women with primary hyperparathyroidism. J Clin Endocrinol Metab. 2003;88:1174–8.
152. Hassani S, Braunstein GD, Seibel MJ, et al. Alendronate therapy of primary hyperparathyroidism. Endocrinologist. 2001;11:459–64.
153. Chow CC, Chan WB, Li JK, et al. Oral alendronate increases bone mineral density in postmenopausal women with primary hyperparathyroidism. J Clin Endocrinol Metab. 2003;88:581–7.
154. Parker CR, Blackwell PJ, Fairbairn KJ, Hosking DJ. Alendronate in the treatment of primary hyperparathyroid-related osteoporosis: a 2-year study. J Clin Endocrinol Metab. 2002;87:4482–9.
155. Khan AA, Bilezikian JP, Kung AW, et al. Alendronate in primary hyperparathyroidism: a double-blind, randomized, placebo-controlled trial. J Clin Endocrinol Metab. 2004;89:3319–25.
156. Eller-Vainicher C, Palmieri S, Cairoli E, et al. Protective effect of denosumab on bone in older women with primary hyperparathyroidism. J Am Geriatr Soc. 2018;66:518–24.
157. Miyaoka M, Imanish Y, Kato E, et al. Effects of denosumab as compared with parathyroidectomy regarding calcium, renal, and bone involvement in osteoporotic patients with primary hyperparathyroidism. Endocrine. 2020;69:642–9.
158. Peacock M, Bilezikian JP, Klassen PS, Guo MD, Turner SA, Shoback D. Cinacalcet hydrochloride maintains long-term normocalcemia in patients with primary hyperparathyroidism. J Clin Endocrinol Metab. 2005;90:135–41.
159. Marcocci C, Chanson P, Shoback D, et al. Cinacalcet reduces serum calcium concentrations in patients with intractable primary hyperparathyroidism. J Clin Endocrinol Metab. 2009;94:2766–72.
160. Peacock M, Bolognese MA, Borofsky M, et al. Cinacalcet treatment of primary hyperparathyroidism: biochemical and bone densitometric outcomes in a five-year study. J Clin Endocrinol Metab. 2009;94:4860–7.
161. Silverberg SJ, Rubin MR, Faiman C, et al. Cinacalcet hydrochloride reduces the serum calcium concentration in inoperable parathyroid carcinoma. J Clin Endocrinol Metab. 2007;92:3803–8.
162. Faggiano A, Di Somma C, Ramundo V, Severino R, Vuolo L, Coppola A, Panico F, Savastano S, Lombardi G, Colao A, Gasperi M. Endocrine. 2011;39(3):283–7, Cinacalcet hydrochloride in combination with alendronate normalizes hypercalcemia and improves bone mineral density in patients with primary hyperparathyroidism. EndocrineEndocrine. 2011;39:283–7.
163. Leere JS, et al. Denosumab and cinacalcet for primary hyperparathyroidism: a randomised, double-blind, placebo-controlled, phase 3 trial. Lancet Diabetes Endocrinol. 2020;8:407–17.

Chapter 7
Genetic Causes of Primary Hyperparathyroidism

Francesca Marini and Maria Luisa Brandi

Introduction

Primary hyperparathyroidism (PHPT) refers to the idiopathic hypersecretion of parathyroid hormone (PTH), caused by a primary defect in growth and/or activity of the parathyroid glands. In the great majority of patients, the condition is caused by occurrence of parathyroid tumors: a single parathyroid adenoma in about 80% of cases, multiple parathyroid adenomas, and/or multiglandular hyperplasia in 15–20% of cases and malignant parathyroid carcinomas in 1% of cases [1]. About 90–95% of all cases of PHPT are sporadic, without any familial history of the disease, mostly caused by a single parathyroid adenoma. The remaining 5–10% of cases occur within familial inherited parathyroid disorders. Compared with their sporadic counterpart, familial PHPT is characterized by multiple, synchronous, or asynchronous development of parathyroid gland overactivity, an earlier age of onset, and a higher rate of postsurgical recurrences. Inherited forms of PHPT can manifest as nonsyndromic diseases, affecting only the parathyroids [familial isolated hyperparathyroidism (FIHP), familial hypocalciuric hypercalcemia syndrome (FHH), and neonatal severe hyperparathyroidism (NSHPT)], or as syndromic disorders in which parathyroid disease is associated with other tumors in endocrine and nonendocrine organs [multiple endocrine neoplasia type 1 (MEN1), multiple endocrine neoplasia type 2A (MEN2A), multiple endocrine neoplasia type 4 (MEN4), and hyperparathyroidism jaw tumor syndrome (HPT-JT)].

F. Marini
Department of Clinical and Experimental Biochemical Sciences, University of Florence, Florence, Italy
e-mail: francesca.marini@unifi.it

M. L. Brandi (✉)
F.I.R.M.O. Foundation, Florence, Italy
e-mail: marialuisa.brandi@unifi.it

M. D. Walker (ed.), *Hypercalcemia*, Contemporary Endocrinology,
https://doi.org/10.1007/978-3-030-93182-7_7

111

These forms of inherited PHPT present in an autosomal dominant pattern of transmission, except for NSHPT; every affected parent has a 50% probability of transmitting the genetic defect to the offspring, independently by sex. Different mutated genes are responsible for variable clinical phenotypes (Table 7.1), characterized by various degrees of PHPT severity, different ages of onset, variable penetrance, different parathyroid pathology, and variable risk of tumor recurrences after surgery. Genetic testing is a key element in order to establish the diagnosis, drive clinical and therapeutic management of patients, and enable the genetic screening of first-degree relatives to identify mutation carriers at early and/or asymptomatic stages of the disease (Fig. 7.1).

Familial Hypocalciuric Hypercalcemia Syndrome

Familial hypocalciuric hypercalcemia (FHH) comprises a group of rare benign, usually asymptomatic, congenital conditions, characterized by lifelong mild to moderate hypercalcemia and a normal or mildly elevated serum PTH, in association with an inappropriately reduced urinary calcium excretion. Parathyroid glands are normal or mildly hyperplastic in the great majority of patients; FHH is caused by a dysregulation in PTH secretion and not due to overgrowth of parathyroid cells. Three clinical variants have been described, characterized by slight clinical differences, and caused by genetic defects in three different genes.

FHH type 1 (FHH1) is the most common variant accounting for about 65% of all FHH cases, caused by a heterozygote inactivating mutation of the calcium-sensing receptor (*CaSR*) gene. This gene encodes the CaSR protein, a G-protein-coupled 7-transmembrane-spanning receptor, expressed in the parathyroids and kidney tubule among other tissues. Within the parathyroid and kidney, it acts as a sensor of small fluctuations in extracellular calcium concentration and regulates the maintenance of calcium ion homeostasis, via induction of PTH secretion and renal tubule calcium reabsorption, in response to a calcium decrease. The loss-of-function-mutated CaSR protein loses its ability to sense extracellular calcium levels, resulting in a constitutive secretion of PTH by the parathyroids, independently of serum calcium values. Over 200 heterogeneous, inactivating and activating, *CaSR* mutations, mostly missense variations, have been reported. Mutations are clustered in the first 300 amino acids of the extracellular domain and in the transmembrane domain of the receptor, encoded by exons 3, 4, and 7. Truncating mutations, presumably not exerting a dominant-negative effect, seem to be associated with less severe hypercalcemia and a minor increase in PTH level, compared with missense inactivating mutations responsible for a protein dominant-negative effect [2].

FHH type 2 (FHH2) is usually associated with high-normal PTH level and mild hypermagnesemia. The FHH2 variant is caused by heterozygote loss-of-function mutations of the *GNA11* gene, which encodes the guanine nucleotide-binding protein (G-protein) alpha 11 (Gα11), a G-protein coupled with CaSR and involved in the activation of phospholipase C and the subsequent second messenger cascade,

Table 7.1 Genes responsible for inherited forms of primary hyperparathyroidism

Disease	Causative gene	Chromosomal position	Type of mutations (Inheritance)	Encoded protein	Role of the encoded protein	Effect of gene mutation on parathyroid glands
Familial hypocalciuric hypercalcaemia type 1 (FHH1)	*CaSR*	3q13.3–q21	Heterozygote, inactivating (AD)	CaSR	Transmembrane sensor of small fluctuations in extracellular calcium concentration	Loss-of-function mutated CaSR is not able to sense variations in extracellular calcium, resulting in a constitutive induction of PTH secretion
Familial hypocalciuric hypercalcaemia type 2 (FHH2)	*GNA11*	19p13.3	Heterozygote, inactivating (AD)	Gα11	The alpha subunit of a G-protein coupled to CaSR receptor, which acts as an activator of phospholipase C and of the second messenger cascade involved in the regulation of PTH secretion	Loss-of-function mutated Gα11 is unable to transmit the CaSR-mediated signal in response to extracellular calcium variations, resulting in a constitutive induction of PTH secretion
Familial hypocalciuric hypercalcaemia type 3 (FHH3)	*AP2S1*	19q13.32	Heterozygote, inactivating (AD)	AP17	The 17-kD α-subunit of adaptor protein complex 2 (AP2), a key component of cell clathrin-dependent endocytosis mechanism, which internalizes the G-protein coupled membrane receptors, like CaSR	Loss-of-function mutated AP2 complex reduces the CaSR-mediated signaling, independently by extracellular variations in calcium levels, resulting in a constitutive induction of PTH secretion
Neonatal severe primary hyperparathyroidism (NSHPT)	*CaSR*	3q13.3–q21	Homozygote, inactivating (AR)	CaSR	Transmembrane sensor of small fluctuations in extracellular calcium concentration	Loss-of-function mutated CaSR is not able to sense variations in extracellular calcium, resulting in a constitutive induction of PTH secretion
Multiple endocrine neoplasia type 1 (MEN1)	*MEN1*	11q13	Heterozygote, inactivating (AD)	menin	Gene transcription, regulation of cell cycle, regulation of apoptosis, DNA repair, etc.	The complete loss of the tumor suppressor function of menin is responsible for uncontrolled parathyroid cell growth and tumorigenesis

(continued)

Table 7.1 (continued)

Disease	Causative gene	Chromosomal position	Type of mutations (Inheritance)	Encoded protein	Role of the encoded protein	Effect of gene mutation on parathyroid glands
Multiple endocrine neoplasia type 4 (MEN4)	CDKN1B	12p13.1	Heterozygote, inactivating (AD)	p27^{Kip1}	Inhibitor of cyclin-dependent kinases and negative regulator of cell growth	Loss-of-function mutated p27^{Kip1} is not able to negatively control cell cycle progression, resulting in an uncontrolled parathyroid cell growth and tumorigenesis
Multiple endocrine neoplasia type 2A (MEN2A)	RET	10q11.21	Heterozygote, activating (AD)	RET	Transmembrane receptor with tyrosine kinase activity	Gain-of-function mutations of RET, affecting one of the extracellular cysteine of the ligand-binding domain, result in a constitutive activation of RET tyrosine kinase activity, which leads to an uncontrolled parathyroid cell growth and tumorigenesis
Hyperparathyroidism jaw tumour syndrome (HPT-JT)	CDC73 [or hyperparathyroidism 2 gene (HRPT2)]	1q25-q31	Heterozygote, inactivating (AD)	Parafibromin	Component of the polymerase associated factor 1 (PAF1) complex, involved in histone ubiquitination and methylation, and regulation of gene transcription	The biallelic loss of nuclear wild type parafibromin results in an uncontrolled parathyroid cell proliferation and tumorigenesis
Familial isolated primary hyperparathyroidism (FIPH)	GCM2	6p24.2	Heterozygote, activating (AD)	GCM2	A master regulator of parathyroid gland development during embryogenesis and a transcription factor involved in regulation of PTH transcription	Gain-of-function mutations of GCM2 could directly increase PTH transcription

Footnotes: *AD* autosomal dominant, *AR* autosomal recessive

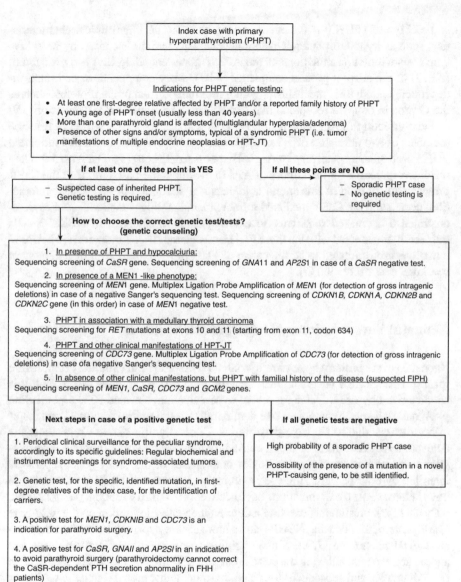

Fig. 7.1 Suggested workup for genetic testing of index cases with primary hyperparathyroidism

which leads to PTH synthesis and secretion. Two FHH2-associated Gα11 missense mutations (p.Thr54Met, p.Leu135Gln) and one in-frame single amino acid deletion (c.598_600delATC, p.Ile200del) have been reported [3, 4]. Inactivating *GNA11* mutations disrupt the G-protein activation, causing an impaired CaSR signal transduction; functional studies demonstrated decreased CaSR sensitivity to changes in extracellular calcium concentrations in HEK293 cells transiently transfected with p.Leu135Gln or p.Ile200del mutations. Up to 10% of patients with a FHH phenotype, and negative for a *CaSR* mutation, are estimated to have a *GNA11* mutation [4].

FHH type 3 (FHH3) is the rarest variant, showing peculiar clinical characteristics, such as hypophosphatemic osteomalacia. This variant is caused by heterozygote loss-of-function mutations of the *AP2S1* gene, encoding the17-kD α-subunit (AP17) of the adaptor protein complex 2 (AP2), a key component of cell clathrin-dependent endocytosis mechanism, which internalizes membrane proteins, such as the G-protein coupled receptors, like CaSR. Three missense *AP2S1* mutations, all of them affecting the arginine residue at codon 15, have been reported in affected members of two unrelated FHH3 families (p.Arg15Cys) and/or in 3 and 4 unrelated FHH3 probands, respectively, (p.Arg15His, or p.Arg15Leu) [5]. The Arg15 is a key residue responsible for the affinity of AP2 to the dileucine-based motif of the CaSR protein. Substitution of this amino acid causes a disruption of AP2-CaSR interaction, decreasing the CaSR-mediated intracellular signaling; functional studies demonstrated a decreased sensitivity to external calcium changes, in HEK293 cells transiently transfected with the three FHH3-associated *AP2S1* mutations [6]. *AP2S1* mutations are estimated to be the cause of FHH in more than 20% of patients not bearing a *CaSR* mutation [5].

Neonatal Severe Primary Hyperparathyroidism

Neonatal severe primary hyperparathyroidism (NSHPT) is an extremely rare, severe form of FHH, which occurs at birth or within the first six months of life, and it is characterized by life-threatening severe hypercalcemia, elevated PTH and alkaline phosphatase levels, hypotonia, bone demineralization, fragility fractures, and respiratory distress due to rib cage deformities. Generally, this disease represents the autosomal recessive form of FHH, caused by homozygote or compound heterozygote germline inactivating mutations of both alleles of the *CaSR* gene, separately inherited by both parents. However, extremely rare cases of NSHPT caused by de novo heterozygote *CaSR* mutations have been reported (p.Arg185Gln, p.Arg227Leu, p.Cys582Tyr), presumably exerting a dominant negative inhibition on the wild-type CaSR protein, thus causing NSHPT and a more severe hypercalcemia, than the classical FHH phenotype [7, 8]. Since avoiding severe neurodevelopmental damage and, in some cases, allowing the survival of NSHPT-affected children depend on an early diagnosis and subsequent total parathyroidectomy, prenatal genetic testing or genetic testing at birth are mandatory when both parents are known to be carriers of a *CaSR* mutation.

Multiple Endocrine Neoplasia Type 1

Multiple endocrine neoplasia type 1 (MEN1) is a rare endocrine cancer syndrome, characterized by the development of multiple tumors in a single patient. The three main tissues affected are the parathyroids, neuroendocrine cells of the gastroenteropancreatic and thoracic tracts, and the anterior pituitary. PHPT is the first clinical manifestation in about 90% of patients, with up to 100% penetrance by the age of 50. It is mainly caused by multigland hyperplasia and/or multiple parathyroid adenomas; all four glands are usually affected during life. The causative gene is the *MEN1* gene, encoding the tumor suppressor nuclear protein menin, which is involved in the regulation of fundamental biological processes, such as the cell cycle, DNA repair, gene transcription, and apoptosis.

A *MEN1* germinal heterozygote inactivating mutation is inherited by the affected parent or, in extremely rare cases, develops de novo at the embryo level. The second wild type *MEN1* allele is usually lost at the somatic level in the parathyroid cells; the latter is the molecular trigger for the development of hyperplasia or adenomas, according to the "Knudson's two hits" hypothesis for tumor suppressor genes. Over 1500 different *MEN1* mutations have been described in MEN1 patients, spread along the entire coding region of the gene. More than 70% of them are truncating mutations (frameshift, nonsense, or splicing-site mutations), generating a truncated menin, missing one or more of the three nuclear localization signals in the 3′ untranslated region (3′-UTR), and being, thus, unable to reach the cell nucleus and exert its biological functions [9, 10]. In-frame mutations (missense or in-frame insertions/deletions) affect only a menin single amino acid, but they have been demonstrated to be a preferential target of ubiquitin-proteasome-driven increased degradation, which shortens their half-life three times more than that of the wild type menin or the benign nonsynonymous polymorphic menin variants (Arg171Gln and Ala541Thr), resulting in a significant reduction of menin activity. About 5–10% of MEN1 patients are estimated to have a large intragenic deletion including more than one exon or even the entire gene. No direct correlation between specific *MEN1* mutation and the clinical phenotype has been demonstrated for any of MEN1 clinical manifestation, including PHPT. PHPT age of onset, presence and severity of hypercalcemia, degree of parathyroid disease, and recurrence rate after parathyroidectomy do not depend on the specific *MEN1* mutation and differ even between members of the same family. Modulatory cofactors, such as epigenetic factors, may together determine the MEN1 individual clinical phenotype and be responsible for the absence of a strict genotype-phenotype correlation in *MEN1* mutated individuals.

Luzi et al. [11] demonstrated a direct regulatory feedback loop between *MEN1*, miR-24-1, and menin, in which this miRNA acts like an oncomir, by inhibiting menin expression via the direct targeting of its mRNA. In tissue samples from MEN1 parathyroid adenomas that still retain one wild type allele of the *MEN1* gene, miR-24-1 was overexpressed together with a normal expression of MEN1 mRNA and the absence of menin expression. Conversely, in MEN1 parathyroid adenomas with the loss of the second wild type copy of *MEN1*, there were no expression of miR-24-1, a low expression of MEN1 mRNA, and no expression of menin. These data suggested that miR-24-1 is involved in MEN1 parathyroid tumorigenesis via an epigenetic regulatory mechanism that inhibits the expression of the wild type menin and mimics the "Knudson's second hit," inducing the development of parathyroid hyperplasia/adenoma before the occurrence of the somatic loss of heterozygosity (LOH) of the second wild type allele of *MEN1*. Data from this study also confirmed the fact that a total lack of menin expression (via the genetic biallelic inactivation or via an epigenetic post-transcriptional "knock-out" of the expression of the wild type protein) is a key step to the development of MEN1 parathyroid tumors.

The same research group [12] further investigated the possible involvement of miRNAs in MEN1 parathyroid tumorigenesis, by comparing the expression profiles of 1890 human miRNAs in MEN1 parathyroid adenomas with or without somatic MEN1 LOH, and with respect to healthy controls. miR-4258 was significantly less expressed in LOH MEN1 parathyroid adenomas compared with the non-LOH samples, while its expression was higher in non-LOH MEN1 parathyroid adenomas compared with the control group. miR-664 was significantly more expressed in non-LOH MEN1 parathyroid adenomas and less expressed in LOH MEN1 parathyroid adenomas, both with respect to the normal parathyroid tissue. miR-1301 was significantly more expressed in LOH MEN1 parathyroid adenomas with respect to healthy controls. This study appears to confirm that epigenetic factors, such as miR-NAs, can be potentially involved in MEN1 parathyroid tumorigenesis and contribute to the development of different MEN1-related PHPT phenotypes. The three miRNAs, identified in this study, showed, in silico, the potential to directly target some genes associated with the development of different inheritable forms of parathyroid tumors (*RET, CDKN1B,* and *CDC73*) and genes suspected to have a role in parathyroid homeostasis and function (*CCND1, RB1, VDR, PRDM2,* and *CDKN2C*), and they could be, thus, involved in the development of PHPT not only in the context of MEN1 syndrome.

Less than 2% of patients with a MEN1 clinical phenotype but without any *MEN1* mutation may represent phenocopies and be carriers of one heterozygote germinal inactivating mutation in *CDKN1A, CDKN1B, CDKN2B,* or *CDKN2C* genes, encoding, respectively, the p21^{Cip1}, p27^{Kip1}, p15^{Ink4b}, and p18^{Ink4c}, cyclin-dependent kinase inhibitors (CDKIs), negative regulators of cell cycle progression, and cell growth [13]. Transcription of these genes is directly regulated by menin, suggesting that *MEN1* and the CDKIs could share a common endocrine tumorigenic pathway. In this light, a non-synonymous c.326T>G, p.Val109Gly polymorphic variant in the *CDKN1B* gene has been investigated regarding a possible role as a genetic cofactor able to influence clinical manifestations in patients bearing a germinal *MEN1* mutation. The presence of the T allele was significantly associated with a higher number of affected endocrine glands in patients over 30 years bearing a *MEN1* truncating mutation [14]. However, no correlation was observed between this polymorphism and the development of PHPT or other MEN1-related endocrine tumors [14, 15].

Multiple Endocrine Neoplasia Type 4

Multiple endocrine neoplasia type 4 (MEN4) is an extremely rare phenocopy of MEN1. MEN4 PHPT is present in about 80% [16], and it is caused by multiple parathyroid hyperplasia or adenomas. MEN4 is caused by heterozygous inactivating mutations in the cyclin-dependent kinase inhibitor 1B (*CDKN1B*) tumor suppressor gene, encoding the p27^{kip1} protein. It is an inhibitor of a broad spectrum of cyclin-dependent kinases (CDKs), mainly the cyclin-dependent kinase 2 (CDK2) during the G1-to-S phase transition of cell cycle. Mutated p27^{kip1} is not able to phosphorylate and inactivate CDK2, and it is, thus, responsible for uncontrolled cell cycle progression in neuroendocrine cells. In these target cells, the lack of p27^{kip1} activity can presumably not be compensated for by other CDKIs, and the loss of a single p27^{kip1} allele alone is sufficient to increase tumor incidence, via the CDK-mediated cell cycle entry. *CDKN1B* acts as a nonconventional tumor suppressor, not following the classical "Knudson's two hits" hypothesis. The condition presumably presents as a consequence of a loss-of-function mutation, a severely reduced nuclear localization of the p27^{kip1} protein, in association with an increased degradation of the mutated protein at cytoplasmatic level.

To date, 19 different *CDKN1B* mutations, affecting the coding region and the 5′ untranslated region (5'-UTR) of the gene, have been identified in MEN4 cases [16]. The 5'-UTR of CDKN1B mRNA contains a U-rich element, which is necessary for the efficient translation of the protein both in proliferating and quiescent cells. No direct genotype-phenotype correlation has been reported. Elston et al. [17] reported a case of apparently sporadic early onset PHPT in a 15-year-old girl, without any family history of PHPT, hypercalcemia, or other endocrine disorders, but presenting with recurrent nephrolithiasis and renal colic, persistent hypercalcemia, and a single gland parathyroid adenoma in the anterior mediastinum. She was a carrier of a novel heterozygote missense mutation in exon 1 of the *CDKN1B* gene (c.378G > C; pGlu126Asp). However, both her mother and her maternal grandfather, carriers of the same heterozygote mutation, showed no signs or symptoms of PHPT and had normal serum values of both PTH and calcium. It is presumed that the index case could be the carrier of one or more other genetic variants in other genes that contribute to the development of the PHPT phenotype. This suggests that the possibility of genetic heterogeneity of MEN4 PHPT, for whom some *CDKN1B* mutations, could be "low-penetrance mutations."

Multiple Endocrine Neoplasia Type 2A

Multiple endocrine neoplasia type 2 (MEN2) is a rare endocrine cancer syndrome, characterized by the development of multiple tumors in a single patient. Only the clinical variant 2A (MEN2A) manifests with PHPT. PHPT in MEN2A is less frequent that in MEN1 and MEN4 (20–30% of cases), and it usually manifests later, during the fourth decade of life. It has a mild clinical presentation, remaining asymptomatic in 42–84% of patients [18]; only about 15% of cases manifest hypercalciuria and nephrocalcinosis. Parathyroid disease in MEN2A may range from single gland involvement (27–54% of cases) up to the involvement of all the four glands, both as marked hyperplasia or benign adenomas.

MEN2 is caused by germinal heterozygote activating mutations of the proto-oncogene REarranged during Transfection (*RET*), encoding the homonym transmembrane tyrosine kinase receptor RET. RET consists of an extracellular portion (composed of four cadherin-like domains, a calcium-binding site, and a cysteine-rich ligand-binding domain), a single-pass transmembrane portion, and an intracellular portion containing two distinct tyrosine kinase domains. The MEN2A variant is specifically caused by a *RET* missense mutation in exon 10, at codons 609, 611, 618, 620, or in exon 11, at codons 630, and 634, encoding the six cysteine residues of the extracellular ligand-binding domain of the receptor. A single amino acid change of one of these cysteine is sufficient to induce constitutive activation (and homodimerization) of the RET receptor, even in the absence of the biological ligand, resulting in constant activation of the intracellular tyrosine kinase activity and signal transduction, with subsequent induction of an uncontrolled parathyroid cell growth. The amino acid substitutions of cysteine at codon 634 (p.Cys634Arg, p.Cys634Tyr, p.Cys634Trp, p.Cys634Ser, p.Cys634Phe, and p.Cys634Gly) together represent the great majority of *RET* mutations in MEN2A (up to 98% of MEN2A cases); the p.Cys634Arg mutation affects, alone, about 85% of all MEN2A patients. The Cys634Arg mutant showed a three- to fivefold higher transforming activity of RET protein, compared with any other cysteine mutant in exon 10, when transfected into NIH-3T3 cells [19]. No significant association was found between the presence of a specific mutation at codon 634 and the risk of PHPT development, although the prevalence of PHPT among individuals with the p.Cys634Arg mutation was slightly higher than that observed in MEN2A patients bearing another mutation of codon 634 [20]. Conversely, the presence of the p.Cys634Arg mutation seemed to correlate with an age-dependent higher penetrance of PHPT, after the age of 35. Beyond 35 years, the relative risk of PHPT development was 1.8 times higher in p.Cys634Arg carriers than in patients bearing any other 634 mutation [20].

Hyperparathyroidism-Jaw Tumor Syndrome

Hyperparathyroidism-jaw tumor syndrome (HPT-JT) is characterized by the development of PHPT, ossifying fibromas of the mandible and/or maxilla, uterine tumors in about 75% of affected women and, more rarely, polycystic bilateral kidney lesions, papillary renal carcinoma, renal hamartomas, and Wilms tumor. Parathyroid tumors are the first clinical manifestation of the syndrome (generally manifesting during late adolescence or young adulthood) in over 95% of cases, affecting up to 100% of mutation carriers. About 75% of HPT-JT PHPT is caused by a single gland benign adenoma showing mild clinical behavior, while 10–15% of patients manifest severe hypercalcemia with hypercalcemic crisis, caused by malignant parathyroid carcinoma.

A recognized cause of HPT-JT is germinal heterozygous inactivating mutations of the cell division cycle 73 (*CDC73*) tumor suppressor gene, encoding a ubiquitously expressed nuclear protein, named parafibromin. The first mutated allele is inherited by the affected parent, while the second wild type copy is inactivated, at the somatic level, in target tissues, leading to the development of multiple tumors. PHPT penetrance is, however, incomplete even in the presence of the CDC73 mutation. Parafibromin is a member of the polymerase-associated factor 1 (PAF1) complex, involved in histone ubiquitination and methylation and in regulation of transcriptional and post-transcriptional events, such as initiation of transcription, transcript elongation, mRNA maturation, and maintenance of poly(A) length at 3'-UTR for mRNA stability. PAF1 complex is responsible for trimethylation of histone H3K4 and methylation of histone H3K79, resulting in chromatin remodeling and, thus, regulation of gene transcription. Parafibromin has also been demonstrated to exert tumor-suppressive functions, such as inhibition of cell cycle G1-to-S phase transition, induction of apoptosis and regulation of the Wnt canonical pathway. Loss of nuclear wild type parafibromin results in an uncontrolled cell proliferation and tumorigenesis.

CDC73 mutations have been reported in about 50% of HPT-JT families and in about 20% of apparently sporadic parathyroid carcinomas. The high incidence of parathyroid carcinoma in HPT-JT (which is instead extremely rare, less than 0.5%, in all the other forms of genetic PHPT) and the fact that somatic homozygote inactivating mutations of the CDC73 gene have been described in a variable percentage of 67–100% of sporadic parathyroid carcinomas suggest a primary role of parafibromin loss in the development of this malignant parathyroid tumor. Over 100 different CDC73 mutations have been described all along the entire coding region of the gene. Over 80% of HPT-JT-associated CDC73 mutations are nonsense or frameshift variants, which encode a truncated parafibromin or cause a rapid loss of the translated protein via nonsense-mediated mRNA decay. Gross intragenic deletions are estimated to represent about 1% of all CDC73 mutations in HPT-JT families [21]. No genotype-phenotype correlation has been reported; however, it has been suggested that mutations causing a gross alteration/disruption of parafibromin could be more likely associated with the classical HPT-JT phenotype, while missense mutations, exerting a more limited effect on parafibromin activity, could be more likely related to the development of FIHP, as an atypical form of HPT-JT affecting only parathyroids [18].

Familial Isolated Primary Hyperparathyroidism

Familial isolated primary hyperparathyroidism (FIHP) consists of PHPT affecting multiple members of the same family and caused by mono- or multiglandular parathyroid lesions in the absence of other endocrine and non-endocrine clinical features. A FIHP-specific causative gene has not been identified yet, and in most FIHP families, the underlying genetic defect remains unknown.

Mutations of CaSR, MEN1, and CDC73 genes have been identified in a significant number of FIHP families, suggesting that many cases of FIHP could represent an early stage of FHH1, MEN1, or HPT-JT, in which only PHPT has already manifested, or nonclassical forms of these diseases affecting only parathyroid glands.

The exome-sequencing analysis of genomic DNA in 8 index cases, from 8 unrelated FIHP pedigrees, followed by the cosegregation analysis of the selected variants in 32 additional FIHP families, allowed identification of three rare gain-of-function missense mutations in the glial cells missing transcription factor 2 (*GCM2*) gene [c.943A > G, p.Asn315Asp; c.1181A > C, p.Tyr394Ser; and c.(751C > G; 1136T > A), p.(Gln251Glu; Leu379Gln)], affecting together about the 20% of the 40 analyzed families [22]. *GCM2* encodes the homonym transcription factor, which exerts a key role in the development of parathyroid glands during embryogenesis; knockout mice for the *Gcm2* gene (the murine homolog of human *GCM2*) have aplasia of the parathyroids. Several inactivating frameshift, nonsense, and missense mutations of the *GCM2* gene have been linked to congenital hypoparathyroidism. Functional studies, by luciferase reporter assays, showed that the p.(Gln251Glu; Leu379Gln) and the p.Tyr394Ser variants have a 18- and 11-fold higher transcriptional activity, respectively, and the p.Asn315Asp variant has a 20% higher transcriptional activity than the wild type *GCM2* allele [22]. Given the fact that the PTH promoter contains a consensus sequence GCM-binding site, it is conceivable that GCM2 could directly activate PTH transcription in cooperation with other transcription factors, such as GATA3 and MAFB, and that *GCM2* gain-of-function mutations could be responsible for PHPT development. However, the exact role of activating *GCM2* mutations in determining penetrance and pathogenesis of FIHP has not yet been clearly established.

Sporadic Primary Hyperparathyroidism

Sporadic PHPT (sPHPT) represents about 90–95% of all PHPT cases and develops later than inherited forms of PHPT, and it is caused by the development of a single-gland adenoma in almost the totality of cases. sPHPT shows genetic heterogeneity; mutations in various genes have been associated with the development of this disease. In many cases, tumor development has been ascribed to somatic or germinal mutations in genes known to control cell growth, some of them the same genes responsible for inherited forms of PHPT.

Somatic homozygote inactivation of the *MEN1* gene (caused by two distinct mutational events at the tissue level) has been observed in 25–40% of sporadic parathyroid tumors [23, 24], while somatic inactivating *CDC73* mutations have been found in only 4% of in sporadic parathyroid adenomas [21] and in 67–100% of sporadic parathyroid carcinomas [25]. Acquired biallelic inactivation of the *CDKN1B* gene, resulting from somatic mutation plus LOH, was also identified in sporadic parathyroid adenomas [26]. Somatic mutation or germinal mutation plus somatic LOH of *CDKN2C*, germline mutation of *CDKN1A*, and germline mutation plus somatic LOH of *CDKN2B* were all identified in patients with sporadic single parathyroid adenoma, no family history of PHPT and no family and personal history of multiple endocrine neoplasia [27]. No mutations of *RET* and *CaSR* genes have been detected in sPHPT.

Cyclin D1 is a positive cell cycle regulator, encoded by the *CCDN1* proto-oncogene, whose overexpression has been identified in 20–40% of sporadic parathyroid adenomas and in up to 90% of sporadic parathyroid carcinomas [28]. Somatic pericentromeric inversions or translocations at chromosome 11q13, containing *CCDN1*, which transcriptionally overactivate this gene by placing it under the direct regulation of the tissue-specific enhancer elements of the *PTH* gene promoter, occur in about 8% of sporadic parathyroid adenomas, and they seem to be one of the mechanisms responsible for cyclin D1 overexpression in sporadic parathyroid tumors. Also copy number variations in the *CCDN1* may lead to parathyroid tumorigenesis, more commonly in malignant parathyroid carcinomas (nearly 70%) than in benign adenomatous counterpart (only 20%) [28]. Interestingly, the 11q13 locus, containing *CCDN1*, is the same location as *MEN1* that, currently, is the main gene whose somatic mutations have been identified most frequently in sporadic parathyroid tumors and nearby to the 11p15.3 locus which contains the *PTH* gene.

The accumulation of nonphosphorylated β-catenin, altering the Wnt/ β-catenin signaling, was demonstrated both in primary sPHPT caused by parathyroid adenomas and in uremic secondary hyperplastic parathyroids. In primary parathyroid tumors, the β-catenin overexpression was caused by a somatic homozygote protein-stabilizing mutation (p.Ser37Ala) in exon 3 of the β-catenin coding gene (*CTNNB1*) [29], while no mutation was detected in secondary hyperplastic glands. The β-catenin target oncogene c-myc was overexpressed in a substantial fraction of both primary parathyroid tumors and secondary hyperplastic glands.

DNA sequencing, by single-gene Sanger's approach or via a whole-exome analysis, on sporadic parathyroid adenoma and blood samples identified low-frequency somatic and germline mutations in novel genes, as potential genetic causes of sPHPT. Cromer et al. identified the gain-of-function somatic heterozygote p.Tyr641Asn mutation in the enhancer of zeste homolog 2 (*EZH2*) gene, affecting a highly conserved residue within the active site of the enzyme and conferring an increased ability of EZH2 to trimethylate the histone H3K27 and deregulate gene expression and cell growth [30]. Another *EZH2* missense mutation, the c.1936T > A, p.Tyr646Asn, affecting a highly conserved residue and predicted to have a pathogenic effect on protein function, was identified in a sporadic parathyroid adenoma [31].

A somatic heterozygote point mutation was identified in the last nucleotide of exon 8 of the protection of telomeres 1 (*POT1*) gene, involved in the maintenance of genome stability. The c.546G > C substitution was predicted to lead either to a single amino acid change (p.Lys85Asn) or to an alternative splicing event skipping the entire exon 8, which encodes part of the two highly conserved oligonucleotide-/oligosaccharide-binding domains, necessary for the telomere protection function of POT1. Thus, this mutation may result in genome instability and contribute to the high mutation rate and LOH observed in the *POT1* mutated parathyroid adenoma sample [32].

Recurrent missense somatic mutations in two highly conserved arginine residues, at codons 786 and 787, of the zinc-finger protein X-linked (*ZFX*) gene on the chromosome X, encoding a zing-finger protein implicated in the regulation of gene transcription, were identified in multiple samples of sporadic parathyroid adenomas [33]. Substitutions of the positively charged arginine with the noncharged glutamine, threonine, or leucine, at positions 786 or 787, alter the DNA-binding affinity and/or specificity of ZFX protein. Mutated *ZFX* may act as an oncogene, in the context of parathyroid tumorigenesis, and confer a selective growth advantage to tumor cells.

Two missense mutations (c.833A > G, p.His278Arg and c.944C > A, p.Ala315Glu), both affecting two highly conserved amino acids and predicted to alter protein function, of the *ASXL3* gene were found in two patients with sPHPT caused by parathyroid adenomas. ASXL3 belongs to a group of vertebrate Asx-like proteins, predicted to act as regulators of gene transcription, whose somatic recurrent mutations have been already identified in specific subset of tumors.

Case

A 39-year-old woman was referred to endocrinology for recurrent hypercalcemia after parathyroidectomy performed five years ago at another hospital. She had been found to be hypercalcemic with labs consistent with primary hyperparathyroidism prior to her initial parathyroidectomy: calcium 10.7 mg/dL (normal 8.5–10.2 mg/dL), PTH 105 pg/mL (normal 15–65 mg/dL), and 24 hour urine calcium 223 mg/24 hours (normal <250 mg/24 hours) at that time. Sestimibi had indicated a left lower adenoma. She underwent focused parathyroidectomy. Intraoperative PTH decreased from 220 →179 →107 → 45 pg/dL before the incision was made and subsequently after excision. Pathology revealed an enlarged hyperplastic parathyroid consistent with an adenoma and weighing 180 milligrams.

After surgery, her serum calcium and PTH normalized. Recurrent hypercalcemia occurred 1 year ago with a similar lab pattern to her initial labs before parathyroidectomy. She has a history of nephrolithiasis at the age of 34 and osteopenia. She takes no medications. Her family history is unknown as she is adopted. On review of systems, she reports her menstrual cycles have become irregular over the last year. Physical exam is normal. Reevaluation of her laboratories indicates serum calcium 10.6 mg/dl and PTH 122 pg/ml. Prolactin is mildly elevated with low-normal gonadatropins. Her other pituitary hormones are normal. The patient is sent for genetic testing for multiple endocrine neoplasia type 1. A pathogenic variant in the MEN1 gene is identified: c.249_252delGTCT (deletion at codons 83–84). Magnetic resonance imaging of the pituitary revealed an 8 mm adenoma.

This case illustrates the importance of considering genetic forms of primary hyperparathyroidism in patients who are <40 years old at the time of diagnosis of primary hyperparathyroidism (Fig. 7.1). While inherited forms of primary hyperparathyroidism represent only 5–10% of cases, a young age of onset should prompt suspicion for this possibility. Penetrence of PHPT is almost 100% before the age of 50 in MEN1. In MEN1, there is asynchronous development of parathyroid adenomas over time. This leads to a high rate of recurrent primary hyperparathyroidism, as observed in this case.

References

1. Carlson D. Parathyroid pathology: hyperparathyroidism and parathyroid tumours. Arch Pathol Lab Med. 2010;134(11):1639–44.
2. Ward BK, Magno AL, Blitvich BJ, Rea AJ, Stuckey BG, Walsh JP, Ratajczak T. Novel mutations in the calcium-sensing receptor gene associated with biochemical and functional differences in familial hypocalciuric hypercalcaemia. Clin Endocrinol (Oxf). 2006;64(5):580–7.
3. Gorvin CM, Cranston T, Hannan FM, Rust N, Qureshi A, Nesbit MA, Thakker RV. A G-protein subunit-alpha11 loss-of-function mutation, Thr54Met, causes familial hypocalciuric hypercalcemia type 2 (FHH2). J Bone Miner Res. 2016;31(6):1200–6.
4. Nesbit MA, Hannan FM, Howles SA, Babinsky VN, Head RA, Cranston T, Rust N, Hobbs MR, Heath H 3rd, Thakker RV. Mutations affecting G-protein subunit $\alpha11$ in hypercalcaemia and hypocalcaemia. N Engl J Med. 2013;368(26):2476–86.
5. Nesbit MA, Hannan FM, Howles SA, Reed AA, Cranston T, Thakker CE, Gregory L, Rimmer AJ, Rust N, Graham U, Morrison PJ, Hunter SJ, Whyte MP, McVean G, Buck D, Thakker RV. Mutations in AP2S1 cause familial hypocalciuric hypercalcemia type 3. Nat Genet. 2013;45(1):93–7.
6. Hendy GN, Cole DEC. Ruling in a suspect: the role of AP2S1 mutations in familial hypocalciuric hypercalcemia type 3. J Clin Endocrinol Metab. 2013;98(12):4666–9.
7. Pearce SHS, Trump D, Wooding C, Besser GM, Chew SL, Grant DB, Heath DA, Hughes IA, Paterson CR, Whyte MP, Thakker RV. Calcium-sensing receptor mutations in familial benign hypercalcemia and neonatal hyperparathyroidism. J Clin Invest. 1995;96:2683–92.
8. Bai M, Pearce SH, Kifor O, Trivedi S, Stauffer UG, Thakker RV, Brown EM, Steinmann B. In vivo and in vitro characterization of neonatal hyperparathyroidism resulting from a de novo, heterozygous mutation in the Ca2+-sensing receptor gene: normal maternal calcium homeostasis as a cause of secondary hyperparathyroidism in familial benign hypocalciuric hypercalcemia. J Clin Invest. 1997;99(1):88–96.
9. Lemos MC, Thakker RV. Multiple endocrine neoplasia type 1 (MEN1): analysis of 1336 mutations reported in the first decade following identification of the gene. Hum Mutat. 2008;29(1):22–32.
10. Concolino P, Costella A, Capoluongo E. Multiple endocrine neoplasia type 1 (MEN1): an update of 208 new germline variants reported in the last nine years. Cancer Genet. 2016;209(1–2):36–41.
11. Luzi E, Marini F, Giusti F, Galli G, Cavalli L, Brandi ML. The negative feedback-loop between the oncomir Mir-24-1 and menin modulates the Men1 tumorigenesis by mimicking the "Knudson's second hit". PLoS One. 2012;7:e39767.
12. Luzi E, Ciuffi S, Marini F, Mavilia C, Galli G, Brandi ML. Analysis of differentially expressed microRNAs in MEN1 parathyroid adenomas. Am J Transl Res. 2017;9:1743–53.
13. Turner JJO, Christie PT, Pearce SHS, Turnpenny PD, Thakker RV. Diagnostic challenges due to phenocopies: lessons from multiple endocrine neoplasia type 1 (MEN1). Hum Mutat. 2010;31:E1089–101.
14. Longuini VC, Lourenço DM Jr, Sekiya T, Meirelles O, Goncalves TD, Coutinho FL, Francisco G, Osaki LH, Chammas R, Alves VA, Siqueira SA, Schlesinger D, Naslavsky MS, Zatz M, Duarte YA, Lebrão ML, Gama P, Lee M, Molatore S, Pereira MA, Jallad RS, Bronstein MD, Cunha-Neto MB, Liberman B, Fragoso MC, Toledo SP, Pellegata NS, Toledo RA. Association between the p27 rs2066827 variant and tumor multiplicity in patients harboring MEN1 germline mutations. Eur J Endocrinol. 2014;171(3):335–42.
15. Circelli L, Ramundo V, Marotta V, Sciammarella C, Marciello F, Del Prete M, Sabatino L, Pasquali D, Izzo F, Scala S, Colao A, Faggiano A, Colantuoni V, Multidisciplinary Group for NeuroEndocrine Tumours of Naples. Prognostic role of the CDNK1B V109G polymorphism in multiple endocrine neoplasia type 1. J Cell Mol Med. 2015;19(7):1735–41.
16. Alrezk R, Hannah-Shmouni F, Stratakis CA. MEN4 and CDKN1B mutations: the latest of the MEN syndromes. Endocr Relat Cancer. 2017;24(10):T195–208.

17. Elston MS, Meyer-Rochow GY, Dray M, Swarbrick M, Conaglen JV. Early onset primary hyperparathyroidism associated with a novel germline mutation in CDKN1B. Case Rep Endocrinol. 2015;2015:510985.
18. Iacobone M, Carnaille B, Palazzo FF, Vriens M. Hereditary hyperparathyroidism--a consensus report of the European Society of Endocrine Surgeons (ESES). Langenbecks Arch Surg. 2015;400(8):867–86.
19. Ito S, Iwashita T, Murakami H, Iwata Y, Sobue-Ku, Takahashi M. Biological properties of RET with cysteine mutations correlate with multiple endocrine neoplasia type 2A, familial thyroid carcinoma, and Hirschsprung's disease phenotype. Cancer Res. 1997;14:2870–2.
20. Schuffenecker I, Virally-Monod M, Brohet R, Goldgar D, Conte-Devolx B, Leclerc L, Chabre O, Boneu A, Caron J, Houdent C, Modigliani E, Rohmer V, Schlumberger M, Eng C, Guillausseau PJ, Lenoir GM. Risk and penetrance of primary hyperparathyroidism in multiple endocrine neoplasia type 2A families with mutations at codon 634 of the RET proto-oncogene. Groupe D'etude des Tumeurs à Calcitonine. J Clin Endocrinol Metab. 1998;83(2):487–91.
21. Newey PJ, Bowl MR, Cranston T, Thakker RV. Cell division cycle protein 73 homolog (CDC73) mutations in the hyperparathyroidism-jaw tumour syndrome (HPT-JT) and parathyroid tumours. Hum Mutat. 2010;31:295–307.
22. Guan B, Welch JM, Sapp JC, Ling H, Li Y, Johnston JJ, Kebebew E, Biesecker LG, Simonds WF, Marx SJ, Agarwal SK. GCM2-activating mutations in familial isolated hyperparathyroidism. Am J Hum Genet. 2016;99(5):1034–44.
23. Heppner C, Kester MB, Agarwal SK, Debelenko LV, Emmert-Buck MR, Guru SC, et al. Somatic mutation of the MEN1 gene in parathyroid tumours. Nat Genet. 1997;16:375–8.
24. Miedlich S, Krohn K, Lamesch P, Müller A, Paschke R. Frequency of somatic MEN1 gene mutations in monoclonal parathyroid tumours in patients with primary hyperparathyroidism. Eur J Endocrinol. 2000;143:47–54.
25. Giusti F, Cavalli L, Cavalli T, Brandi ML. Hereditary hyperparathyroidism syndromes. J Clin Densitom. 2013;16(1):69–74.
26. Costa-Guda J, Marinoni I, Molatore S, Pellegata NS, Arnold A. Somatic mutation and germline sequence abnormalities in CDKN1B, encoding p27Kip1, in sporadic parathyroid adenomas. J Clin Endocrinol Metab. 2011;96(4):E701–6.
27. Costa-Guda J, Soong CP, Parekh VI, Agarwal SK, Arnold A. Germline and somatic mutations in cyclin-dependent kinase inhibitor genes CDKN1A, CDKN2B, and CDKN2C in sporadic parathyroid adenomas. Horm. Cancer. 2013;4(5):301–7.
28. Zhao L, Sun LH, Liu DM, He XY, Tao B, Ning G, Liu JM, Zhao HY. Copy number variation in CCND1 gene is implicated in the pathogenesis of sporadic parathyroid carcinoma. World J Surg. 2014;38:1730–7.
29. Björklund P, Akerström G, Westin G. Accumulation of nonphosphorylated beta-catenin and c-myc in primary and uremic secondary hyperparathyroid tumors. J Clin Endocrinol Metab. 2007;92(1):338–44.
30. Cromer MK, Starker LF, Choi M, Udelsman R, Nelson-Williams C, Lifton RP, Carling T. Identification of somatic mutations in parathyroid tumors using whole-exome sequencing. J Clin Endocrinol Metab. 2012;97(9):E1774–81.
31. Wei Z, Sun B, Wang ZP, He JW, Fu WZ, Fan YB, Zhang ZL. Whole-exome sequencing identifies novel recurrent somatic mutations in sporadic parathyroid adenomas. Endocrinology. 2018;159(8):3061–8.
32. Newey PJ, Nesbit MA, Rimmer AJ, Attar M, Head RT, Christie PT, Gorvin CM, Stechman M, Gregory L, Mihai R, Sadler G, McVean G, Buck D, Thakker RV. Whole-exome sequencing studies of nonhereditary (sporadic) parathyroid adenomas. J Clin Endocrinol Metab. 2012;97(10):E1995–2005.
33. Soong CP, Arnold A. Recurrent ZFX mutations in human sporadic parathyroid adenomas. Onco Targets Ther. 2014;1(5):360–6.

Chapter 8
Familial Hypocalciuric Hypercalcemia and Disorders of the Calcium-Sensing Receptor

Susan Shey and Dolores Shoback

Epidemiology

Precise rates of FHH in the general population are difficult to obtain. Two estimates that have been published are substantially different. Among patients with hypercalcemia, Varghese et al. estimated that ~2% of all cases are due to FHH [1]. A study of six known FHH kindreds in the Greater Glasgow and Lanarkshire areas of West Scotland reported a minimum prevalence of 1 in 78,000 based off the clinical features of asymptomatic hypercalcemia with hypocalciuria and an autosomal dominant pattern of inheritance [2]. In an unbiased electronic health record (EHR) cohort (DiscovEHR), composed of 51,289 individuals from a single US healthcare system who consented to whole-genome sequencing, genetic prevalence for FHH1 was determined to be 74 cases per 100,000 [3]. If one extrapolates, that would be ~1/1350 individuals in a community with the demographics of that cohort [predominantly northern European descent (50,387), with 57 American Indian/Alaska Native, 137 Asian, 570 Black/African American, 40 Native Hawaiian/Pacific Islander, and 3 Uncategorized/Other individuals, as self-reported]. More studies with genetic testing and careful clinical phenotyping of different cohorts worldwide would be of considerable interest to address the true prevalence with greater

S. Shey
Division of Endocrinology and Metabolism, University of California,
San Francisco, CA, USA
e-mail: Susan.Shey@ucsf.edu

D. Shoback (✉)
Division of Endocrinology and Metabolism, University of California,
San Francisco, CA, USA

Endocrine Research Unit, Department of Veterans Affairs Medical Center,
San Francisco, CA, USA
e-mail: Dolores.shoback@ucsf.edu

© The Author(s), under exclusive license to Springer Nature
Switzerland AG 2022
M. D. Walker (ed.), *Hypercalcemia*, Contemporary Endocrinology,
https://doi.org/10.1007/978-3-030-93182-7_8

precision in different populations. Because FHH often is asymptomatic and affected individuals may not come to medical attention to be diagnosed, it is likely the prevalence is higher than older studies have suggested. The most common variant of FHH due to inactivating *CASR* mutations (FHH1) accounts for 65% of FHH cases. Approximately 13–26% of patients without *CASR* mutations have been reported to have a *GNA11* mutation (FHH3), and up to 10% of patients with neither *CASR* nor *AP2S1* mutations have *GNA11* mutations (FHH2) [4]. Thus, there remains a small proportion of patients with the FHH phenotype and inheritance who remain without a clear genetic diagnosis.

Pathophysiology

The majority of FHH cases are due to heterozygous inactivating mutations of the *CASR* on chromosome 3q13.3-21, which encodes the CaSR [3]. The CaSR protein is a ~120–160 kDa, 1078 amino acid, G-protein-coupled receptor (GPCR) that is expressed as a multimeric complex on the membranes of cells almost ubiquitously throughout the body, playing a key role in regulating molecular and cellular functions such as gene expression, cell proliferation, differentiation, and apoptosis [5]. The CaSR is expressed in many tissues, including the parathyroid glands, kidneys, bone, thyroid C cells, pancreas, gastrointestinal tract, brain, lung, muscle, skin, breast, and placenta [6]. In particular, CaSRs in the parathyroid chief cells and in several portions of the nephron play central roles in calcium regulation in the body.

In the setting of hypercalcemia, CaSRs in parathyroid cell membranes sense increased extracellular calcium concentrations which trigger activation of the phospholipase C pathway, elevating intracellular calcium levels, protein kinase C activity, and several other signaling pathways. The culmination of CaSR activation is the inhibition of PTH release and biosynthesis [7]. The mutations in *CASR* in cases of FHH1 produce CaSR molecules that, when expressed in heterologous cell systems, display decreased sensitivity to raising the extracellular calcium concentration, due to a calcium set point that is shifted to the right (see Fig. 8.1) [45]. The calcium set point is the calcium concentration at which PTH secretion is half-maximal [8]. This shifted set point in turn leads to higher levels of circulating PTH and concomitantly higher levels of serum calcium.

Usually in response to hypercalcemia, renal CaSRs couple to the inhibition of tubular calcium and magnesium reabsorption. In FHH1, mutant CaSRs instead promote increased renal tubular calcium reabsorption and decreased urinary calcium excretion [43]. In a study of three patients from FHH kindreds with biochemical evidence of FHH who underwent total parathyroidectomy, these individuals became hypocalcemic, but their renal calcium excretion levels were persistently low, even when given calcium infusions. This supported the fact that their low urinary calcium levels were due to the mutant renal CaSRs, rather than a reflection of increased PTH secretion [9]. This study is limited by the era in which it was undertaken, as the genes responsible for FHH had not yet been identified. These patients had the FHH phenotype but had not been genotyped. The abnormal renal calcium handling of

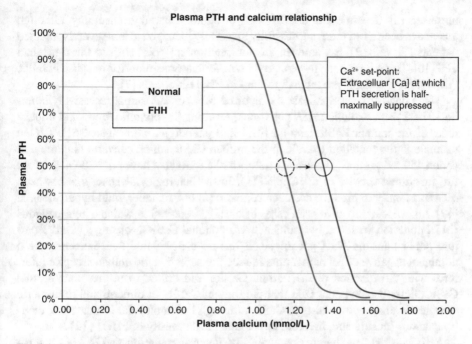

Fig. 8.1 Depicted is the relationship between plasma ionized calcium (mmol/L) and plasma PTH (% of maximal secretion), represented by a steep, inverse sigmoid curve. The calcium set point is the extracellular calcium concentration at which PTH maximum secretion is decreased by 50%. In FHH (red line), this curve is shifted to the right in comparison to normal (blue line). This means in FHH, there is a higher calcium set point and higher levels of calcium are needed to suppress PTH. (Reprinted from Lee and Shoback [14], Copyright 2018, with permission from Elsevier Ltd)

FHH occurs primarily in the thick ascending limb of the loop of Henle in the nephron, as treatment with furosemide, which works on calcium and sodium transport in the thick ascending limb of the loop of Henle, has been shown to abolish the relative hypocalciuria in FHH when compared to PHPT [10].

Etiology

FHH1 is due to heterozygous mutations in *CASR*, and its inheritance is autosomal dominant with high penetrance. *CASR* was first mapped, and the cDNA encoding the CaSR was identified in the early 1990s. Since then, over 200 loss-of-function mutations in *CASR* have been reported from laboratories around the world. Homozygous loss-of-function *CASR* mutations lead to neonatal severe hyperparathyroidism (NSHPT), which typically presents in the first weeks of life with life-threatening hypercalcemia (usually with serum calcium levels of at least 15 mg/dL, but can be as high as 30 mg/dL) [6, 11, 49], significantly elevated PTH levels, parathyroid gland hyperplasia, skeletal demineralization, multiple fractures (including rib fractures), hypotonia, and respiratory distress with high mortality if left untreated [6]. Treatment is usually total or subtotal parathyroidectomy, although there have been a few cases successfully medically managed in less severely affected patients [7]. NSHPT has an even greater calcium set point shift to the right than FHH [8]. There have been more than 25 *CASR* mutations reported to cause NSHPT [11]. NSHPT patients are typically found in FHH1 kindreds [7].

There have also been at least six reported cases of autosomal recessively inherited FHH1 from biallelic *CASR* mutations, resulting in only mild functional impairment of the mutant CaSRs and an FHH-like phenotype rather than NSHPT. One example is the mutation Q459R in the human CaSR which converts glutamine at codon 459 to arginine. This leads to abnormal CaSRs that have only 30–50% of the full functional activity of the CaSR [11]. In the heterozygous state, this has been seen in a family to produce normocalcemia, or in one member, mild hypercalcemia [47]. Likewise, there have been cases of NSHPT reported in which a heterozygous *CASR* mutation presumably results in nonfunctional CaSRs, causing a NSHPT picture rather than the FHH phenotype. It has been postulated that there may be a dominant negative effect of that mutant receptor such that the mutant receptor interferes with the function of the normal CaSRs transcribed from the other normal CaSR allele. It is hypothesized that the mutant CaSRs in dimeric and multimeric complexes along with wild-type CaSRs, through intermolecular interactions, modify calcium-sensing and therefore the biochemical severity of FHH1 [12].

FHH2 results from heterozygous loss-of-function mutations in *GNA11* on chromosome 19q13.3. This gene encodes the G-protein subunit α11 (Gα11), a downstream protein involved in CaSR signal transduction (see Fig. 8.2). To date, there are

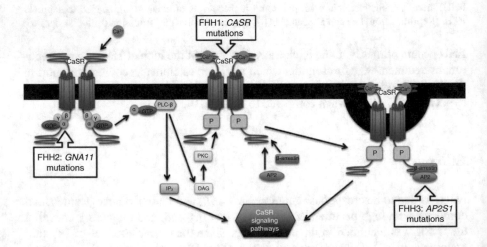

Fig. 8.2 A model of the calcium-sensing receptor, downstream pathways, and FHH1–FHH3 gene mutations. AP2 adaptor protein 2; β-arrestin, Ca2+ calcium ion, CaSR calcium-sensing receptor, DAG diacylglycerol, GDP guanosine diphosphate, GTP guanosine triphosphate, IP3 inositol triphosphate, P phosphothreonine, PKC protein kinase C, PLC-β phospholipase C β, *AP2S1* adaptor-related protein complex 2 subunit sigma 1 gene, *CASR* calcium-sensing receptor gene, *GNA11* G protein subunit alpha 11 gene. (Reprinted from Lee and Shoback [14], Copyright 2018, with permission from Elsevier Ltd)

three *GNA11* gene mutations resulting in FHH2 that have been identified [7]. Each of these mutations causes mild impairment in CaSR signal transduction in vitro and a mild clinical phenotype in affected humans [11].

FHH3 is due to a heterozygous loss-of-function mutation in *AP2S1*, the adaptor-related protein complex 2 subunit sigma 1 gene, which maps to chromosome 19p13.3. This gene encodes AP2σ2, the σ2 subunit of adaptor-related protein 2, which is a complex responsible for clathrin-mediated endocytosis of the CaSR and in membrane trafficking of the receptor (see Fig. 8.2) [44]. *AP2S1* gene mutations, expressed in heterologous cell systems, lead to decreased CaSR cell membrane expression and signal transduction [11, 44]. So far, three mutations have been identified [11].

Clinical Presentation

The first FHH kindred was described in 1966, with 19 family members and noted to have asymptomatic hypercalcemia with normal PTH levels; 3 members had a history of failed subtotal parathyroidectomy [13]. In 1972, this disorder was termed "familial benign hypercalcemia" by *Foley* et al. [48]. Since then, many more FHH kindreds have been identified, and the disease has been divided into three genetically distinct entities with subtle biochemical variations. Now because it is clear that not all FHH patients are asymptomatic, the word "benign" in the disease name is not used.

Today, much as in PHPT, most cases of FHH are incidentally detected due to elevated serum calcium levels seen on routine labs. It is thought that FHH is present from birth, but it can be diagnosed at any age, depending on when the patient has serum calcium levels checked or if family screening is being done. The majority of FHH patients do not experience the typical symptoms and complications associated with hypercalcemia as can be seen in patients with PHPT [14]. Before the availability of genetic testing, a study of 14 kindreds (characterized by autosomal dominant inheritance of asymptomatic hypercalcemia, normal PTH levels, low urinary calcium excretion, and failure of subtotal parathyroidectomy to normalize calcium) showed normal lumbar spine and forearm bone mineral density (BMD) in patients with FHH and that FHH patients had comparable fracture risk to their normocalcemic relatives [15, 57].

There have been reports of chondrocalcinosis and pancreatitis in patients with FHH1 in particular [16]. CaSRs are expressed in the human pancreas, with the highest expression in the exocrine ducts, and have been theorized to play multiple roles in the pancreas, with abnormal CaSRs possibly leading in some way to pancreatitis [17]. There are also studies, however, which dispute the connection between FHH and pancreatitis. Patients with FHH1 have been reported to have rates of nephrolithiasis and osteopenia comparable to those in the general population [18]. Patients with FHH3 tend to have more severe phenotypic and biochemical profiles compared to FHH1 and FHH2, with symptomatic hypercalcemia (>20% of cases), low bone mineral density (>50% of cases), and childhood cognitive deficits (>75% of cases) [19]. Increased cognitive disorders have particularly been associated with the Arg15Leu mutation in AP2S1 in FHH3 [19, 40].

Diagnosis

Although often a family history of hypercalcemia is unknown at the initial visit of an individual patient, especially as FHH tends to be asymptomatic, an accurate family history asking in detail about calcium disorders, complications of hypercalcemia, and parathyroidectomy history should be obtained. A positive family history can be very useful in making the diagnosis, especially if the onset of the hypercalcemia is early in childhood [50]. A known family history was shown to be the most important predictor for having a *CASR* mutation in a previous study. In that same study, a personal history of an unsuccessful parathyroidectomy was also shown to be a valuable predictor of molecularly confirmed FHH1; 23% of patients who underwent unsuccessful parathyroidectomies with persistent hypercalcemia had verified *CASR* mutations (testing for FHH2 and FHH3 was not done in that study) [20].

FHH is classically characterized by longstanding, mild to moderate hypercalcemia with an inappropriately normal to elevated PTH and low urinary calcium excretion. Serum calcium levels usually do not exceed greater than 10% above than the upper limit of normal (usually less than 12 mg/dL) and do not progress throughout life [21, 22]. Eighty percent of FHH patients have normal intact PTH levels, while 20% have mildly elevated PTH levels [23]. Serum phosphorus levels are usually low to normal [22]. Serum magnesium levels are usually high-normal to mildly elevated [24]. Interestingly, the renal dysfunction that can be seen in PHPT is not present in FHH, despite lifelong hypercalcemia [50, 55]. Both 25OH vitamin D and $1,25(OH)_2$ vitamin D levels are usually within the normal range in FHH [25]. There can be biochemical differences between FHH1, FHH2, and FHH3. In general, patients with FHH1 and FHH2 have similar phenotypes, but patients with FHH3 tend to have higher serum calcium and magnesium levels without differences in serum phosphorus and PTH levels [26, 38]. The clinical and biochemical phenotypes of FHH are shown in Table 8.1.

About 95% of FHH patients demonstrate low urinary calcium excretion [26]. When patients on normal calcium diets demonstrate marked hypocalciuria in a 24-hour urine collection, FHH should be suspected, although other etiologies for low urine calcium excretion to consider in the differential diagnosis are low dietary calcium intake, thiazide diuretic use, vitamin D deficiency, chronic kidney disease, and lithium use [27]. The calcium-to-creatinine clearance ratio (CCCR), equivalent to the fractional excretion of calcium, is an important measurement used in differentiating PHPT from FHH. The measurement requires a concurrently assessed

Table 8.1 Characteristics of patients with familial hypocalciuric hypercalcemia 1–3 and primary hyperparathyroidism

	Serum Ca	PTH	Urine Ca excretion	Serum phos	Serum Mg	eGFR	Possible symptoms
FHH1	↑	– to ↑	↓	– to ↓	– to ↑	–	Usually asymptomatic
FHH2	↑	– to ↑	↓	– to ↓	– to ↑	–	Usually asymptomatic
FHH3	↑↑	– to ↑	↓↓	– to ↓	↑	–	Low BMD, neuropsychiatric abnormalities
PHPT	↑ to ↑↑↑ (depending on the severity of the disease)	↑ to ↑↑↑ (depending on the severity of the disease)	– to ↑ to ↑↑↑ (depending on the severity of the disease)	– to ↓	–	– to ↓	Hypercalcemia symptoms, low BMD, renal stones or can be asymptomatic

↑ = increased; ↓ = decreased; – = unaffected

serum calcium, serum creatinine, 24-hour urine calcium, and 24-hour urine creatinine, which are usually a routine part of the workup for PHPT to ensure the correct diagnosis is made [28]. Spot urine calcium and creatinine can also be used to determine the CCCR [51].

$$CCCR = \frac{\text{Urine calcium} \times \text{Serum creatinine}}{\text{Urine creatinine} \times \text{Serum calcium}}$$

Traditionally it has been recommended that a CCCR cutoff of <0.01 is suggestive of FHH, while >0.02 is suggestive of PHPT, and CCCRs of 0.01–0.02 are in an area of uncertainty. Variable cutoff values to differentiate PHPT from FHH have been proposed, but none of them are perfect, considering the overlap between the two diseases [46]. In general, CCCR is a sensitive tool, but has low specificity. While 80% of PHPT patients have a CCCR >0.01, up to 20% of FHH patients can also have a CCCR >0.01 [46]. Of note, FHH3 patients have been noted to have more severe hypocalciuria with reduced CCCR compared to FHH1 patients [26, 38].

If there is still suspicion that a patient has FHH, especially with CCCR <0.02, the individual should be referred for genetic testing to solidify the diagnosis and prevent unnecessary parathyroidectomy in the case of FHH [29, 36]. In very rare cases, there have been reports of coexisting FHH and PHPT, where a parathyroid lesion with pathology suggestive of a parathyroid adenoma was surgically removed. At least in one case, hypercalcemia was detected again a week postoperatively, and the patient was ultimately confirmed to have a *CASR* mutation in keeping with the diagnosis of FHH [30, 37].

Parathyroid localization studies are not recommended in FHH, unless there is suspicion for coexisting PHPT. Patients with FHH have been reported to have normal to mildly hyperplasic parathyroid glands on pathology. In an older study, FHH glands were noted to have increased parathyroid parenchymal area compared to normal subjects, but smaller than PHPT patients; the authors suggested that the mild hyperplasia may be a reflection of the PTH oversecretion in FHH [31, 41]. Another study of the pathology in FHH reported that parathyroid glands from patients with FHH are larger than those from normal subjects. Unlike the pure parenchymal cell hyperplasia with few adipocytes seen in PHPT, glands from patients with FHH can exhibit lipohyperplasia with a lipid/parenchymal distribution closer to that of normal parathyroid cells [32, 41].

Of note, in patients who have negative genetic testing for FHH, but have a preexisting autoimmune disease with neither a prior personal or family history of hypercalcemia nor hyperfunctioning parathyroid glands, suspicion may be raised for the possibility of very rare autoimmune hypocalciuric hypercalcemia (AHH), which has been documented in only a few case reports [39]. AHH, caused by inactivating CaSR autoantibodies, mimics the biochemical profile of FHH, although PTH levels have been reported to be significantly more elevated in AHH than in FHH [33].

Management/Treatment

It is very important to differentiate FHH from PHPT as management of the two is very different. Unlike in PHPT, parathyroidectomy is not beneficial in FHH. Patients with FHH who undergo subtotal parathyroidectomies may have an initial decline of serum calcium after surgery, but within a few days postoperatively will have a recurrence of the hypercalcemia [26]. With the potentially lifelong complications that can occur from parathyroidectomies (recurrent nerve injury and hypoparathyroidism), surgery is not recommended as treatment for FHH [4].

The majority of FHH patients will live asymptomatically with mild to moderate hypercalcemia through their lifetimes and do not need treatment. There have been a growing number of case reports which support the use of calcimimetics for treatment in FHH patients who are symptomatic or have complications related to hypercalcemia. Calcimimetics are allosteric agonists of the CaSR that enhance its affinity for calcium in parathyroid cells and in the kidney, resulting in decreased PTH secretion and increased renal calcium excretion [42]. These changes lead to a lowering of serum calcium, but not always a normalization of the serum calcium levels. In vitro studies have shown that the calcimimetic cinacalcet, in particular, can allosterically modulate CaSR signaling function. Cinacalcet has been also shown in vitro to overcome CaSR signaling abnormalities in cells expressing the mutant molecules involved in causing FHH2 and FHH3 [34].

Currently, the only oral calcimimetic available is cinacalcet. In the United States, this drug is FDA-approved for secondary hyperparathyroidism in patients with endstage renal disease receiving dialysis, for the nonsurgical management of PHPT in patients unwilling or unable to undergo surgery, and for the management of hypercalcemia in patients with parathyroid carcinoma. It has been reported in a small number of studies to reduce serum calcium and PTH levels, increase renal calcium clearance, and improve symptoms of hypercalcemia in FHH1/FHH2/FHH3 [34, 35, 52–54, 56]. The longest study to date has followed patients for up to 3 years and saw sustained improvement in calcium and PTH levels with good tolerability of cinacalcet.

Case

A 41-year-old female presented with a serum calcium level of 11.0 mg/dL. She denied any hypercalcemic symptoms. She reported a history of serum calcium levels as high as 13 mg/dL with elevated urinary calcium levels which led to a 3.5 gland parathyroidectomy when she was 24 years old. She was not taking any prescribed medications or supplements. Her family history included a father with hypercalcemia and kidney stones, who had also had a 3.5 gland parathyroidectomy; a brother, sister, and daughter with hypercalcemia; and a son with hypercalcemia and a history of three episodes of pancreatitis. Her review of symptoms was negative. Her physical exam was unremarkable. On further evaluation, her serum calcium levels were 10.3–11.6 mg/dL with intact PTH levels of 30–60 pg/mL (normal, 15–65 pg/mL). Her renal function and 25OH vitamin D levels were normal. Her 24-hour urine calcium was 183 mg/day with CCCR 0.017. Her DXA scan showed normal bone mineralization, and renal ultrasound did not show nephrolithiasis. CaSR gene sequencing showed a heterozygous *CASR* mutation (R220W with a tryptophan for arginine substitution in the human *CASR*) previously reported in FHH and confirming the diagnosis in this patient and her family members.

This clinical case emphasizes that asymptomatic hypercalcemia with inappropriately normal PTH levels is found in FHH1 and that the history of failed subtotal parathyroidectomies in multiple family members is a strong clue. Interestingly, this patient did have a strong family history of hypercalcemia, and her father and son both had complications of hypercalcemia, which is unusual for FHH1. Of note, this patient did not have impressively low urine calcium excretion, and this is noted in a small percentage of FHH patients. The challenges of arriving at the correct diagnosis in this kindred illustrate the importance of performing genetic evaluation to make the definitive diagnosis of FHH early, as it will impact future management of the patient's and her family's hypercalcemia.

References

1. Varghese J, Rich T, Jimenez C. Benign familial hypocalciuric hypercalcemia. Endocr Pract. 2011;17 Suppl 1:13–7.
2. Hinnie J, Bell E, McKillop E, Gallacher S. The prevalence of familial hypocalciuric hypercalcemia. Calcif Tissue Int. 2001;68(4):216–8.

3. Dershem R, et al. Familial hypocalciuric hypercalcemia type 1 and autosomal-dominant hypocalcemia type 1: prevalence in a large healthcare population. Am J Hum Genet. 2020;106(6):734–47.
4. Hovden S, Gorvin CM, Metpally RPR, Krishnamurthy S, Smelser DT, Hannan FM, et al. AP2S1 and GNA11 mutations - not a common cause of familial hypocalciuric hypercalcemia. Eur J Endocrinol. 2017;176(2):177–85.
5. Hannan FM, Kallay E, Chang W, Brandi ML, Thakker RV. The calcium-sensing receptor in physiology and in calcitropic and noncalcitropic diseases. Nat Rev Endocrinol. 2018;15(1):33–51.
6. Brown EM, Hebert SC. The First Annual Bayard D. Catherwood Memorial Lecture. Ca2+-receptor-mediated regulation of parathyroid and renal function. Am J Med Sci. 1996;312(3):99–109.
7. Janicic N, Pausova Z, Cole DE, Hendy GN. Insertion of an Alu sequence in the Ca(2+)-sensing receptor gene in familial hypocalciuric hypercalcemia and neonatal severe hyperparathyroidism. Am J Hum Genet. 1995;56(4):880–6.
8. Pollak MR, Brown EM, Chou YH, Hebert SC, Marx SJ, Steinmann B, et al. Mutations in the human Ca(2+)-sensing receptor gene cause familial hypocalciuric hypercalcemia and neonatal severe hyperparathyroidism. Am J Med. 1984;76(6):1021–6.
9. Attie MF, Gill JR, Stock JL, Spiegel AM, Downs RW Jr, Levine MA, et al. Urinary calcium excretion in familial hypocalciuric hypercalcemia. Persistence of relative hypocalciuria after induction of hypoparathyroidism. J Clin Invest. 1983;72(2):667–76.
10. Watanabe H, Sutton RA. Renal calcium handling in familial hypocalciuric hypercalcemia. Kidney Int. 1983;24(3):353–7.
11. Vannucci L, Brandi ML. Familial hypocalciuric hypercalcemia and neonatal severe hyperparathyroidism. Front Horm Res. 2019;51:52–62.
12. Ward BK, Magno AL, Walsh JP, Ratajczak T. The role of the calcium-sensing receptor in human disease. Clin Biochem. 2012;45(12):943–53.
13. Marx SJ, Goltzman D. Evolution of our understanding of the hyperparathyroid syndromes: a historical perspective. J Bone Miner Res. 2019;34(1):22–37.
14. Lee JY, Shoback DM. Familial hypocalciuric hypercalcemia and related disorders. Best Pract Res Clin Endocrinol Metab. 2018;32(5):609–19.
15. Christensen SE, Nissen PH, Vestergaard P, Heickendorff L, Rejnmark L, Brixen K, et al. Skeletal consequences of familial hypocalciuric hypercalcaemia vs. primary hyperparathyroidism. Clin Endocrinol. 2009;71(6):798–807.
16. Al-Salameh A, Cetani F, Pardi E, Vulpoi C, Pierre P, de Calan L, et al. A novel mutation in the calcium-sensing receptor in a French family with familial hypocalciuric hypercalcaemia. Eur J Endocrinol. 2011;165(2):359–63.
17. Rácz GZ, Kittel A, Riccardi D, Case RM, Elliott AC, Varga G, et al. Extracellular calcium sensing receptor in human pancreatic cells. Gut. 2002;51(5):705–11.
18. Marx SJ. Calcimimetic use in familial hypocalciuric hypercalcemia-a perspective in endocrinology. J Clin Endocrinol Metab. 2017;102(11):3933–6.
19. Hannan FM, Babinsky VN, Thakker RV. Disorders of the calcium-sensing receptor and partner proteins: insights into the molecular basis of calcium homeostasis. J Mol Endocrinol. 2016;47(3):R127–42.
20. Nissen PH. Molecular genetic analysis of the calcium sensing receptor gene in patients clinically suspected to have familial hypocalciuric hypercalcemia: phenotypic variation and mutation spectrum in a Danish population. J Clin Endocrinol Metab. 2007;92(11):4373–9.
21. Leech C, Lohse P, Stanojevic V, Lechner A, Göke B, Spitzweg C. Identification of a novel inactivating R465Q mutation of the calcium-sensing receptor. Biochem Biophys Res Commun. 2006;342(3):996–1002.
22. Eldeiry LS, Ruan DT, Brown EM, Gaglia JL, Garber JR. Primary hyperparathyroidism and familial hypocalciuric hypercalcemia: relationships and clinical implications. Endocr Pract. 2012;18(3):412–7.

23. Firek AF, Kao PC, Heath H 3rd. Plasma intact parathyroid hormone (PTH) and PTH-related peptide in familial benign hypercalcemia: greater responsiveness to endogenous PTH than in primary hyperparathyroidism. J Clin Endocrinol Metab. 1991;72(3):541–6.

24. Marini F, Cianferotti L, Giusti F, Brandi ML. Molecular genetics in primary hyperparathyroidism: the role of genetic tests in differential diagnosis, disease prevention strategy, and therapeutic planning. A 2017 update. Clin Cases Miner Bone Metab. 2017;14(1):60–70.

25. Christensen SE, Nissen PH, Vestergaard P, Heickendorff L, Rejnmark L, Brixen K, et al. Plasma 25-hydroxyvitamin D, 1,25-dihydroxyvitamin D, and parathyroid hormone in familial hypocalciuric hypercalcemia and primary hyperparathyroidism. Eur J Endocrinol. 2008;159(6):719–27.

26. Cetani F, Saponaro F, Borsari S, Marcocci C. Familial and hereditary forms of primary hyperparathyroidism. Front Horm Res. 2019;51:40–51.

27. O'Connell K, Yen TW, Shaker J, Wilson SD, Evans DB, Wang TS. Low 24-hour urine calcium levels in patients with sporadic primary hyperparathyroidism: is further evaluation warranted prior to parathyroidectomy? Am J Surg. 2015;210(1):123–8.

28. Bilezikian JP, Brandi ML, Eastell R, Silverberg SJ, Udelsman R, Marcocci C, et al. Guidelines for the management of asymptomatic primary hyperparathyroidism: summary statement from the Fourth International Workshop. J Clin Endocrinol Metab. 2014;99(10):3561–9.

29. Eastell R, Brandi ML, Costa AG, D'Amour P, Shoback DM, Thakker RV. Diagnosis of asymptomatic primary hyperparathyroidism: proceedings of the Fourth International Workshop. J Clin Endocrinol Metab. 2014;99(10):3570–9.

30. Papadakis M, Meurer N, Margariti T, Meyer A, Weyerbrock N, Dotzenrath C. A novel mutation of the calcium-sensing receptor gene in a German subject with familial hypocalciuric hypercalcemia and primary hyperparathyroidism. Hormones (Athens). 2016;15(4):557–9.

31. Thorgeirsson U, Costa J, Marx SJ. The parathyroid glands in familial hypocalciuric hypercalcemia. Hum Pathol. 1981;12(3):229–37.

32. Fukumoto S, Chikatsu N, Okazaki R, Takeuchi Y, Tamura Y, Murakami T, et al. Inactivating mutations of calcium-sensing receptor results in parathyroid lipohyperplasia. Diagn Mol Pathol. 2001;10(4):242–7.

33. Miñambres I, Corcoy R, Weetman AP, Kemp EH. Autoimmune hypercalcemia due to autoantibodies against the calcium-sensing receptor. J Clin Endocrinol Metab. 2020;105(7):dgaa219.

34. Gorvin CM, Hannan FM, Cranston T, Valta H, Makitie O, Schalin-Jantti C, et al. Cinacalcet rectifies hypercalcemia in a patient with familial hypocalciuric hypercalcemia type 2 (FHH2) caused by a germline loss-of-function Gα11 mutation. J Bone Miner Res. 2018;33(1):32–41.

35. Mayr B, Schnabel D, Dörr HG, Schöfl C. Genetics in endocrinology: gain and loss of function mutations of the calcium-sensing receptor and associated proteins: current treatment concepts. Eur J Endocrinol. 2016;174(5):R189–208.

36. Szalat A, Shpitzen S, Tsur A, Zalmon Koren I, Shilo S, Tripto-Shkolnik L, et al. Stepwise CaSR, AP2S1, and GNA11 sequencing in patients with suspected familial hypocalciuric hypercalcemia. Endocrine. 2017;55(3):741–7.

37. Forde HE, Hill AD, Smith D. Parathyroid adenoma in a patient with familial hypocalciuric hypercalcaemia. BMJ Case Rep. 2014;2014:bcr2014206473.

38. Vargas-Poussou R, Mansour-Hendili L, Baron S, Bertocchio JP, Travers C, Simian C, et al. Familial hypocalciuric hypercalcemia types 1 and 3 and primary hyperparathyroidism: similarities and differences. J Clin Endocrinol Metab. 2016;101(5):2185–95.

39. Pallais JC, Kifor O, Chen YB, Slovik D, Brown EM. Acquired hypocalciuric hypercalcemia due to autoantibodies against the calcium-sensing receptor. N Engl J Med. 2004;351:362–9.

40. Nesbit MA, Hannan FM, Howles SA, Babinsky VN, Head RA, Cranston T, et al. Mutations affecting G-protein subunit α11 in hypercalcemia and hypocalcemia. N Engl J Med. 2013;368(26):2476–86.

41. Law WM Jr, Carney JA, Heath H. Parathyroid glands in familial benign hypercalcemia (familial hypocalciuric hypercalcemia). Am J Med. 1984;76(6):1021–6.

42. Babinsky VN, Hannan FM, Gorvin CM, Howles SA, Nesbit MA, Rust N, et al. Allosteric modulation of the calcium-sensing receptor rectifies signaling abnormalities associated with G-protein α-11 mutations causing hypercalcemic and hypocalcemic disorders. J Biol Chem. 2016;291(20):10876–85.

43. Mastromatteo E, Lamacchia O, Campo MR, Conserva A, Baorda F, Cinque L, et al. A novel mutation in calcium-sensing receptor gene associated to hypercalcemia and hypercalciuria. BMC Endocr Disord. 2014;14:81.

44. Hannan FM, Howles SA, Rogers A, Cranston T, Gorvin CM, Babinsky VN, et al. Adaptor protein-2 sigma subunit mutations causing familial hypocalciuric hypercalcaemia type 3 (FHH3) demonstrate genotype-phenotype correlations, codon bias and dominant-negative effects. Hum Mol Genet. 2015;24(18):5079–92.

45. Pollak MR, Brown EM, Chou YH, Hebert SC, Marx SJ, Steinmann B, et al. Mutations in the human Ca(2+)-sensing receptor gene cause familial hypocalciuric hypercalcemia and neonatal severe hyperparathyroidism. Cell. 1993;75(7):1297–303.

46. Bhangu JS, Selberherr A, Brammen L, Scheuba C, Riss P. Efficacy of calcium excretion and calcium/creatinine clearance ratio in the differential diagnosis of familial hypocalciuric hypercalcemia and primary hyperparathyroidism. Head Neck. 2019;41(5):1372–8.

47. Lietman SA, Tenenbaum-Rakover Y, Jap TS, Yi-Chi W, De-Ming Y, Ding C, et al. A novel loss-of-function mutation, Gln459Arg, of the calcium-sensing receptor gene associated with apparent autosomal recessive inheritance of familial hypocalciuric hypercalcemia. J Clin Endocrinol Metab. 2009;94(11):4372–9.

48. Foley TP Jr, Harrison HC, Arnaud CD, Harrison HE. Familial benign hypercalcemia. J Pediatr. 1972;81(6):1060–7.

49. Sadacharan D, Mahadevan S, Rao SS, Kumar AP, Swathi S, Kumar S, et al. Neonatal severe primary hyperparathyroidism: a series of four cases and their long-term management in India. Indian J Endocrinol Metab. 2020;24(2):196–201.

50. Marx SJ, Spiegel AM, Levine MA, Rizzoli RE, Lasker RD, Santora AC, et al. Familial hypocalciuric hypercalcemia: the relation to primary parathyroid hyperplasia. N Engl J Med. 1982;307(7):416–26.

51. Foley KF, Boccuzzi L. Urine calcium: laboratory measurement and clinical utility. Lab Med. 2010;41(11):683–6.

52. Rasmussen AQ, Jørgensen NR, Schwarz P. Clinical and biochemical outcomes of cinacalcet treatment of familial hypocalciuric hypercalcemia: a case series. J Med Case Rep. 2011;5:564.

53. Alon US, VandeVoorde RG. Beneficial effect of cinacalcet in a child with familial hypocalciuric hypercalcemia. Pediatr Nephrol. 2010;25(9):1747–50.

54. Festen-Spanjer B, Haring CM, Koster JB, Mudde AH. Correction of hypercalcaemia by cinacalcet in familial hypocalciuric hypercalcaemia. Clin Endocrinol. 2008;68(2):324–5.

55. Nair CG, Babu M, Jacob P, Menon R, Mathew J, Unnikrishnan. Renal dysfunction in primary hyperparathyroidism; effect of parathyroidectomy: a retrospective cohort study. Int J Surg. 2016;36(Pt A):383–7.

56. Timmers HJ, Karperien M, Hamdy NA, de Boer H, Hermus AR. Normalization of serum calcium by cinacalcet in a patient with hypercalcaemia due to a de novo inactivating mutation of the calcium-sensing receptor. J Intern Med. 2006;260(2):177–82.

57. Law WM, Wahner HW, Heath H. Bone mineral density and skeletal fractures in familial benign hypercalcemia (hypocalciuric hypercalcemia). Mayo Clin Proc. 1984;59(12):811–5.

Chapter 9
Overview of Hypercalcemia of Malignancy and Humoral Hypercalcemia of Malignancy

Azeez Farooki

Overview of the Mechanisms of Hypercalcemia of Malignancy

Hypercalcemia of malignancy (HCM) is common in patients with cancer, occurring in up to 30% of patients with disseminated solid tumors, including most often lung cancer, renal cell carcinoma, and breast carcinoma, as well as several types of hematologic malignancies [1]. Indeed, hypercalcemia almost always arises in the context of advanced cancer, its clinical presentation varying by degree and rapidity of onset, ranging from asymptomatic hypercalcemia detected on routine blood work to rapidly developing confusion and orthostasis. When patients do not have a cancer diagnosis and present with severe PTH-independent hypercalcemia, HCM should be considered in the differential diagnosis as it can cause acute, severe hypercalcemia.

Parathyroid hormone (PTH)-independent HCM is characterized by suppressed PTH and may be mediated through various mechanisms: via humoral HCM, wherein tumors secrete PTH-related peptide (PTHrP); via local osteolytic lesions; and via overproduction of 1,25-dihydroxyvitamin D (calcitriol). More than one mechanism may be operating simultaneously and need to be targeted for treatment, especially in patients who are refractory to standard calcium-lowering treatments. Notably, when primary hyperparathyroidism coexists with HCM, the PTH value may be non-suppressed (>20 pg/mL). Furthermore, PTHrP may be slightly elevated in normocalcemic malignancy [2] but is markedly elevated in cases of humoral HCM. Among the hypercalcemic patients with solid tumors in the seminal Burtis study, 80% had plasma PTHrP concentration above normal.

Local osteolysis resulting from metastatic bone lesions or advanced cancer involving the bone (multiple myeloma) is a major mechanism of HCM, occurring in

A. Farooki (✉)
Division of Endocrinology, Memorial Sloan Kettering Cancer Center, New York, NY, USA
e-mail: farookia@mskcc.org

© The Author(s), under exclusive license to Springer Nature Switzerland AG 2022
M. D. Walker (ed.), *Hypercalcemia*, Contemporary Endocrinology, https://doi.org/10.1007/978-3-030-93182-7_9

approximately 10–20% of patients with multiple myeloma at diagnosis (see Chap. 10) [3]. When local osteolytic lesions mediate HCM, a "vicious cycle" hypothesis has been proposed, in which osteolysis from metastatic bone lesions or advanced multiple myeloma cells invade the bone and then activate bone remodeling on nearby osteoblasts and osteoclasts via locally secreted stimulatory factors (such as PTHrP, bone morphogenetic protein [BMP], transforming growth factor beta [TGF-β], insulin-like growth factor [IGF], vascular endothelial growth factor [VEGF], endothelin-1 [ET1], and wingless-related integration site [WNT]), in turn causing the release of growth factors stored in the bone matrix, stimulating the tumor cells, and fueling the cycle [4]. In this context, PTHrP acts as a paracrine factor rather than an endocrine "humor" as in humoral hypercalcemia. Among solid tumors, prostate cancer has the lowest rate of hypercalcemia, likely because it features osteoblastic metastases that can consume calcium [5].

In other hematologic malignancies, hypercalcemia is usually linked to overproduction of calcitriol, which is thought to be driven by increased activity of 1-alpha-hydroxylase in macrophages or by PTHrP- or hypophosphatemia-mediated stimulation. A retrospective case-control study found that the prevalence of hypercalcemia in non-Hodgkin-lymphoma is 1.3–7.4% and in diffuse large B-cell lymphoma (DLBCL) is 18% at diagnosis. This mechanism has also been described in Hodgkin lymphoma, lymphomatosis/granulomatosis, pancreatic neuroendocrine tumor [6], ovarian dysgerminomas, and, very recently, various solid tumor types [7].

Humoral hypercalcemia of malignancy (HHM), the primary focus of this chapter, involves systemic PTHrP production by the tumor and endocrine secretion into the systemic circulation. This mechanism has been described in many tumor types: squamous cell carcinomas (lung, head, and neck), renal carcinoma, bladder carcinoma, breast carcinoma, ovarian carcinoma, prostate carcinoma, colorectal carcinoma, non-Hodgkin lymphoma, chronic myelogenous leukemia, and other blood cancers [8]. These patients typically have advanced cancer and a poor prognosis although there are exceptions, such as with some neuroendocrine tumors [9–11].

An often-cited breakdown of its causes attributing 80% of HCM as PTHrP-mediated is based on two relatively small studies [12, 13] which evaluated 50 and 38 consecutive patients with HCM, respectively. The more recent study by Burtis et al., in 1990, showed PTHrP elevation and biochemical evidence of PTHrP activity (elevated urinary cyclic AMP excretion) in 30 of 38 patients, 9 with metastatic bone disease and 6 without radiologic evaluation; the contribution of metastatic bone disease to hypercalcemia is unknown. Solid tumors produce PTHrP much more commonly than hematologic cancers. A recent retrospective series by Donovan et al., only including patients with elevated PTHrP ($n = 138$), reports that PTHrP-mediated hypercalcemia is most often found in solid tumors (83%, with breast and lung cancers the most common), 9% of cases were related to hematologic malignancy (most often non-Hodgkin lymphoma), and another 9% were related to benign causes [8]. The median survival was 52 days for patients with solid tumors and 326 days for patients with hematologic cancers.

Humoral Hypercalcemia of Malignancy: History, Pathophysiology, and Detection

Humoral HCM is systemic PTHrP-mediated hypercalcemia. Secretion of a "PTH-like" substance into the systemic circulation was first hypothesized by Fuller Albright in 1941 based on his clinical observation of a case of renal cell carcinoma with bone metastases that featured both hypercalcemia and hypophosphatemia [14]. If bone lysis was the cause of hypercalcemia, elevations in both calcium and phosphate would be expected; the case suggested that the tumor could be producing a factor inducing both hypercalcemia and phosphaturia, similar to the physiologic effects of parathyroid hormone.

In the 1980s, patients with HCM were found to frequently have increased nephrogenous cyclic adenosine monophosphate (cAMP) and a novel circulating protein similar to PTH that led to increased adenylate cyclase activity in rat osteosarcoma cells [15]. In 1987, this protein – which was named parathyroid hormone-related peptide (PTHrP) given its structural and functional similarity to PTH [1] – was purified from a patient with squamous cell carcinoma of the lung and humoral HCM [10]. The genes for PTH and PTHrP are found on chromosomes 11 and 12, respectively, and gene duplication of PTH is thought to be the teleologic origin of PTHrP. PTHrP is homologous with PTH at the first 13 amino acids of the amino terminal end [16], and both can activate the PTH1 receptor; thereafter the peptide sequences diverge. PTHrP exists in several isoforms created by differential splicing and posttranslational processing, ranging in size from 60 to 173 amino acids. The initial PTHrP messenger ribonucleic acid translation products are PTHrP-(1–139), PTHrP-(1–141), and PTHrP-(1–173); these undergo posttranslational cleavage by prohormone convertases to yield various mature secretory forms of PTHrP.

The pathophysiology of PTHrP-induced HCM involves increased resorption of bone and increased distal tubular renal calcium reabsorption. Like PTH, PTHrP activates cAMP and other second messengers (inositol phosphate, protein kinases A and C, and phospholipase C) [17], inducing expression of RANKL in osteoblasts, which then binds the RANK receptor in osteoclasts, inducing osteoclast maturation and proliferation. In humans, continuous PTHrP infusion appears to uncouple bone turnover to some extent, increasing bone resorption (serum CTX) while decreasing bone formation (P1NP), thereby creating calcium efflux from bone without a corresponding calcium influx, contributing to hypercalcemia [18].

The extent to which PTHrP induces calcitriol production is unclear. Although one study associated PTHrP-mediated hypercalcemia with suppressed serum calcitriol [19], in healthy volunteers continuous, PTHrP administration is associated with increased serum calcitriol, albeit to a lesser extent versus PTH [20, 21]. Elevated calcitriol levels have been reported in patients with solid tumors and HCM in case reports and a retrospective study of patients with hypercalcemia of malignancy [7]. When the cohort was divided into elevated calcitriol and normal calcitriol groups, PTHrP elevation was significantly more common in patients with elevated calcitriol compared to those without elevated calcitriol (76% vs 52%; $p = 0.025$). The study found no correlation between PTHrP and calcitriol, however.

Detection of PTHrP can be challenging and the current assays require standardization. Given their divergent amino acid sequences, immunoassays for PTH cannot detect PTHrP [22]. Assays for PTHrP detect its fragments, and the results of assays from different manufacturers are not comparable. PTHrP is also unstable in plasma and requires collection in tubes containing protease inhibitors and EDTA (ethylenediaminetetraacetic acid), as well as separation within 30 minutes. The C-terminal of PTHrP is more stable and easier to assay than the N-terminal, but assays measuring C-terminal fragments are impacted by renal function, producing falsely higher values in patients with renal insufficiency. N-terminal fragments are less influenced by renal function and yield fewer false positive results. Overall, existing PTHrP assays lack the clinical sensitivity and specificity that are present with other peptide hormone commercial assays.

Rare Causes of Hypercalcemia of Malignancy: HTLV-1/ATLL and Non-parathyroid Tumors

A rare cause of PTHrP-mediated hypercalcemia is adult T-cell leukemia/lymphoma (ATLL) induced by human T-cell leukemia virus type 1 (HTLV-1) [23]. HTLV and HIV, both retroviruses, are frequent co-pathogens. Worldwide, 10–20 million people are infected with HTLV-1, which is endemic to Japan, the Caribbean, Central and South America, and Africa, with seroprevalence 1–37% [24]. The estimated lifetime risk of developing ATLL in a person positive for HTLV-1 is 2–7%, and ATLL has a variable average age at onset depending on geographical region (from age 40 to 60 years) [25].

In the acute form of ATLL, patients present with organomegaly, lymphadenopathy, and leukemia. Severe and refractory hypercalcemia has been shown to complicate ATLL in over 50% of cases and is a chief cause of early mortality due to complications such as renal failure and pancreatitis [26]. Standard therapies for hypercalcemia, including bisphosphonates, may be ineffective. Severe hypercalcemia requiring hemodialysis has been reported, and treatment with denosumab has also been successful [27]. In the lymphoma form, patients present with organomegaly, raised LDH, and occasional hypercalcemia [28].

While elevated PTHrP has been found in patients with ATLL and without hypercalcemia, in general PTHrP is a driver of hypercalcemia in ATLL [29]. Indeed, PTHrP secreted from ATL cells is a frequent contributing factor to hypercalcemia [30], the pathogenesis of which is also driven by elevated serum M-CSF levels, expression of RANKL on ATL cells, and ATL infiltration into the bone marrow. Notably, these patients can develop osteolytic bone lesions that contribute to hypercalcemia via local osteolysis, similar to the mechanism in multiple myeloma [31, 32].

In rare cases PTH is secreted from primary and metastatic non-parathyroid tumors; the ten cases reported in the literature include two small cell lung carcinomas and one case each of squamous cell lung carcinoma, thymoma, ovarian tumor, neuroectodermal cancer, thyroid papillary carcinoma, metastatic rhabdomyosarcoma, pancreatic malignancy, and gastric carcinoma [33–43]. Cultured cells from the squamous cell carcinoma were calcium-sensitive, implying that some of these cases could respond to treatment with cinacalcet, a calcium-sensing receptor agonist.

Treatment of PTHrP-Mediated Hypercalcemia of Malignancy

The usual clinical presentation of PTHrP-mediated hypercalcemia is in patients known to have advanced cancer who present with PTH-independent hypercalcemia. Patients with PTHrP-mediated hypercalcemia often have cachexia [44]. In a hypercalcemic patient without systemic signs of cancer, humoral HCM is very unlikely, and the differential diagnosis should focus on other causes of PTH-independent hypercalcemia, such as granulomatous disease or vitamin D intoxication.

When determining the clinical approach to HCM, it is useful to consider the mechanisms driving hypercalcemia (Table 9.1). The biochemical profile from

Table 9.1 Mechanisms contributing to hypercalcemia of malignancy

	Calcitriol production	PTHrP production (humoral hypercalcemia of malignancy)	Local osteolysis (advanced cancer involving the bone)
Bone resorption	+	+++	+++
GI calcium absorption	+++	a	−
Renal calcium reabsorption	−	+++	−
Hypophosphatemia (less calcium binding = ↑serum calcium)	−	++	−
Therapy specific to a given abnormality[b]	Corticosteroids or other inhibitor of 1-alpha-hydroxylase; Limit dietary calcium intake	Intravenous bisphosphonates or denosumab; Calcitonin; Frequent NS hydration with furosemide; Oral phosphorus therapy	Intravenous bisphosphonates or denosumab[c]; Calcitonin

[a]Potential indirect effect: only if high PTHrP stimulates 1,25-dihydroxyvitamin D production
[b]Note that corticosteroids and phosphorus may be helpful regardless of causative etiology
[c]Intravenous bisphosphonates and denosumab are FDA approved for hypercalcemia of malignancy and are also approved to reduce the risk of skeletal-related events in patients with solid tumors metastatic to bone and multiple myeloma

Table 9.2 Baseline laboratory evaluation for patients

	Normal range (CU)	Normal range (SI)	Case 1 (CU)	Case 1 (SI)	Case 2 (CU)	Case 2 (SI)
Ca	8.5–10.5 mg/dL	2.13–2.63 mmol/L	11.6 mg/dL	2.90 mmol/L	12.0 mg/dL	3.0 mmol/L
P	2.5–4.2 mg/dL	0.81–1.36 mmol/L	1.4 mg/dL	0.45 mmol/L	1.5 mg/dL	0.48 mmol/L
PTH	12–88 pg/mL	12–88 ng/L	11.2 pg/mL	11.2 ng/L	<4.0 pg/mL	11.2 ng/L
PTHrP	14–27 pg/mL	14–27 ng/L	28 pg/mL	28 ng/L	132 pg/mL	132 ng/L
1,25(OH)$_2$D	18–72 pg/mL	46.8–187.2 pmol/L	327 pg/mL	850.2 pmol/L	234 pg/mL	608.4 pmol/L
25(OH)D	30–100 ng/dL	74.88–249.60 nmol/L	19 ng/dL	47.42 nmol/L	14 ng/dL	34.94 nmol/L
ACE	9–67 U/L	0.15–1.12 uat/L	58 U/L	0.97 µKat/L	34 U/L	0.57 µKat/L
BSAP	14.2–42.7 U/L	0.24–0.71 uKat/L	19.9 U/L	0.33 µKat/L	8.3 U/L	0.14 µKat/L
CTX	40–465 pg/ml	40–465 ng/L	–	–	67 pg/mL	67 ng/L
Urine NTX	3–63 BCE	3–63 BCE	12 BCE	12 BCE	–	–
24-hour urine calcium	50–150 mg/day	1.25–3.75 mmol/day	–	–	60 mg/day	1.50 mmol/d

CU conventional units, *SI* International System of Units, *Ca* calcium, *P* phosphorous, *PTH* parathyroid hormone, *PTHrP* parathyroid hormone-related peptide, *ACE* angiotensin-converting enzyme, *BSAP* bone-specific alkaline phosphatase, *CTx* C-telopeptide, *urine NTx* urine N-telopeptide, *24 urine Ca* 24-hour urine calcium

laboratory evaluation typically provides insight into the mechanism (Table 9.2; see cases). Intravenous hydration with normal saline should always be initiated in patients with HCM for serum calcium >12 mg/dL or for lower calcium values with evidence of volume depletion. Patients with serum calcium <12 mg/dL may be followed carefully and advised to hydrate vigorously and avoid calcium supplements, thiazide diuretics, or calcium-fortified foods. Calcitonin, dosed subcutaneously, is effective in rapidly treating acute moderate-to-severe symptomatic hypercalcemia, but its efficacy wanes after 48 hours due to tachyphylaxis. As with granulomatous disease–mediated hypercalcemia, calcitriol-mediated hypercalcemia is most effectively treated with corticosteroids or other inhibitors of 1-alpha-hydroxylase (ketoconazole, rifampin).

Parenteral antiresorptives (intravenous bisphosphonates and denosumab) are the mainstay therapy for humoral hypercalcemia given the contribution of bone resorption mechanisms (calcitriol elevation has the least dependency on bone resorption).

These drugs lower calcium with 24–48 hours after administration. Depending on the success of cancer therapy, parenteral antiresorptives frequently need to be re-dosed to maintain control of serum calcium. Although they are approved for reduction of skeletal-related events in patients with solid tumors metastatic to bone and multiple myeloma, at a frequency of once-monthly dosing, more frequent dosing for uncontrolled hypercalcemia is allowable.

In the context of HCM patients with limited life expectancy, aiming for albumin-corrected calcium levels <12.0 mg/dL is acceptable (although normal calcium levels are preferable), provided that the patient can maintain vigorous oral hydration and calcium levels can be monitored on a regular basis. Although endocrinologists often follow patients with chronically high calcium values (usually in primary hyperparathyroidism), oncologists and other healthcare professionals may need reassurance that these calcium values may be tolerated without the need for hospital admission. For patients who fail to respond to intravenous bisphosphonates, weekly dosing of denosumab 120 mg (the same dose approved once-monthly to decrease skeletal-related events in patients with solid tumors and multiple myeloma) has shown improvement in one study [45].

In refractory cases, it may be necessary to target multiple causative mechanisms to achieve lower calcium (see case 1 and case 2 below). Given that inflammatory cytokines can play a role in local osteolysis due to metastatic bone disease, cortico-steroids can also be considered for highly refractory patients [46]. In a rat model of bisphosphonate- and calcitonin-refractory hypercalcemia, administration of an anti-PTHrP antibody led to increased fractional excretion of calcium and a marked decrease of blood calcium level, highlighting the importance of the renal mecha-nism [47]. Regular administration of intravenous fluids and furosemide (e.g., twice-weekly) is the main method available in the clinic to overcome the effect of PTHrP on renal calcium reabsorption; however patients who are hypercalcemic and volume-depleted should not receive furosemide. Long before the advent of intrave-nous bisphosphonates, therapy with oral and intravenous phosphorus was success-fully used to lower serum calcium levels in HCM [48]. Since PTHrP-mediated hypercalcemia often also causes severe hypophosphatemia, the author frequently utilizes oral phosphorus repletion in refractory HCM cases (see case 1 and case 2). Humoral HCM also responds to cancer therapies such as chemotherapy, chemoem-bolization, radiation, and surgery. Dialysis may be required in patients with severe hypercalcemia refractory to other treatments, as well as those with congestive heart failure or severe renal dysfunction who cannot receive aggressive hydration due to their underlying comorbidities. Chapter 5 provides a further discussion of the treat-ment of hypercalcemia (Fig. 9.1).

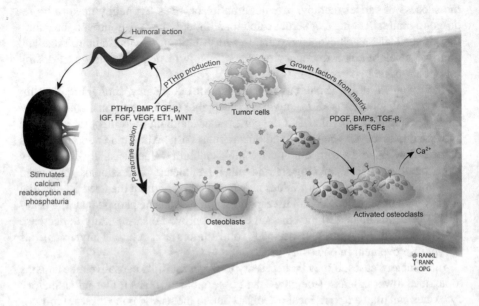

Fig. 9.1 Vicious cycle of metastatic bone disease. OB osteoblast, OC osteoclast. Tumor cells can produce PTHrP in a paracrine or endocrine (humoral) manner. The paracrine secretion of PTHrP along with other cytokines causes activation of bone turnover ("local osteolysis"), thereby liberating bone-derived growth factors which in turn stimulate tumor growth (a vicious cycle). PTHrP may be secreted in a humoral fashion by tumors cells in bone or elsewhere, causing renal calcium reabsorption and phosphaturia as well as activation of bone resorption. PTHrP secreted in a humoral manner may be measured with PTHrP assays

Conclusions

Hypercalcemia of malignancy occurs commonly in patients with many types of cancer. The pathophysiology may involve multiple mechanisms. It may be refractory to standard measures such as FDA-approved oncologic doses of zoledronic acid and denosumab, leading to substantially impaired quality of life for patients experiencing the symptoms of hypercalcemia and repeated inpatient admissions. Given that multiple mechanism may contribute to hypercalcemia in this context, therapy should be tailored to each likely driver of HCM as clinically feasible, including elevated bone resorption, increased calcitriol production, PTHrP-driven renal calcium retention, and hypophosphatemia. Calcitriol levels should be checked for elevation in patients with solid tumors and lymphoma; if elevated levels are found, granulomatous disease should be ruled out. Patients with elevated calcitriol should avoid vitamin D supplements and calcium-fortified foods. Corticosteroid therapy may also be attempted. Elevated PTHrP may cause renal calcium retention; frequent IV fluids along with furosemide to induce calciuresis may be beneficial. Significant hypophosphatemia should also be diagnosed and treated with the aim of improving hypercalcemia.

Cases of Refractory Hypercalcemia of Malignancy with Contribution from PTHrP Elevation and Other Mechanisms

Case 1

A 41-year-old woman was referred to endocrinology clinic for refractory hypercalcemia. She had a history of breast cancer with pathological examination consistent with invasive ductal carcinoma (*BRACA1+*, *ER+*, *PR–*, *Her2/neu–*). She underwent bilateral mastectomy and received multiple lines of chemotherapies. Her course was complicated by biopsy-proven liver metastasis and bone metastases. At the time of presentation, she was enrolled in an investigational protocol with cyclophosphamide and a poly(ADP-ribose) polymerase (PARP) inhibitor and had suffered from hypercalcemia for 6 months despite receiving multiple courses of intravenous (IV) fluid hydration, monthly denosumab (120 mg), and two doses of IV zoledronic acid (4 mg) within a 6-month time period. Approximately 2.5 weeks prior to endocrine consultation, her peak corrected serum calcium was equal to 13.9 mg/dL (8.5–10.5 mg/dL) (SI: 3.48 mmol/L [2.13–2.63 mmol/L]) in the setting of normal renal function and volume status. The patient, however, was also taking calcium carbonate 600 mg once-daily for bone health, which was discontinued a few days prior to endocrinology evaluation.

On initial evaluation, elevations in serum calcium equal to 11.6 mg/dL (8.5–10.5 mg/dL) (SI: 2.90 mmol/L [2.13–2.63 mmol/L]) and $1,25(OH)_2D$ level of 327 pg/mL (18–72 pg/mL) (SI: 850.2 pmol/L [46.8–187.2 pmol/L]) were noted (Table 9.2, Case 1). Calcium levels were often above 12.0 mg/dL (SI: 3 mmol/L). Her $1,25(OH)_2D$ levels had been increasing steadily from 177 pg/mL (SI: 460.2 pmol/L) 1 month earlier and 248 pg/mL (SI: 644.8 pmol/L) 10 days earlier. Phosphorus was low at 1.4 mg/dL (2.5–4.2 mg/dL) (SI: 0.45 mmol/L [0.81–1.36 mmol/L]). The patient had normal angiotensin-converting enzyme at 58 U/L (9–67 U/L) (SI: 0.97 μKat/L [0.15–1.12 μKat/L]), suppressed PTH at 11.2 pg/mL (12–88 pg/mL) (SI: 11.2 ng/L [12–88 ng/L]), a 25(OH)D level of 19 ng/dL (30–100 ng/dL) (SI: 47.42 nmol/L [74.88–249.60 nmol/L]), "low" urine N-terminal telopeptide (NTx) at 12 nmol BCE/mmol creatinine (3–63 nmol BCE/mmol creatinine), and normal bone-specific alkaline phosphatase (BSAP) at 19.9 U/L (14.2–42.7 U/L) (SI: 0.33 μKat/L [0.24–0.71 μKat/L]). Of note, the patient also had slightly elevated PTHrP at 28 pg/mL (14–27 pg/mL) (SI: 28 ng/L [14–27 ng/L]), which had increased from 18 pg/mL (SI: 18 ng/L) 1 month earlier. Phosphorus levels remained <2 mg/dL (2.5–4.2 mg/dL) (SI: 0.65 mmol/L [0.81–1.36 mmol/L]) despite repletion; fractional excretion of phosphate was calculated at 33%, indicating phosphaturesis. Fibroblast growth factor 23 (FGF-23) level was normal. The patient declined collection of a 24-hour urine for calcium. She had a repeat whole-body PET/CT scan, which revealed diffuse osseous metastases (right sacrum and throughout the axial and appendicular skeleton). There was no evidence of granulomatous disease on imaging.

Given the elevated 1,25(OH)$_2$D levels from presumed increased 1-alpha-hydroxylase activity likely related to breast cancer, prednisone 40 mg daily was started. After 5 days of prednisone 40 mg daily, repeat serum calcium normalized from 11.6 mg/dL (SI: 2.9 mmol/L) to 10.3 mg/dL (SI: 2.58 mmol/L), at which time a prednisone taper was started. Once the patient reached a prednisone dose of 15 mg daily after 5 weeks, repeat calcium level was slightly increased again to 11.1 mg/dL (8.5–10.5 mg/dL) (SI: 2.78 mmol/L [2.13–2.63 mmol/L]). The patient's repeat 1,25(OH)$_2$D level remained elevated, but stable at 306 pg/mL (18–72 pg/mL) (SI: 795.6 pmol/L [46.8–187.2 pmol/L]). The patient transferred her oncology care outside the institution; anticancer therapy was changed, serum calcium remained mildly elevated between 10 and 11 mg/dL (SI: 2.50–2.75 mmol/L), and the phosphate requirement improved.

Questions for Discussion

1. What mechanisms were responsible for hypercalcemia in this patient with metastatic breast cancer?

   Answer: This patient likely had HCM due to (1) extrarenal production of calcitriol from tumor-associated macrophages and/or PTHrP stimulation and (2) increased bone resorption resulting from the following:

   • Osteolysis mediated by "local" cytokines stimulating bone resorption in the context of metastatic bone disease
   • Osteolysis mediated by systemically measured PTHrP (humoral HCM)
   • Increased distal tubular calcium reabsorption and proximal tubular-mediated phosphaturia (due to PTHrP)

   Workup for hypercalcemia in patients with malignancy should start by excluding PTH-dependent hypercalcemia. In this patient's case, PTH was suppressed and was unlikely contributing to the hypercalcemia. The rest of the diagnostic workup should include phosphorus, PTHrP, 25-hydroxyvitamin D, and 1,25-dihydroxyvitamin D levels. Other causes of PTH-independent hypercalcemia, such as granulomatous disease not related to cancer, vitamin A toxicity, hyperthyroidism, and milk alkali syndrome, should be excluded.

   This patient had marked elevation in calcitriol, which the Memorial Sloan Kettering retrospective data suggest may be associated with refractory hypercalcemia in solid tumor patients [7]. Although this patient's calcitriol level was clearly inappropriately elevated, it is important to note that a "high normal" calcitriol level in the face of PTH-independent hypercalcemia is also inappropriate. PTHrP is thought to only weakly stimulate calcitriol production and was minimally elevated. Thus, this case suggests a source of calcitriol such as tumor-associated macrophages, which has been described in lymphoma [49]. Increased intestinal calcium absorption induced by high serum calcitriol concentrations is probably the main mechanism of hypercalcemia. Elevated calcitriol has been shown to increase bone resorption and possibly inhibit bone mineralization [50].

This patient also had hypophosphatemia. Patients with calcitriol-mediated hypercalcemia do not typically have hypophosphatemia, and therefore PTHrP was probably the mechanism of hypophosphatemia (via inhibition of proximal tubular phosphate transport).

2. What other management strategies might be employed?

Answer: Given the multiple mechanisms contributing to hypercalcemia, and the fact that this patient was refractory to standard antiresorptive therapies given at approved oncologic doses (monthly zoledronic acid and denosumab), a multipronged treatment approach was used.

First, to reduce calcitriol production in a manner analogous to therapy of granulomatous diseases causing hypercalcemia, steroid therapy was started at a dose of 20–30 mg per day of prednisone. As second-line therapy for those unable to take steroids, a general inhibitor of P450 enzymes, such as ketoconazole, can be used also to decrease calcitriol production via inhibition of 1-alpha-hydroxylase. As gastrointestinal absorption of calcium is markedly increased due to elevated calcitriol levels, patients should be advised to avoid both calcium and vitamin D supplements; hypocalcemia resulting from antiresorptive therapy is not a concern in the context of refractory hypercalcemia. Furthermore, some patients with cancer receive highly calcium-fortified supplements such as Ensure or Boost – these should be avoided, and low-calcium nutritional supplements should be advised. A low-calcium diet is also prudent. However, significant dietary calcium restriction should also be accompanied by a low-oxalate diet to lower the risk for calcium oxalate kidney stones. In addition to their effects inhibiting 1-alpha-hydroxylase and decreasing calcium absorption, steroids have long been known to ameliorate HCM, probably due to a reduction of inflammatory mediators in the bone microenvironment which activate osteoclast activity.

Second, to address the increased bone resorption due to metastatic bone disease and PTHrP, denosumab was continued at 120 mg subcutaneously monthly. It is important to note that weekly denosumab at 120 mg may be given in the setting of hypercalcemia refractory to monthly intravenous bisphosphonates and may result in more efficacious reductions in serum calcium [51], as would be expected with the increased dosing schedule and the slightly higher antiresorptive potency of denosumab. Given that refractory hypercalcemia is an acute situation compromising quality of life and that many such patients have a limited life expectancy, concern for long-term adverse effects (e.g., osteonecrosis of the jaw or atypical femur fracture) with more intensive dosing schedules should not drive treatment decisions. Furthermore, in refractory cases, antiresorptive therapy should not be stopped under the premise it is ineffective.

Third, addressing the PTHrP-driven hypophosphatemia may also ameliorate hypercalcemia. Before the advent of bisphosphonates, intravenous and/or oral phosphate was demonstrated to improve HCM [48, 52]. Calcium phosphate is thought to complex in the blood and be eliminated via the reticuloendothelial system. Furthermore, some patients with PTHrP-driven hypercalcemia have dangerously low phosphorus levels, and these patients should be treated regardless of the severity of the hypercalcemia, although keeping the calcium-phosphorus product to <40 is advisable.

3. Should the patient's 25-hydroxyvitamin D level be repleted?

    Answer: The deficient vitamin D level should not be treated since there could be accelerated conversion to 1,25-dihydroxyvitamin D, exacerbating the hypercalcemia.

Case 2

A 52-year-old woman was referred for refractory hypercalcemia. She had a history of clear cell carcinoma of the ovary. The patient underwent resection and received multiple chemotherapies and immunotherapy, which was followed by a recurrence. Upon initial presentation, the patient's hypercalcemia was refractory to zoledronic acid 4 mg × 2 doses followed by denosumab 120 mg dosed weekly × 3 doses, with serum calcium in the 12–13 mg/dL (SI: 3.0–3.25 mmol/L) range.

On initial evaluation, calcium was consistently elevated to 12 mg/dL or higher (8.5–10.5 mg/dL) (SI: 3 mmol/L [2.13–2.63 mmol/L]) (Table 9.2, case 2). Phosphorus was low at 1.5 mg/dL (2.5–4.2 mg/dL) (SI: 0.48 mmol/L [0.81–1.36 mmol/L]). The patient had normal angiotensin-converting enzyme at 34 U/L (9–67 U/L) (SI: 0.57 µKat/L [0.15–1.12 µKat/L]), suppressed PTH <4.0 pg/mL (12–88 pg/mL) (SI: <4 ng/L [12–88 ng/L]), low 25(OH)D level at 14 ng/dL (30–100 ng/dL) (SI: 34.94 nmol/L [74.88–249.6 nmol/L]), elevated 1,25(OH)$_2$D level at 234 pg/mL (18–72 pg/mL) (SI: 608.4 pmol/L [46.8–187.2 pmol/L]), suppressed serum CTx at 67 pg/mL (40–465 pg/mL) (SI: 67 [40–465 ng/L]), and normal bone-specific alkaline phosphatase (BSAP) at 8.3 U/L (premenopausal range <14.3 U/L) (SI: 0.14 µKat/L [premenopausal range <0.24 µKat/L]). The patient also had a markedly elevated PTHrP at 132 pg/mL (14–27 pg/mL) (SI: 132 ng/L [14–27 ng/L]). Her 24-hour urine levels for calcium, sodium, and phosphorus were 60 mg/24 h (SI: 1.5 mmol/d), 328 mEq/24 h (SI: 328 mmol/d), and 1360 mg/24 h (SI: 43.93 mmol/d), respectively. On imaging, there was no evidence of osseous metastases or granulomatous disease.

This patient had intermittent GI bleeding related to her tumor, and thus prednisone therapy could not be attempted to reduce calcitriol levels. The patient was advised to avoid both dietary calcium (especially calcium-fortified foods such as Ensure) and vitamin D. Ketoconazole therapy was attempted as an alternative strategy to reduce both 1-alpha-hydroxylase activity and calcitriol levels [53, 54]; however, the patient's liver function tests were elevated, and ketoconazole appeared to be poorly tolerated. Denosumab was also continued.

She was given weekly hydration with 2–3 liters of normal saline in addition to intravenous furosemide 40 mg. This strategy succeeded in temporarily reducing the calcium level, but there was a rapid rise in serum calcium over the next few days. The patient was given furosemide to take at home daily, along with vigorous hydration with 1 liter of normal saline self-administered via gravity through her port (4 hours for 1 liter).

Treatment of hypophosphatemia was also started in an attempt to ameliorate the hypercalcemia. Ultimately, through the above measures and a change in anticancer therapy, this patient's calcium normalized.

Questions for Discussion

1. What mechanisms were responsible for hypercalcemia?
   Answer: This patient likely had HCM due to (1) extrarenal calcitriol production of calcitriol from tumor-associated macrophages and/or PTHrP stimulation; (2) increased bone resorption (due to markedly elevated PTHrP levels); and (3) increased distal tubular calcium reabsorption and proximal tubular-mediated phosphaturia (due to PTHrP).
2. What other management strategies might be employed?
   Answer: Since this patient was refractory to standard antiresorptive therapies given at approved oncologic doses (monthly zoledronic acid and denosumab), a multipronged treatment approach was necessary.

First, this patient was not a good candidate for prednisone use to reduce calcitriol production, and therefore ketoconazole, a general inhibitor of P450 enzymes, was attempted [53, 54]. The patient, however, was unable to tolerate it at the necessary doses. Of note, ketoconazole at high doses may cause hypogonadism, hypoadrenalism, hepatotoxicity, and adverse effects (e.g., headache, sedation, nausea, and vomiting).

Second, to address the increased bone resorption due to PTHrP, denosumab was continued at 120 mg subcutaneously monthly. The patient had suppressed levels of bone turnover markers as would be expected after denosumab 120 mg. It is important to note that weekly denosumab 120 mg may be given in the setting of hypercalcemia refractory to monthly intravenous bisphosphonates and may result in more efficacious reduction of serum calcium [51], as would be expected with the increased dosing schedule and the slightly higher antiresorptive potency of denosumab. Given that refractory hypercalcemia is an acute situation compromising quality of life and that many such patients have a limited life expectancy, concern for long-term adverse effects (e.g., osteonecrosis of the jaw or atypical femur fracture) with more intensive dosing schedules should not drive treatment decisions.

Third, another management strategy would be trying to overcome PTHrP-mediated renal calcium retention. The patient's low 24-hour urine calcium value in the setting of hypercalcemia was most certainly driven by PTHrP. This may be treated via intermittent furosemide IV (along with vigorous normal saline hydration) and/or oral furosemide. Furosemide should only be administered in the setting of vigorous hydration and adequate volume status, which is problematic for some hypercalcemic patients to achieve via oral hydration due to nausea.

Of note, PTHrP is not thought to stimulate calcitriol production to the same extent as the parathyroid hormone [19]. Ectopic calcitriol production in solid tumors has rarely been described [7, 55]. Thus, the etiology of this patient's marked calcitriol elevation is unclear.

Treatment of hypophosphatemia was also started in an attempt to ameliorate the hypercalcemia. Before the advent of bisphosphonates, intravenous and/or oral phosphate was demonstrated to improve HCM [48, 52]. Calcium phosphate is thought to complex in the blood and be eliminated via the reticuloendothelial system. Furthermore, some patients with PTHrP-driven hypercalcemia have dangerously low phosphorus levels which should be treated regardless of the severity of the hypercalcemia.

Ultimately, through the above measures and a change in anticancer therapy, this patient's calcium normalized.

3. Should the patient's 25-hydroxyvitamin D level be repleted?
   Answer: As in case 1, the deficient vitamin D level should not be treated since there could be accelerated conversion to 1,25-dihydroxyvitamin D, exacerbating the hypercalcemia.

Acknowledgments The author would like to thank Hannah Rice, ELS, for editorial assistance.

References

1. Stewart AF. Clinical practice. Hypercalcemia associated with cancer. N Engl J Med. 2005;352(4):373–9.
2. Takahashi S, Hakuta M, Aiba K, Ito Y, Horikoshi N, Miura M, et al. Elevation of circulating plasma cytokines in cancer patients with high plasma parathyroid hormone-related protein levels. Endocr Relat Cancer. 2003;10(3):403–7.
3. Kyle RA, Rajkumar SV. Multiple myeloma. N Engl J Med. 2004;351(18):1860–73.
4. Roodman GD. Mechanisms of bone metastasis. N Engl J Med. 2004;350(16):1655–64.
5. Jick S, Li L, Gastanaga VM, Liede A. Prevalence of hypercalcemia of malignancy among cancer patients in the UK: analysis of the Clinical Practice Research Datalink database. Cancer Epidemiol. 2015;39(6):901–7.
6. Zhu V, de Las MA, Janicek M, Hartshorn K. Hypercalcemia from metastatic pancreatic neuroendocrine tumor secreting 1,25-dihydroxyvitamin D. J Gastrointest Oncol. 2014;5(4):E84–7.
7. Chukir T, Liu Y, Hoffman K, Bilezikian JP, Farooki A. Calcitriol elevation is associated with a higher risk of refractory hypercalcemia of malignancy in solid tumors. J Clin Endocrinol Metab. 2020;105(4):e1115–23.

8. Donovan PJ, Achong N, Griffin K, Galligan J, Pretorius CJ, McLeod DS. PTHrP-mediated hypercalcemia: causes and survival in 138 patients. J Clin Endocrinol Metab. 2015;100(5):2024–9.
9. Papazachariou IM, Virlos IT, Williamson RC. Parathyroid hormone-related peptide in pancreatic neuroendocrine tumours associated with hypercalcaemia. HPB (Oxford). 2001;3(3):221–5.
10. Abraham P, Ralston SH, Hewison M, Fraser WD, Bevan JS. Presentation of a PTHrP-secreting pancreatic neuroendocrine tumour, with hypercalcaemic crisis, pre-eclampsia, and renal failure. Postgrad Med J. 2002;78(926):752–3.
11. Kanakis G, Kaltsas G, Granberg D, Grimelius L, Papaioannou D, Tsolakis AV, et al. Unusual complication of a pancreatic neuroendocrine tumor presenting with malignant hypercalcemia. J Clin Endocrinol Metab. 2012;97(4):E627–31.
12. Stewart AF, Horst R, Deftos LJ, Cadman EC, Lang R, Broadus AE. Biochemical evaluation of patients with cancer-associated hypercalcemia: evidence for humoral and nonhumoral groups. N Engl J Med. 1980;303(24):1377–83.
13. Burtis WJ, Brady TG, Orloff JJ, Ersbak JB, Warrell RP Jr, Olson BR, et al. Immunochemical characterization of circulating parathyroid hormone-related protein in patients with humoral hypercalcemia of cancer. N Engl J Med. 1990;322(16):1106–12.
14. Albright F. Case records of the Massachusetts General Hospital (case 27461). N Engl J Med. 1941;225:789–91.
15. Rodan SB, Noda M, Wesolowski G, Rosenblatt M, Rodan GA. Comparison of postreceptor effects of 1-34 human hypercalcemia factor and 1-34 human parathyroid hormone in rat osteosarcoma cells. J Clin Invest. 1988;81(3):924–7.
16. Fraher LJ, Hodsman AB, Jonas K, Saunders D, Rose CI, Henderson JE, et al. A comparison of the in vivo biochemical responses to exogenous parathyroid hormone-(1-34) [PTH-(1-34)] and PTH-related peptide-(1-34) in man. J Clin Endocrinol Metab. 1992;75(2):417–23.
17. Orloff JJ, Wu TL, Stewart AF. Parathyroid hormone-like proteins: biochemical responses and receptor interactions. Endocr Rev. 1989;10(4):476–95.
18. Horwitz MJ, Tedesco MB, Sereika SM, Prebehala L, Gundberg CM, Hollis BW, et al. A 7-day continuous infusion of PTH or PTHrP suppresses bone formation and uncouples bone turnover. J Bone Miner Res. 2011;26(9):2287–97.
19. Schilling T, Pecherstorfer M, Blind E, Leidig G, Ziegler R, Raue F. Parathyroid hormone-related protein (PTHrP) does not regulate 1,25-dihydroxyvitamin D serum levels in hypercalcemia of malignancy. J Clin Endocrinol Metab. 1993;76(3):801–3.
20. Horwitz MJ, Tedesco MB, Sereika SM, Hollis BW, Garcia-Ocana A, Stewart AF. Direct comparison of sustained infusion of human parathyroid hormone-related protein-(1-36) [hPTHrP-(1-36)] versus hPTH-(1-34) on serum calcium, plasma 1,25-dihydroxyvitamin D concentrations, and fractional calcium excretion in healthy human volunteers. J Clin Endocrinol Metab. 2003;88(4):1603–9.
21. Horwitz MJ, Tedesco MB, Sereika SM, Syed MA, Garcia-Ocana A, Bisello A, et al. Continuous PTH and PTHrP infusion causes suppression of bone formation and discordant effects on 1,25(OH)2 vitamin D. J Bone Miner Res. 2005;20(10):1792–803.
22. Broadus AE, Mangin M, Ikeda K, Insogna KL, Weir EC, Burtis WJ, et al. Humoral hypercalcemia of cancer. Identification of a novel parathyroid hormone-like peptide. N Engl J Med. 1988;319(9):556–63.
23. Siegel R, Gartenhaus R, Kuzel T. HTLV-I associated leukemia/lymphoma: epidemiology, biology, and treatment. Cancer Treat Res. 2001;104:75–88.
24. Goncalves DU, Proietti FA, Ribas JG, Araujo MG, Pinheiro SR, Guedes AC, et al. Epidemiology, treatment, and prevention of human T-cell leukemia virus type 1-associated diseases. Clin Microbiol Rev. 2010;23(3):577–89.
25. Iwanaga M, Watanabe T, Yamaguchi K. Adult T-cell leukemia: a review of epidemiological evidence. Front Microbiol. 2012;3:322.
26. Hagler KT, Lynch JW Jr. Paraneoplastic manifestations of lymphoma. Clin Lymphoma. 2004;5(1):29–36.

27. Japp EA, Meron MK, Zonszein J. A dramatic response to denosumab: protracted hypocalcemia related to human T-cell lymphotropic virus type 1-associated adult T-cell leukemia/lymphoma. AACE Clin Case Rep. 2019;5(3):e210–e3.
28. Laher AE, Ebrahim O. HTLV-1, ATLL, severe hypercalcaemia and HIV-1 co-infection: an overview. Pan Afr Med J. 2018;30:61.
29. Watanabe T, Yamaguchi K, Takatsuki K, Osame M, Yoshida M. Constitutive expression of parathyroid hormone-related protein gene in human T cell leukemia virus type 1 (HTLV-1) carriers and adult T cell leukemia patients that can be trans-activated by HTLV-1 tax gene. J Exp Med. 1990;172(3):759–65.
30. Nosaka K, Miyamoto T, Sakai T, Mitsuya H, Suda T, Matsuoka M. Mechanism of hypercalcemia in adult T-cell leukemia: overexpression of receptor activator of nuclear factor kappaB ligand on adult T-cell leukemia cells. Blood. 2002;99(2):634–40.
31. Shimoyama M. Diagnostic criteria and classification of clinical subtypes of adult T-cell leukaemia-lymphoma. A report from the Lymphoma Study Group (1984-87). Br J Haematol. 1991;79(3):428–37.
32. Katsuya H, Ishitsuka K, Utsunomiya A, Hanada S, Eto T, Moriuchi Y, et al. Treatment and survival among 1594 patients with ATL. Blood. 2015;126(24):2570–7.
33. Schmelzer HJ, Hesch RD, Mayer H. Parathyroid hormone and PTHmRNA in a human small cell lung cancer. Recent Results Cancer Res. 1985;99:88–93.
34. Yoshimoto K, Yamasaki R, Sakai H, Tezuka U, Takahashi M, Iizuka M, et al. Ectopic production of parathyroid hormone by small cell lung cancer in a patient with hypercalcemia. J Clin Endocrinol Metab. 1989;68(5):976–81.
35. Nielsen PK, Rasmussen AK, Feldt-Rasmussen U, Brandt M, Christensen L, Olgaard K. Ectopic production of intact parathyroid hormone by a squamous cell lung carcinoma in vivo and in vitro. J Clin Endocrinol Metab. 1996;81(10):3793–6.
36. Rizzoli R, Pache JC, Didierjean L, Burger A, Bonjour JP. A thymoma as a cause of true ectopic hyperparathyroidism. J Clin Endocrinol Metab. 1994;79(3):912–5.
37. Nussbaum SR, Gaz RD, Arnold A. Hypercalcemia and ectopic secretion of parathyroid hormone by an ovarian carcinoma with rearrangement of the gene for parathyroid hormone. N Engl J Med. 1990;323(19):1324–8.
38. Strewler GJ, Budayr AA, Clark OH, Nissenson RA. Production of parathyroid hormone by a malignant nonparathyroid tumor in a hypercalcemic patient. J Clin Endocrinol Metab. 1993;76(5):1373–5.
39. Wong K, Tsuda S, Mukai R, Sumida K, Arakaki R. Parathyroid hormone expression in a patient with metastatic nasopharyngeal rhabdomyosarcoma and hypercalcemia. Endocrine. 2005;27(1):83–6.
40. VanHouten JN, Yu N, Rimm D, Dotto J, Arnold A, Wysolmerski JJ, et al. Hypercalcemia of malignancy due to ectopic transactivation of the parathyroid hormone gene. J Clin Endocrinol Metab. 2006;91(2):580–3.
41. Vacher-Coponat H, Opris A, Denizot A, Dussol B, Berland Y. Hypercalcaemia induced by excessive parathyroid hormone secretion in a patient with a neuroendocrine tumour. Nephrol Dial Transplant. 2005;20(12):2832–5.
42. Kandil E, Noureldine S, Khalek MA, Daroca P, Friedlander P. Ectopic secretion of parathyroid hormone in a neuroendocrine tumor: a case report and review of the literature. Int J Clin Exp Med. 2011;4(3):234–40.
43. Nakajima K, Tamai M, Okaniwa S, Nakamura Y, Kobayashi M, Niwa T, et al. Humoral hypercalcemia associated with gastric carcinoma secreting parathyroid hormone: a case report and review of the literature. Endocr J. 2013;60(5):557–62.
44. Hong N, Yoon HJ, Lee YH, Kim HR, Lee BW, Rhee Y, et al. Serum PTHrP predicts weight loss in cancer patients independent of hypercalcemia, inflammation, and tumor burden. J Clin Endocrinol Metab. 2016;101(3):1207–14.
45. Hu MI, Glezerman IG, Leboulleux S, Insogna K, Gucalp R, Misiorowski W, et al. Denosumab for treatment of hypercalcemia of malignancy. J Clin Endocrinol Metab. 2014;99(9):3144–52.

46. Goldner W. Cancer-related hypercalcemia. J Oncol Pract. 2016;12(5):426–32.
47. Onuma E, Azuma Y, Saito H, Tsunenari T, Watanabe T, Hirabayashi M, et al. Increased renal calcium reabsorption by parathyroid hormone-related protein is a causative factor in the development of humoral hypercalcemia of malignancy refractory to osteoclastic bone resorption inhibitors. Clin Cancer Res. 2005;11(11):4198–203.
48. Goldsmith RS, Ingbar SH. Inorganic phosphate treatment of hypercalcemia of diverse etiologies. N Engl J Med. 1966;274(1):1–7.
49. Hewison M, Kantorovich V, Liker HR, Van Herle AJ, Cohan P, Zehnder D, et al. Vitamin D-mediated hypercalcemia in lymphoma: evidence for hormone production by tumor-adjacent macrophages. J Bone Miner Res. 2003;18(3):579–82.
50. Lieben L, Masuyama R, Torrekens S, Van Looveren R, Schrooten J, Baatsen P, et al. Normocalcemia is maintained in mice under conditions of calcium malabsorption by vitamin D-induced inhibition of bone mineralization. J Clin Invest. 2012;122(5):1803–15.
51. Hu MI, Glezerman I, Leboulleux S, Insogna K, Gucalp R, Misiorowski W, et al. Denosumab for patients with persistent or relapsed hypercalcemia of malignancy despite recent bisphosphonate treatment. J Natl Cancer Inst. 2013;105(18):1417–20.
52. Thalassinos N, Joplin GF. Phosphate treatment of hypercalcaemia due to carcinoma. Br Med J. 1968;4(5622):14–9.
53. Conron M, Beynon HL. Ketoconazole for the treatment of refractory hypercalcemic sarcoidosis. Sarcoidosis Vasc Diffuse Lung Dis. 2000;17(3):277–80.
54. Adams JS, Sharma OP, Diz MM, Endres DB. Ketoconazole decreases the serum 1,25-dihydroxyvitamin D and calcium concentration in sarcoidosis-associated hypercalcemia. J Clin Endocrinol Metab. 1990;70(4):1090–5.
55. Kallas M, Green F, Hewison M, White C, Kline G. Rare causes of calcitriol-mediated hypercalcemia: a case report and literature review. J Clin Endocrinol Metab. 2010;95(7):3111–7.

Chapter 10
Myeloma-Related Hypercalcemia and Bone Disease

Divaya Bhutani, Rajshekhar Chakraborty, and Suzanne Lentzsch

Introduction

Multiple myeloma (MM) is characterized by growth of malignant clonal plasma cells and by clinical manifestations commonly referred to as "CRAB" features, namely, hypercalcemia, renal dysfunction, anemia, and bone disease [1]. Development of MM is always preceded by a premalignant phase known as monoclonal gammopathy of unknown significant (MGUS) and/or smoldering multiple myeloma [2]. Development of one of the CRAB features is considered a sign of progression to symptomatic multiple myeloma.

Epidemiology and Diagnosis

MM is the most common hematologic malignancy with about 32,000 new cases diagnosed in United States in 2020 [3]. Malignant transformation and growth of plasma cells leads to various manifestations of the disease. Common presenting sings of the disease include anemia because of bone marrow dysfunction, renal dysfunction related to excess production of monoclonal immunoglobulins, bone disease, and hypercalcemia. Useful initial diagnostic tests to evaluate for myeloma include a complete blood count, serum protein electrophoresis, immunofixation, serum free light chain analysis, serum creatinine, and calcium. Suggestive results should prompt referral to a specialist for further testing including but not limited to

D. Bhutani · R. Chakraborty · S. Lentzsch (✉)
Division of Hematology Oncology, Columbia University Irving Medical Center, New York, NY, USA
e-mail: db3203@cumc.columbia.edu; rc3360@cumc.columbia.edu; sl3440@cumc.columbia.edu

© The Author(s), under exclusive license to Springer Nature Switzerland AG 2022
M. D. Walker (ed.), *Hypercalcemia*, Contemporary Endocrinology, https://doi.org/10.1007/978-3-030-93182-7_10

bone marrow aspiration and biopsy. In addition, patients with suspected MM should have imaging studies for skeletal evaluation as discussed below. Hypercalcemia in MM develops due to increased bone resorption resulting in lytic bone disease and as a consequence of the interaction of proliferating malignant plasma cells and the bone microenvironment. Bone disease is present in about 80% of the patients at the time of diagnosis [4]. The incidence of hypercalcemia at the time of diagnosis of MM is about 21% [5], highest among the various malignancies leading to hypercalcemia [6]. Development of bone disease in MM leads to an increased incidence of skeletal-related events (SREs) such as bone fractures and mortality as well [7]. Patients with MM presenting with an early skeletal-related event (SRE) have up to a 2.5-fold increase in mortality as compared to patients without an early SRE [7].

Pathophysiology of Bone Disease in Multiple Myeloma

Bone remodeling is a continuous dynamic process essential for sustaining skeletal health. The process is mediated by the basic multicellular unit (BMU) which consists of osteocytes, osteoblasts, and osteoclasts. Under normal physiologic conditions, the process of osteoclast-mediated bone resorption is balanced by osteoblast-mediated bone formation with the whole process integrated by the interaction among various components of the BMU [8]. Development of bone disease in MM is the result of interaction of a malignant plasma cell clone with the bone microenvironment that includes various bone components such as osteocytes, osteoblasts, osteoclasts, bony matrix, and immune cells. The malignant plasma cells increase osteoclast-mediated bone resorption and suppress osteoblast-mediated bone formation. The various components involved in the process are described below and summarized in Fig. 10.1.

1. *Osteoclast activation*: The development of excessive bone resorption in patients with MM is mediated by osteoclast activation driven by various molecular mechanisms described below.

    (a) RANK/RANKL/OPG pathway: Osteoprotegerin (OPG) is a tumor necrosis factor or TNF-related protein secreted by bone marrow stromal cells and osteoblasts that regulates bone formation and inhibits bone resorption [9]. Receptor activator of nuclear factor κ B (RANK) is a transmembrane receptor expressed on the surface of osteoclast precursors, and RANK ligand (RANKL) is a cytokine produced by bone marrow stromal cells of osteoblastic lineage and activated T lymphocytes. The binding of RANKL to RANK leads to development of osteoclasts from precursor cells as well as activation of osteoclast function [10]. OPG is a decoy receptor for RANKL and prevents binding of RANKL to RANK thus preventing osteoclastogenesis. The expression of RANKL is increased by glucocorticoids, vitamin D, parathyroid hormone (PTH), and prostaglandin E2 leading to increased activity of osteoclasts and bone resorption. OPG expression is enhanced by

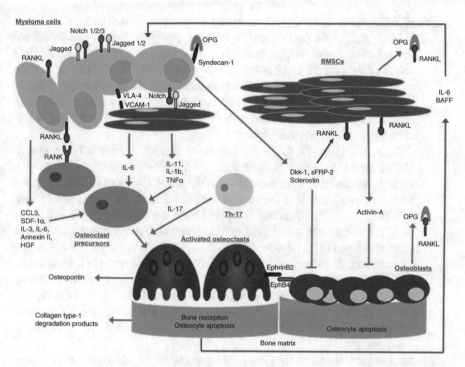

Fig. 10.1 Pathogenesis of myeloma bone disease: malignant plasma cells express RANKL [12], and interaction of plasma cells with T lymphocytes and bone marrow stromal cells also leads to increased production of RANKL by these cells [13]. Increased expression of syndecan-1 on MM cells binds to OPG, leading to internalization and degradation. This further alters the RANKL/OPG ratio favoring osteoclastogenesis. Activation of notch signaling leads to osteocyte apoptosis, which increases osteoclast precursor recruitment and RANKL production as well. CCL-3 (chemokine ligand 3) and other chemokine ligands secreted by malignant plasma cells bind to their receptors on osteoclasts, activating them. CCL-3 also promotes MM cell growth, survival, and proliferation. IL-6 is produced primarily by the bone marrow stromal cells and acts as a growth factor for both the malignant plasma cells and the osteoclasts. IL-17, osteopontin, annexin-2, TNF-alpha, B-cell activating factor (BAFF), and matrix metalloproteinase (MMP-13) also activate osteoclasts. MM cells produce soluble factors that inhibit osteoblastogenesis such as DKK1, sFRP-2, and sclerostin. Activin A secreted by BMSCs also impedes osteoblast production while at the same time activates osteoclasts. (Reproduced by permission from Springer Nature, Ref. [58])

factors such as estradiol, TNF-alpha, and transforming growth factor beta (TGF-beta) leading to increased bone mass [11]. Development of MM leads to disruption in the balance of RANKL and OPG with increased RANKL and decreased OPG expression, thus causing excessive bone resorption and development of myeloma bone disease. Malignant plasma cells themselves express RANKL [12], but in addition, interaction of plasma cells with T lymphocytes and bone marrow stromal cells also results in increased production of RANKL by these cells [13]. MM cells also induce upregulation of syndecan-1 on MM cells that binds to OPG. OPG is then internalized by the MM cells and degraded [14].

(b) NOTCH pathway: NOTCH receptors are expressed on malignant plasma cells as well as on osteocytes. Development of MM leads to bidirectional activation of the NOTCH pathway in both osteocytes and malignant plasma cells as they interact in the bone marrow microenvironment [15]. Activation of the NOTCH signaling in osteocytes leads to their apoptosis resulting in osteoclast precursor recruitment and increased RANKL production by both MM and bone marrow stromal cells (BMSCs). This in turn increases osteoclastogenesis and bone resorption.

(c) CCL-3 and CCL-20: CCL-3 (chemokine ligand 3), formerly known as MIP-1 alpha (macrophage inflammatory protein-1 alpha), is a chemokine secreted by malignant plasma cells that binds to CCR1 and CCR5 expressed on osteoclasts leading to their activation [16]. Another member of this family known as CCL-20 and its receptor CCR6 are also overexpressed in the bone marrow microenvironment of MM patients, leading to increased osteoclast activation [17]. Levels of CCL-3 and CCL-20 are significantly higher as compared to patient with lower degree of bone disease [17]. In addition, CCL-3 promotes MM cell growth, survival, proliferation, and downstream activation of the MAP kinase pathway in the MM cells [18]. Blockage of CCL-3 binding to its receptor decreases myeloma bone disease in a preclinical model [19], thus making it an attractive target for therapy of myeloma bone disease.

(d) Interleukins: IL-6 and IL-3 levels are elevated in the bone marrow microenvironment of patients with MM and contribute to bone resorption. IL-6 is produced primarily by the bone marrow stromal cells and acts as a growth factor for both the malignant plasma cells and the osteoclasts [20]. Elevated IL-6 levels have been shown to correlate with MM proliferation and osteoclastogenesis [21], although a clinical trial of anti-IL-6 antibody failed to demonstrate any anti-myeloma or anti-osteoclast effects [22]. Multiple other factors have been described to cause osteoclast activation, including IL-17, osteopontin, annexin 2, TNF-alpha, and B-cell activating factor (BAFF) (Fig. 10.1).

(e) MMP-13/PD-1H pathway: Matrix metalloproteinase 13 (MMP-13) is a critical osteoclastogenic factor that is highly secreted by MM cells. MMP-13 induces osteoclast fusion and bone resorption independent of its proteolytic activity [23] and by binding to the checkpoint inhibitor programmed death-1 homolog (PD-1H/VISTA), a surface receptor that is expressed in osteoclasts at high levels [24]. Binding of MMP-13 to PD-1H/VISTA induces osteoclast fusion and bone resorption activity, whereas knockdown or knockout of PD-1H/VISTA largely blocks MMP-13-mediated effects on osteoclasts in vivo and in vitro [25]. Given the checkpoint role of PD-1H/VISTA in cancer immunosuppression, targeting the interaction of MMP-13 and PD-1H may represent a novel therapeutic strategy to treat MM bone disease and modulate the MM immune environment (Fig. 10.2).

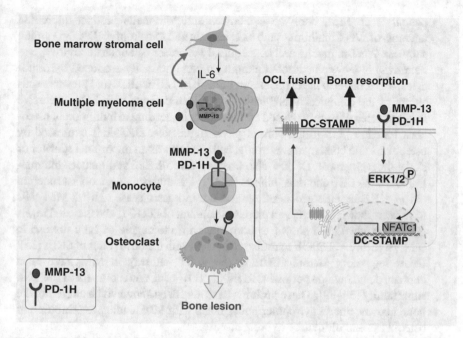

Fig. 10.2 MMP-13 binds PD-1H expressed on OCL precursors inducing osteoclast formation and activation. OCL fusion and cytoskeleton reorganization is induced by the MMP-13/PD-1H axis. MMP-13 secreted by MM cells binds to PD-1H on the OCL cell surface. The binding enhances RANKL-triggered activation of c-Src and subsequently ERK1-/ERK2-mediated upregulation of NFATc1 and DC-STAMP and enhances cell fusion. In addition, PD-1H directly associates with cytoskeleton protein c-Src and activates Rac1, thereby regulating cytoskeleton reorganization. (The figure was created with BioRender.com)

2. *Osteoblast inhibition*: In addition to osteoclast activation, myeloma bone disease is also characterized by inhibition of osteoblast activity. This uncoupling exacerbates the imbalance between bone resorption and formation.

   - *WNT Pathway*
   - The primary pathway of bone homeostasis is the canonical branch of the WNT (wingless-type) signaling pathway. Mutations leading to abnormalities in this pathway were initially described in a low bone mass disorder known as osteoporosis-pseudoglioma (OPPG) syndrome [26]. OPPG is characterized by a loss-of-function mutation in low-density lipoprotein receptor-related protein 5 (LRP5), which encodes for a WNT co-receptor. At the same time, a gain-of-function mutation was described in this gene leading to increased bone mass in otherwise healthy patients [27]. Further work has shown that WNT signaling is the cardinal pathway involved in skeletal development [28], joint formation [29], and bone homeostasis [30]. Canonical WNT signaling leads the mesenchymal stem cell towards osteoblastic differentiation and leads to increased secretion of OPG in the bone microenvironment. At the same time, WNT3a inhibits osteoclastogenesis leading to increased bone mass [31]. In

patients with MM, both the osteocytes and MM cells produce increased amounts of WNT inhibitors such as sclerostin and Dickkopf-1 (DKK-1) which suppress WNT signaling and consequently decrease osteoblast activity.

- Sclerostin is a cysteine knot-containing protein normally produced by osteocytes, and it binds to the extracellular domain of LRP5/LRP6 and prevents activation of the canonical WNT pathway [32]. In patients with MM, excessive levels of sclerostin are produced by the MM cells, leading to inhibition of osteoblast function [33]. In the normal physiologic state, DKK-1 is expressed by osteoblasts and bone marrow stromal cells and acts as an important regulator of skeletal development. DKK-1 also binds to LRP5/LRP6 and induces internalization of the LRP and thus inhibits the WNT pathway and osteoblast function [34]. DKK1 has emerged as a key mediator of bone disease in MM. MM cells have been shown to secrete an increased amount of DKK-1, and elevated levels of DKK-1 have been shown to correlate with the degree of lytic disease in MM. High levels of DKK-1 are also correlated with increased rates of SREs [35].
- Other regulatory factors affecting the WNT pathway in MM have been described and include periostin, RUNX1, TGF-beta, and members of the TNF superfamily [36–39]. These proteins have also been shown to be altered in the bone marrow microenvironment of patients with MM leading to inhibition of osteoblasts and ultimately to bone disease.

Clinical Presentation of Bone Disease in Multiple Myeloma

The most common presentation of myeloma bone disease (MBD) is lytic bone lesions, which are seen in about 70–80% of patients at the time of diagnosis. Development of these lesions is a risk factor for development of SREs which include bone fractures, hypercalcemia, and spinal cord compression. Development of SREs in MM is associated with both increased morbidity and mortality in patients with MM [40]. Traditionally, skeletal survey has been used to evaluate the bone disease in these patients, but with the advent of modern imaging techniques, it has become clear that this method misses lytic bone lesions in about 25% of patients [41]. Low-dose non-contrast CT has become the standard imaging modality for assessment of MBD; in addition, positron emission tomography/computed tomography (PET/CT) and magnetic resonance imaging have been shown to be highly sensitive methods [42]. Further, PET/CT also offers the advantage of response assessment by comparison of fluorodeoxyglucose (FDG) uptake before and after therapy. Hypercalcemia is seen in about 20% of patients with MM at the time of diagnosis and is related to the degree of bone disease. Typical presentation of hypercalcemia includes renal dysfunction driven by hypovolemia related to hypercalcemia-induced diuresis. Treatment of hypercalcemia in these patients includes use of intravenous (IV) hydration to correct hypovolemia as well as calcitonin and bisphosphonates to reduce osteoclast activity and to lower the calcium level (see Chap. 5). In addition, prompt initiation of therapy for MM including use of steroids, such as dexamethasone, can be effective for hypercalcemia in this disease.

Effect of Myeloma Bone Disease on Survival of Patients with Multiple Myeloma

In addition to the obvious morbidity related to the bone disease, presence of advanced bone disease in MM has been associated with decreased overall survival as well. Two large registry studies from the United Kingdom and Sweden have demonstrated an increase in death rates among patients with MM presenting with fracture. There are even greater rates of mortality that are almost twice as high (as compared to MM patients without fracture) in patients who develop a bone fracture during the course of MM [43, 44].

Management of Myeloma Bone Disease

1. *Bisphosphonates:* Bisphosphonates have been extensively studied for therapy of MBD and are recommended for treatment of the majority of patients with MM. Nitrogen-containing bisphosphonates inhibit osteoclast activation primarily by inhibiting the enzyme farnesyl pyrophosphate (FPP) synthase in the mevalonate pathway (cholesterol biosynthetic pathway) [45]. This leads to disruption of protein prenylation, which creates cytoskeletal abnormalities in the osteoclast and detachment of the osteoclast from the bone perimeter, leading to reduced bone resorption [45]. Multiple, prospective randomized trials have compared bisphosphonates to placebo [46] and various bisphosphonates to each other [47] in patients with multiple myeloma. A meta-analysis of 24 randomized trials (with 7293 patients) showed the following effects of bisphosphonates as compared to placebo in patients with MM [48]. The results are summarized below:

   (a) Decreased risk of pathologic vertebral fractures (RR 0.74, 95% CI 0.62–0.89)
   (b) Reduced risk of skeletal-related events (RR 0.74, 95% CI 0.63–0.88)
   (c) Improvement in skeletal pain (RR 0.75, 95% CI 0.60–0.95)
   (d) No improvement in progression-free survival of multiple myeloma (HR 0.75, 95% CI 0.57–1.00)
   (e) Possible improvement in overall survival seen only in patients who received zoledronic acid (placebo vs zoledronic acid HR 0.67, 95% CI 0.46–0.91)
   (f) Increased risk of osteonecrosis of the jaw (RR 4.61, 95% CI 0.99–21.35)
   (g) Increased risk of hypocalcemia (RR 2.19, 95% CI 0.49–9.74)

   In this analysis, there was no significant difference among various bisphosphonates in terms of rates of skeletal events, but a few studies comparing the various bisphosphonates have shown differences among them. A large prospective trial (MRC myeloma IX) [47] compared zoledronic acid (4 mg intravenously every 21–28 days) to oral clodronic acid (1600 mg per day), and results showed that patients receiving zoledronic acid had significantly reduced rates of SREs (27% vs 35%) and reduced rates of vertebral fractures (5% vs. 9%). Rates of osteonecrosis of the jaw (ONJ) were higher in the zoledronic acid group (4% vs. <1%). In addition, the study also showed an improvement in overall survival and progression-free survival in patients receiving zoledronic acid, although it must be noted that the improvement in overall survival was related to reduced incidence of infections in this arm. A retrospective registry study of patients treated at veteran affairs medical centers [49] compared outcomes of patients who had received intravenous zoledronic acid vs. pamidronate in 1018 patients and showed nearly a 25% reduction in SREs in patients receiving zoledronic acid. Based on these studies, zoledronic acid 4 mg intravenously given every 3–4 weeks is currently recommended for patients with myeloma bone disease. Pamidronate 30 or 90 mg intravenously given every 4 weeks is an alternative as well.

Frequency of Bisphosphonate Administration: The majority of studies have tested zoledronic acid administered intravenously at a frequency of every 4 weeks. Given the risk of ONJ related to bisphosphonates, reduced frequency of administration has been tested as an alternative to monthly administration to reduce adverse effects. A prospective trial compared zoledronic acid given monthly vs. every 3 months intravenously in patients with bone metastases. Patients with MM ($N = 278$) constituted a subgroup of the study, and results showed no significant differences in outcomes in SREs between the two groups [50]. There was a trend towards lower incidence of ONJ in patients who received every 3-month versus monthly intravenous zoledronic acid (1% vs 2%, $P = 0.08$), but it did not reach statistical significance.

Duration of Treatment: The data regarding the optimal duration of therapy with bisphosphonates is limited in patients with MM, as some studies have used a fixed duration of therapy (ranging from 2 to 3 years), and other studies, such as the MRC myeloma IX trial, used therapy until disease progression. In this trial, patients who received zoledronic acid for 2 or more years showed improved overall survival compared with patients receiving clodronic acid [47]. Overall treatment duration of 1–2 years is recommended based on the existing data [51]. In addition, patients who achieve a complete or very good partial remission (VGPR) of MM with therapy also tend to have fewer SREs, and duration of bisphosphonate therapy can be curtailed to 1 year in those patients. Patients who achieve less than VGPR should receive a longer duration of therapy, and therapy with bisphosphonates should be restarted in patients who develop a relapse of MM.

Prevention and Management of Adverse Effects of Bisphosphonates: Hypocalcemia can develop in patients on bisphosphonates especially in the setting of vitamin D deficiency. A serum 25-hydroxyvitamin D level should be checked prior to starting bisphosphonates and calcium, and vitamin D supplementation is recommended in patients receiving bisphosphonates to prevent hypocalcemia.

Monitoring of renal function is important in patients, as bisphosphonates can induce renal damage [52]. Use of bisphosphonates is not recommended in patients with a creatinine clearance less than 30 ml/min, and reduced dosing should be used in patients with creatinine clearance between 30 and 60 ml/min.

ONJ is an uncommon, but a debilitating adverse effect of bisphosphonate use. A combined analysis of three prospective trials ($N = 5723$) comparing denosumab vs. zoledronic acid in patients with bone metastases (related to solid tumors and multiple myeloma) showed an incidence of 1.8% in patients on denosumab and 1.3% on zoledronic acid [53]. The incidence is higher in those with a longer duration of therapy, with use of intravenous bisphosphonates as compared to oral bisphosphonates, and in those who undergo invasive dental procedures, such as extractions while receiving bisphosphonates. Patients should have a dental evaluation prior to starting bisphosphonates, and bisphosphonates should be withheld 3 months before and after an invasive dental procedure.

2. *Denosumab*: Denosumab is a fully human and highly specific monoclonal IgG2 antibody against RANK ligand. It prevents the interaction of RANK with RANK ligand. This leads to decreased osteoclast activity and less bone resorption. Denosumab was compared to zoledronic acid in a large prospective double blind study [54] of patients with newly diagnosed multiple myeloma. Denosumab was shown to be non-inferior to zoledronic acid for prevention of first SRE (HR 0.98, CI 0.85–1.14). Patients in the denosumab arm had less renal toxicity as compared to those receiving zoledronic acid. Among patients with a creatinine clearance between 30 and 60 ml/min, the incidence of renal toxicity was reduced by 50% in the denosumab group (13% vs. 26%) as compared to those receiving zoledronic acid. In addition, the denosumab group also had improvement in multiple myeloma progression-free survival (median PFS 46.1 vs. 35.4 months) as compared to zoledronic acid. Patients with a creatinine clearance less than 30 ml/min were excluded from the trial; studies performed in patients with osteoporosis [55] have shown the overall safety of this drug in patients with low creatinine clearance, though hypocalcemia is not infrequent in this population.

   The recommended dose of denosumab in patients with multiple myeloma is 120 mg subcutaneous once a month given continuously. Discontinuation of denosumab in patients with osteoporosis can lead to rebound activation of osteoclast activity leading to bone loss and vertebral fracture. Currently, data on the discontinuation of denosumab specifically in patients with MM is not available, as the drug was given continuously until unacceptable toxicity in clinical trials. If the decision is made to discontinue the drug, a single of dose of intravenous bisphosphonate or a year of oral bisphosphonate therapy should be administered 6 months after stopping the drug to prevent excessive osteoclast activation [56]. Denosumab, like bisphosphonates, is associated with the adverse events of hypocalcemia and ONJ, and similar measures as above should be used to prevent and manage these.

3. *Other Measures:* Pain control in patients with MBD can be of paramount importance for maintaining quality of life and activity, and use of opioids and muscle relaxants can be helpful adjunctive measures. Kyphoplasty and vertebroplasty

can be effective in patients with pain related to vertebral fractures and may help in improving functional status as well [57]. In some patients with localized bone pain, RT and/or surgical intervention can also be helpful in improving the symptoms. Orthopedic evaluation of patients at risk of developing pathologic fractures is very important, as in some cases, prophylactic surgery can prevent these fractures.

Summary

Lytic bone disease is quite common and can cause significant symptom burden in patients with MM. In addition, patients with advanced bone disease may have significant effects on quality of life and overall survival. Effective evaluation and management of MBD is important in patients with MM to prevent complications. The use of bisphosphonates and denosumab has been a major advance in management of MBD. Overall bisphosphonates remain the drug of choice for most patients, but denosumab is the preferred option for patients with renal dysfunction. Care must to taken to monitor for potential adverse events especially ONJ in patients on these medications.

References

1. Palumbo A, Anderson K. Multiple myeloma. N Engl J Med. 2011;364(11):1046–60.
2. Landgren O, Kyle RA, Pfeiffer RM, et al. Monoclonal gammopathy of undetermined significance (MGUS) consistently precedes multiple myeloma: a prospective study. Blood. 2009;113(22):5412–7.
3. https://seer.cancer.gov/statfacts/html/mulmy.html.
4. Kyle RA, Gertz MA, Witzig TE, et al. Review of 1027 patients with newly diagnosed multiple myeloma. Mayo Clin Proc. 2003;78(1):21–33.
5. Kastritis E, et al. Frequency and prognostic significance of hypercalcemia in patients with multiple myeloma: an analysis of the database of the Greek Myeloma Study Group. Blood. 2011;118(21):5083.
6. Gastanaga VM, Schwartzberg LS, Jain RK, et al. Prevalence of hypercalcemia among cancer patients in the United States. Cancer Med. 2016;5(8):2091–100.
7. Terpos E, Berenson J, Cook RJ, Lipton A, Coleman RE. Prognostic variables for survival and skeletal complications in patients with multiple myeloma osteolytic bone disease. Leukemia. 2010;24(5):1043–9.
8. Xiao W, Wang Y, Pacios S, Li S, Graves DT. Cellular and molecular aspects of bone remodeling. Front Oral Biol. 2016;18:9–16.
9. Simonet WS, Lacey DL, Dunstan CR, et al. Osteoprotegerin: a novel secreted protein involved in the regulation of bone density. Cell. 1997;89(2):309–19.
10. Boyle WJ, Simonet WS, Lacey DL. Osteoclast differentiation and activation. Nature. 2003;423(6937):337–42.
11. Takayanagi H. Osteoimmunology: shared mechanisms and crosstalk between the immune and bone systems. Nat Rev Immunol. 2007;7(4):292–304.

12. Heider U, Langelotz C, Jakob C, Zavrski I, Fleissner C, Eucker J, Possinger K, Hofbauer LC, Sezer O. Expression of receptor activator of nuclear factor kappaB ligand on bone marrow plasma cells correlates with osteolytic bone disease in patients with multiple myeloma. Clin Cancer Res. 2003;9(4):1436–40. PMID: 12684416.
13. Giuliani N, Colla S, Sala R, et al. Human myeloma cells stimulate the receptor activator of nuclear factor-kB ligand (RANKL) in T lymphocytes: a potential role in multiple myeloma bone disease. Blood. 2002;100:4615–21.
14. Standal T, Seidel C, Hjertner Ø, et al. Osteoprotegerin is bound, internalized, and degraded by multiple myeloma cells. Blood. 2002;100(8):3002–7.
15. Delgado-Calle J, Anderson J, Cregor MD, et al. Bidirectional notch signaling and osteocyte-derived factors in the bone marrow microenvironment promote tumor cell proliferation and bone destruction in multiple myeloma. Cancer Res. 2016;76(5):1089–100.
16. Terpos E, Politou M, Viniou N, Rahemtulla A. Significance of macrophage inflammatory protein-1 alpha (MIP-1alpha) in multiple myeloma. Leuk Lymphoma. 2005;46(12):1699–707.
17. Palma BD, Guasco D, Pedrazzoni M, et al. Osteolytic lesions, cytogenetic features and bone marrow levels of cytokines and chemokines in multiple myeloma patients: role of chemokine (C-C motif) ligand 20. Leukemia. 2016;30(2):409–16.
18. Lentzsch S, Gries M, Janz M, et al. Macrophage inflammatory protein 1-alpha (MIP-1 alpha) triggers migration and signaling cascades mediating survival and proliferation in multiple myeloma (MM) cells. Blood. 2003;101(9):3568–73.
19. Fu R, Liu H, Zhao S, et al. Osteoblast inhibition by chemokine cytokine ligand3 in myeloma-induced bone disease. Cancer Cell Int. 2014;14(1):132.
20. Klein B, Tarte K, Jourdan M, et al. Survival and proliferation factors of normal and malignant plasma cells. Int J Hematol. 2003;78:106–13.
21. Kyrtsonis MC, Dedoussis G, Baxevanis C, et al. Serum interleukin-6 (IL-6) and interleukin-4 (IL-4) in patients with multiple myeloma (MM). Br J Haematol. 1996;92:420–2.
22. van Zaanen HC, Lokhorst HM, Aarden LA, et al. Chimaeric anti-interleukin 6 monoclonal antibodies in the treatment of advanced multiple myeloma: a phase I dose-escalating study. Br J Haematol. 1998;102:783–90.
23. Fu J, Li S, Feng R, Ma H, Sabeh F, Roodman GD, Wang J, Robinson S, Guo XE, Lund T, Normolle D, Mapara MY, Weiss SJ, Lentzsch S. Multiple myeloma-derived MMP-13 mediates osteoclast fusogenesis and osteolytic disease. J Clin Invest. 2016;126(5):1759–72.
24. Fu J, Li S, Yang C, et al. Checkpoint inhibitor PD-1H/VISTA functions as MMP-13 receptor on osteoclasts and mediates MMP-13 induced osteoclast activation in multiple myeloma. Blood. 2019;134(Supplement_1):3165.
25. Fu J, Li S, Ma H, et al. Checkpoint inhibitor PD-1H/VISTA mediated MMP-13 induced osteoclast activation and multiple myeloma bone disease. Blood. 2020;136(Supplement 1): 15–6.
26. Gong Y, et al.; Osteoporosis-Pseudoglioma Syndrome Collaborative Group. LDL receptor–related protein 5 (LRP5) affects bone accrual and eye development. Cell. 2001;107:513–23.
27. Boyden LM, et al. High bone density due to a mutation in LDL-receptor–related protein 5. N Engl J Med. 2002;346:1513–21.
28. Day TF, Guo X, Garrett-Beal L, Yang Y. Wnt/β-catenin signaling in mesenchymal progenitors controls osteoblast and chondrocyte differentiation during vertebrate skeletogenesis. Dev Cell. 2005;8:739–50.
29. Niemann S, et al. Homozygous WNT3 mutation causes tetra-amelia in a large consanguineous family. Am J Hum Genet. 2004;74:558–63.
30. Bennett CN, et al. Wnt10b increases postnatal bone formation by enhancing osteoblast differentiation. J Bone Miner Res. 2007;22:1924–32.
31. Wei W, et al. Biphasic and dosage-dependent regulation of osteoclastogenesis by β-catenin. Mol Cell Biol. 2011;31:4706–19.
32. Sutherland MK, Geoghegan JC, Yu C, et al. Sclerostin promotes the apoptosis of human osteoblastic cells: a novel regulation of bone formation. Bone. 2004;35(4):828–35.

33. Colucci S, Brunetti G, Oranger A, et al. Myeloma cells suppress osteoblasts through sclerostin secretion. Blood Cancer J. 2011;1(6):e27.
34. Gavriatopoulou M, Dimopoulos MA, Christoulas D, et al. Dickkopf-1: a suitable target for the management of myeloma bone disease. Expert Opin Ther Targets. 2009;13(7):839–48.
35. Tian E, Zhan F, Walker R, et al. The role of the Wnt-signaling antagonist DKK1 in the development of osteolytic lesions in multiple myeloma. N Engl J Med. 2003;349(26):2483–94.
36. Terpos E, Christoulas D, Kastritis E, et al. High levels of periostin correlate with increased fracture rate, diffuse MRI pattern, abnormal bone remodeling and advanced disease stage in patients with newly diagnosed symptomatic multiple myeloma. Blood Cancer J. 2016;6(10):e482.
37. Giuliani N, Colla S, Morandi F, et al. Myeloma cells block RUNX2/CBFA1 activity in human bone marrow osteoblast progenitors and inhibit osteoblast formation and differentiation. Blood. 2005;106(7):2472–83.
38. Takeuchi K, Abe M, Hiasa M, et al. Tgf-Beta inhibition restores terminal osteoblast differentiation to suppress myeloma growth. PLoS One. 2010;5(3):e9870.
39. D'Souza S, del Prete D, et al. Gfi1 expressed in bone marrow stromal cells is a novel osteoblast suppressor in patients with multiple myeloma bone disease. Blood. 2011;118(26):6871–80.
40. Terpos E, Berenson J, Cook RJ, Lipton A, Coleman RE. Prognostic variables for survival and skeletal complications in patients with multiple myeloma osteolytic bone disease. Leukemia. 2010;24:1043–9.
41. Hillengass J, Moulopoulos LA, Delorme S, et al. Findings of whole body computed tomography compared to conventional skeletal survey in patients with monoclonal plasma cell disorders — a study of the International Myeloma Working Group. Blood. 2016;128:4468.
42. Hillengass J, Usmani S, Rajkumar SV, et al. International myeloma working group consensus recommendations on imaging in monoclonal plasma cell disorders. Lancet Oncol. 2019;20:e302–12.
43. McIlroy G, Mytton J, Evison F, Yadav P, Drayson MT, Cook M, Pratt G, Cockwell P, Pinney JH. Increased fracture risk in plasma cell dyscrasias is associated with poorer overall survival. Br J Haematol. 2017;179(1):61–5.
44. Thorsteinsdottir S, Gislason G, Aspelund T, Sverrisdottir I, Landgren O, Turesson I, Björkholm M, Kristinsson SY. Fractures and survival in multiple myeloma: results from a population-based study. Haematologica. 2020;105(4):1067–73.
45. Russell RG. Bisphosphonates: mode of action and pharmacology. Pediatrics. 2007;119 Suppl 2:S150–62.
46. Berenson JR, Lichtenstein A, Porter L, et al. Efficacy of pamidronate in reducing skeletal events in patients with advanced multiple myeloma. Myeloma Aredia Study Group. N Engl J Med. 1996;334(8):488–93.
47. Morgan GJ, Child JA, Gregory WM, et al. Effects of zoledronic acid versus clodronic acid on skeletal morbidity in patients with newly diagnosed multiple myeloma (MRC Myeloma IX): secondary outcomes from a randomised controlled trial. Lancet Oncol. 2011;12:743–52.
48. Mhaskar R, Kumar A, Miladinovic B, Djulbegovic B. Bisphosphonates in multiple myeloma: an updated network metaanalysis. Cochrane Database Syst Rev. 2017;12:CD003188.
49. Sanfilippo KM, Gage B, Luo S, et al. Comparative effectiveness on survival of zoledronic acid versus pamidronate in multiple myeloma. Leuk Lymphoma. 2015;56(3):615–21.
50. Himelstein AL, Foster JC, Khatcheressian JL, et al. Effect of longer-interval vs standard dosing of zoledronic acid on skeletal events in patients with bone metastases: a randomized clinical trial. JAMA. 2017;317(1):48–58.
51. Terpos E, Zamagni E, Lentzsch S, et al. Treatment of multiple myeloma-related bone disease: recommendations from the Bone Working Group of the International Myeloma Working Group. Lancet Oncol. 2021;22(3):e119–30.
52. Weide R, Koppler H, Antras L, et al. Renal toxicity in patients with multiple myeloma receiving zoledronic acid vs. ibandronate: a retrospective medical records review. J Cancer Res Ther. 2010;6(1):31–5.

53. Saad F, Brown JE, Van Poznak C, et al. Incidence, risk factors, and outcomes of osteonecrosis of the jaw: integrated analysis from three blinded active-controlled phase III trials in cancer patients with bone metastases. Ann Oncol. 2012;23(5):1341–7.
54. Raje N, Terpos E, Willenbacher W, et al. Denosumab versus zoledronic acid in bone disease treatment of newly diagnosed multiple myeloma: an international, double-blind, double-dummy, randomised, controlled, phase 3 study. Lancet Oncol. 2018;19:370–81.
55. Jamal SA, Ljunggren O, Stehman-Breen C, et al. Effects of denosumab on fracture and bone mineral density by level of kidney function. J Bone Miner Res. 2011;26:1829–35.
56. Tsourdi E, Langdahl B, Cohen-Solal M, et al. Discontinuation of denosumab therapy for osteoporosis: a systematic review and position statement by ECTS. Bone. 2017;105:11–7.
57. Kyriakou C, Molloy S, Vrionis F, et al. The role of cement augmentation with percutaneous vertebroplasty and balloon kyphoplasty for the treatment of vertebral compression fractures in multiple myeloma: a consensus statement from the International Myeloma Working Group (IMWG). Blood Cancer J. 2019;9:27.
58. Terpos E, Ntanasis-Stathopoulos I, Gavriatopoulou M, Dimopoulos MA. Pathogenesis of bone disease in multiple myeloma: from bench to bedside. Blood Cancer J. 2018;8(1):7.

Chapter 11
Hypercalcemia Due to Malignancy-Related Production of 1,25-Dihydroxyvitamin D

Hannah McMullen and Marcella Donovan Walker

Introduction and Epidemiology

Hypercalcemia of malignancy accounts for about 35% of cases of hypercalcemia overall, and its relative frequency is even higher among inpatients [1]. Up to 44% of patients with cancer will ultimately be affected by hypercalcemia of malignancy [2]. Notably, incidence of hypercalcemia is low in the early stages of malignancy and higher in advanced stage cancer [3]. There are several mechanisms by which malignancy induces hypercalcemia. Ectopic production of parathyroid hormone-related protein (PTHrP) and osteolytic metastases cause the majority of cases of hypercalcemia of malignancy (see Chaps. 9 and 10), while ectopic production of 1,25-dihydroxyvitamin D by malignancies is relatively rare [4]. Estimates suggest this mechanism is responsible for only 1% of cases of hypercalcemia of malignancy [3, 5].

Associated Malignancies

A very limited number of cancers cause hypercalcemia via production of 1,25-dihydroxyvitamin D, but it is the mechanism of hypercalcemia in the vast majority of cases of Hodgkin lymphoma and non-Hodgkin lymphoma-related

H. McMullen
Columbia University, Vagelos College of Physicians and Surgeons, New York, NY, USA
e-mail: hlm2138@cumc.columbia.edu

M. D. Walker (✉)
Division of Endocrinology, Columbia University Irving Medical Center, New York, NY, USA
e-mail: mad2037@columbia.edu

M. D. Walker (ed.), *Hypercalcemia*, Contemporary Endocrinology,
https://doi.org/10.1007/978-3-030-93182-7_11

hypercalcemia. In contrast, PTHrP production has been observed rarely in Hodgkin and non-Hodgkin lymphoma [6]. Most solid tumors induce hypercalcemic states via mechanisms other than 1,25-dihydroxyvitamin D production, such as osteolytic metastases or PTHrP production (discussed extensively in Chaps. 9 and 10). There are, however, scarce case reports of solid malignancies that have been associated with the production of 1,25-dihydroxyvitamin D. These include ovarian dysgerminoma, ovarian cystadenocarcinoma, pancreatic neuroendocrine tumor, squamous cell lung carcinoma, and squamous cell tongue carcinoma [7–10]. A recent large case series reported associations with breast cancer, renal cell cancer, prostate cancer, head and neck squamous cell carcinoma, bladder cancer, melanoma, sarcoma, and others [6, 11]. To date, no specific solid malignancies have been shown to have a strong correlation with this mechanism [11].

Mechanism of 1,25-Dihydroxyvitamin D Production

1-Alpha-hydroxylase (CYP27B1) is the enzyme responsible for conversion of 25-hydroxyvitamin D (calcidiol) to the physiologically active form of 1,25-dihydroxyvitamin D (calcitriol). In the normal state, this largely takes place in the peritubular capillary endothelial cells of the kidney [12, 13]. The activity of this enzyme is normally tightly regulated by parathyroid hormone (PTH). Under normal physiological conditions, elevated serum 1,25-dihydroxyvitamin D provides negative feedback to the parathyroid glands. This leads to a decrease in secretion of parathyroid hormone (PTH) and thus a decrease in the production of 1-alpha-hydroxylase with a subsequent decline in 1,25-dihydroxyvitamin D and serum calcium [13].

Conversely, elevated PTH induces the 1-alpha-hydroxylase. 1,25-Dihydroxyvitamin D acts via its receptor to increase the expression of calcium channels as well as the calcium shuttling protein, calbindin, in the intestine and kidney [12]. Further, it increases bone resorption and release of calcium from the skeleton. These actions increase serum calcium levels. In addition to regulation via PTH, 1,25-dihydroxyvitamin D regulates its own production by inhibiting the 1-alpha-hydroxylase in the kidney and increasing the expression of the gene encoding 24-alpha-hydroxylase, which is responsible for the conversion of 25-hydroxyvitamin D to the inactive metabolite, 24,25-dihydroxyvitamin D as well as 1,25-dihydroxyvitamin D to 1,24,25-trihydroxyvitamin D [13].

In the case of hypercalcemia of malignancy mediated by production of 1,25-dihydroxyvitamin D, malignant lymphocytes and/or surrounding macrophages are thought to directly perform this conversion via expression of 1-alpha-hydroxylase. Although this production of 1,25-dihydroxyvitamin D has been attributed to the malignant lymphocytes, there is no robust evidence for this attribution beyond observation of production by lymphoma and plasma cells in vitro [9]. At least one case has been reported where the activity of 1-alpha-hydroxylase was directly identified in the surrounding tissue macrophages but not the malignant lymphocytes themselves, suggesting lymphocyte-induced expression of 1-alpha-hydroxylase in

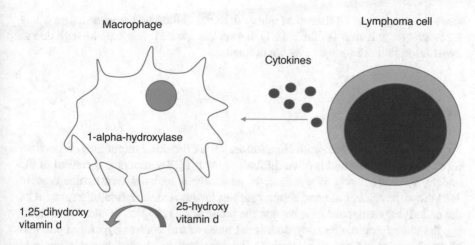

Fig. 11.1 Proposed mechanism of hypercalcemia mediated by malignancy-associated production of 1,25-dihydroxyvitamin D

these tissues (see Fig. 11.1); this closely mirrors the mechanism observed in granu-lomatous diseases such as sarcoidosis (see Chap. 13) [9, 14, 15]. Further investiga-tion is needed to identify the precise cellular source of the ectopically produced 1,25-dihydroxyvitamin D in malignancy. The significantly elevated serum 1,25-dihydroxyvitamin D levels then induce a state of hypercalcemia via the nor-mal physiological mechanisms, primarily driven by increased intestinal calcium absorption with some contribution from increased bone resorption [3, 16]. In con-trast to normal physiological conditions, however, the expression of 1-alpha-hydroxylase in malignancy is not responsive to the normal feedback control.

Clinical and Biochemical Presentation

In general, hypercalcemia of malignancy, including 1,25-dihydroxyvitamin D-induced hypercalcemia, is frequently a late-stage manifestation of malignancy. Thus, malig-nancy is often clinically apparent by the time hypercalcemia develops [17]. Like other causes of hypercalcemia of malignancy, 1,25-dihydroxyvitamin D-induced hypercal-cemia can be characterized by marked hypercalcemia that is symptomatic. One series suggests the majority of patients had calcium levels >12 mg/dl [6]. The symptoms and signs of hypercalcemia are dependent on the degree of hypercalcemia and rate of rise and are described in Chap. 2. The biochemical pattern of 1,25-dihydroxyvitamin D-induced hypercalcemia of malignancy is characterized by a suppressed PTH and high 1,25-dihydroxyvitamin D levels and elevated urinary calcium. In one series, mean calcitriol levels were two times the upper limit of normal but ranged up to 5.4 times the upper limit of normal [6]. Inappropriately normal 1,25-dihydroxyvitamin D levels may also be consistent with a 1,25-dihydroxyvitamin D-medicated process since the suppressed PTH level in other etiologies should be associated with a low 1,25-dihydroxyvitamin D (Table 11.1). Serum phosphate levels may be high due to hyperabsorption or in some cases are normal.

Treatment

Hypercalcemia associated with Hodgkin and non-Hodgkin lymphoma is an indicator of poor prognosis and is often difficult to treat [6]. Treatment and control of the underlying malignancy, if possible, is generally associated with a decrease in 1,25-dihydroxyvitamin D and serum calcium levels. A description of treatment of the underlying malignancies is beyond the scope of this chapter. In addition to treating the underlying malignancy, additional measures to control hypercalcemia and alleviate symptoms are often needed. The approach to treating hypercalcemia is covered in detail in Chap. 5. While corticosteroids are the most effective treatment for 1,25-dihydroxyvitamin D-associated hypercalcemia, the etiology may or may not be apparent on initial presentation [3, 6]. Further, there may be a delay in results from 1,25-dihydroxyvitamin D assays. Therefore, other measures to control hypercalcemia are usually necessary. Given the degree of hypercalcemia, dehydration is typically present, and the initial approach to treatment usually involves aggressive hydration.

The minimal effective or optimal dosing of glucocorticoids is unclear. Hydrocortisone 200–300 mg/day for 3–5 days and then prednisone 10–20 mg/day for 7 days or prednisone 40–60 mg/day for 10 days is recommended by some sources [3]. The onset of response to corticosteroid treatment is usually 2 days, but the full hypocalcemic effect may not be observed until 7–10 days [3]. Higher doses are sometimes needed. Corticosteroids have specific actions that ameliorate 1,25-dihydroxyvitamin D-mediated hypercalcemia independent of its tumoral cytotoxic effects [6]. Glucocorticoids decrease absorption of calcium from the gastrointestinal tract by reducing duodenal expression of the active calcium ion transporter Transient receptor potential vanilloid subfamily member 6 (TRPV6) and calbindin [18]. Glucocorticoids also increase urinary calcium excretion and directly inhibit 1-alpha-hydroxylase activity. [6, 19]. Ketoconazole, which inhibits P450 enzymes, also decreases calcitriol production. Its use may be limited by its hepatotoxic effects.

Hypercalcemia related to excessive 1,25-dihydroxyvitamin D is also responsive to general strategies to treat hypercalcemia of any etiology. Agents that reduce mobilization of calcium from the bone, including intravenous bisphosphonates, denosumab, subcutaneous calcitonin, or those that increase the excretion of urinary calcium such as loop diuretics, are also effective supplementary treatments. A recent case series suggested that patients with solid tumors associated with elevated 1,25-dihydroxyvitamin D levels responded less well to anti-resorptive treatment than those without elevated 1,25-dihydroxyvitamin D [11]. Specifically, these patients have been reported to have higher rates of incomplete response to bisphosphonate therapy, even when bisphosphonates were initiated early in the disease

Table 11.1 Biochemical patterns in hypercalcemia of malignancy of different etiologies

	Serum calcium	Serum phosphate	Serum PTH	PTHrP	25-Hydroxyvitamin D	1,25-Dihydroxyvitamin D
1,25-Dihydroxyvitamin D-mediated	↑	↑	↓	↓	↔	↑
PTHrP-mediated	↑	↓	↓	↑	↔	↓
Osteolytic metastases	↑	↔ or ↑	↓	↓	↔	↓

course [11]. Because the main mechanism of 1,25-dihydroxyvitamin D-mediated hypercalcemia is hyperabsorption of calcium from the gastrointestinal tract, dietary modifications such as limiting dietary calcium intake may be helpful as an adjunctive treatment. Avoidance of supplemental vitamin D intake to limit substrate is also recommended [3, 6]. However, it should be noted that these strategies are less effective than steroids for hypercalcemia of malignancy due to excess 1,25-dihydroxyvitamin D production.

Summary

In summary, excessive production of 1,25-dihydroxyvitamin D is a rare cause of hypercalcemia of malignancy but should be suspected in patients with lymphoma. Although there is evidence that this is attributable to macrophages and/or malignant lymphocytes themselves acting independently of the body's physiologic tight PTH-regulated production of 1,25-dihydroxyvitamin D, the precise mechanism and cell type responsible remains to be fully elucidated. Identification of hypercalcemia of malignancy due to elevated 1,25-dihydroxyvitamin D is clinically important because it is a poor prognostic indicator and often refractory to traditional treatments for hypercalcemia such as bisphosphonates (Table 11.1).

References

1. Mundy GR, Ibbotson KJ, D'Souza SM, Simpson EL, Jacobs JW, Martin TJ. The hypercalcemia of cancer. N Engl J Med. 1984;310(26):1718–27.
2. Mirrakhimov A. Hypercalcemia of malignancy: an update on pathogenesis and management. N Am J Med Sci. 2015;7(11):483.
3. Asonitis N, Angelousi A, Zafeiris C, Lambrou GI, Dontas I, Kassi E. Diagnosis, pathophysiology and management of hypercalcemia in malignancy: a review of the literature. Horm Metab Res. 2019;51(12):770–8.
4. Glezerman IG, Sternlicht H. Hypercalcemia of malignancy and new treatment options. Ther Clin Risk Manag. 2015;11:1779.
5. Grill V. Hypercalcemia of malignancy. Rev Endocr Metab Disord. 2000;1(4):253–63.
6. Seymour J, Gagel R. Calcitriol: the major humoral mediator of hypercalcemia in Hodgkin's disease and non-Hodgkin's lymphomas. Blood. 1993;82(5):1383–94.

7. Van Lierop AH, Bisschop PH, Boelen A, Van Eeden S, Engelman AF, Nieveen Van Dijkum EJ, et al. hypercalcaemia due to a calcitriol-producing neuroendocrine tumour. J Surg Case Rep. 2019;2019(12):rjz346.
8. Nemr S, Alluri S, Sundaramurthy D, Landry D, Braden G. Hypercalcemia in lung cancer due to simultaneously elevated PTHrP and ectopic calcitriol production: first case report. Case Rep Oncol Med. 2017;2017:1–3.
9. Donovan PJ, Sundac L, Pretorius CJ, D'Emden MC, McLeod DSA. Calcitriol-mediated hypercalcemia: causes and course in 101 patients. J Clin Endocrinol Metabol. 2013;98(10):4023–9.
10. Hibi M, Hara Fujio, Tomishige H, Nishida Y, Kato T, Okumura N, Hashimoto T, Kato R. 1,25-dihydroxyvitamin Dmediated hypercalcemia in ovarian dysgerminoma. Pediatric hematology. Oncology. 2008;25(1):73–8.
11. Chukir T, Liu Y, Hoffman K, Bilezikian JP, Farooki A. Calcitriol elevation is associated with a higher risk of refractory hypercalcemia of malignancy in solid tumors. J Clin Endocrinol Metabol. 2020;105(4):e1115–e23.
12. Lambers TT, Bindels RJM, Hoenderop JGJ. Coordinated control of renal Ca2+ handling. Kidney Int. 2006;69(4):650–4.
13. Kumar R, Tebben PJ, Thompson JR. Vitamin D and the kidney. Arch Biochem Biophys. 2012;523(1):77–86.
14. Hewison M, Kantorovich V, Liker HR, Van Herle AJ, Cohan P, Zehnder D, et al. Vitamin D-mediated hypercalcemia in lymphoma: evidence for hormone production by tumor-adjacent macrophages. J Bone Miner Res. 2003;18(3):579–82.
15. Fuss M, Pepersack T, Gillet C, Karmali R, Corvilain J. Calcium and vitamin D metabolism in granulomatous diseases. 1992;11(1):28–36.
16. Shivnani S, Shelton J, Richardson J, Maalouf N. Hypercalcemia of malignancy with simultaneous elevation in serum parathyroid hormone—related peptide and 1,25-dihydroxyvitamin D in a patient with metastatic renal cell carcinoma. Endocr Pract. 2009;15(3):234–9.
17. Shallis RMRR, Reagan JL. Mechanisms of hypercalcemia in non-Hodgkin lymphoma and associated outcomes: a retrospective review. Clin Lymphoma Myeloma Leuk. 2018;18:e123–e9.
18. Huybers S, Naber THJ, Bindels RJ, Hoenderop JG. Prednisolone-induced Ca2+ malabsorption is caused by diminished expression of the epithelial Ca2+ channel TRPV6. Am J Physiol Gastrointest Liver Physiol. 2007;292(1):G92.
19. Suzuki Y, Ichikawa Y, Saito E, Homma M. Importance of increased urinary calcium excretion in the development of secondary hyperparathyroidism of patients under glucocorticoid therapy. Metabolism. 1983;32(2):151–6.

Chapter 12
Vitamin D Intoxication

Sajal Patel, Beatriz Martinez Quintero, and Robert A. Adler

Overview of Vitamin D Metabolism

Vitamin D exists primarily in two forms in nature: vitamin D2 (ergocalciferol), which is produced by plants/fungi through solar ultraviolet B radiation of ergosterol, and vitamin D3 (cholecalciferol), which is produced in the skin of animals/lanolin through radiation of 7-dehydrocholesterol [1, 2].

In humans, the primary source of vitamin D may be obtained through endogenous production of vitamin D3 [3, 4]. However, vitamin D is also ingested in the form of both vitamin D2 (such as fortified dairy products and breakfast cereals) and D3 (such as eggs yolks and oily fish). They are also sold as over-the-counter supplements and in prescription strength doses [1].

Regardless of form, due to its lipophilic nature, ingested vitamin D is incorporated into chylomicrons and travels through the lymphatic system to enter venous blood [3, 5, 6]. Once there, it is either stored in adipose tissue or taken up by the liver for further processing [5, 6]. Vitamin D stored in fat cells allows for a large reservoir, and the whole-body half-life is about 2 months [5]. The endogenous production of vitamin D3 is regulated by enzymatic processing of excess into inactive metabolites [2, 7].

Vitamins D2 and D3 function as prohormones that undergo a two-step enzymatic hydroxylation process. The first hydroxylation step occurs in the liver, where vitamins D2 and D3 are converted to 25-hydroxyvitamin D2 or D3 [25(OH)D] via the 25-hydroxylase enzyme. The second step occurs in the kidney where 1α-hydroxylase

S. Patel · B. M. Quintero · R. A. Adler (✉)
Endocrinology and Metabolism Section, Central Virginia Veterans Affairs Health Care System, Richmond, VA, USA

Division of Endocrinology, Metabolism, and Diabetes Mellitus, Virginia Commonwealth University, Richmond, VA, USA
e-mail: Sajal.Patel@vcuhealth.org; bmartinez1@iuhealth.org; Robert.adler@va.gov

© The Author(s), under exclusive license to Springer Nature
Switzerland AG 2022
M. D. Walker (ed.), *Hypercalcemia*, Contemporary Endocrinology,
https://doi.org/10.1007/978-3-030-93182-7_12

converts 25(OH)D to the biologically active form 1,25-dihydroxyvitamin D2 or D3 (calcitriol) [1]. Other tissues also contain this final enzyme, but they produce calcitriol primarily for local use and do not contribute significantly to the whole-body pool [4].

In the serum, endogenously produced vitamin D and the metabolites of both endogenous and ingested vitamin D bind to vitamin D-binding protein (VDBP), which allows for its delivery to target cells as well as maintaining a large pool of easily accessible hormone. Binding affects the metabolites' half-lives as well as the rate of uptake in target cells [5, 6]. 25(OH)D has the strongest affinity to VDBP and also has the longest plasma half-life (approximately 3 weeks). Calcitriol has a short circulating plasma half-life (approximately 4–20 h) but is more rapidly taken up by tissues due to its weaker binding affinity [4–6]. At physiologic levels, only calcitriol exerts target tissue effects [5].

Calcitriol and other metabolites exert effects in target cells via binding to vitamin D receptors (VDR), which are nuclear receptors [7]. These effects are wide ranging with both calcemic and non-calcemic effects. Calcemic effects, which are much better understood, are through increased absorption of both calcium and phosphorus in the gastrointestinal tract [3, 7]. In the absence of adequate vitamin D, only 10–15% of dietary calcium and 60% of phosphorus are absorbed. Vitamin D repletion improves absorption by 30–40% and 80%, respectively [3]. Potential non-calcemic effects include promotion of cell differentiation, inhibition of cell proliferation, inhibition of angiogenesis, stimulation of insulin production, inhibition of renin production, and stimulation of immune modulatory effects in both the innate and adaptive immune systems [3, 4, 8, 9]. Vitamin D deficiency has been associated with increased all-cause mortality, cardiovascular disease, reduced bone density with increased fracture risk, metabolic syndrome, malignancy, autoimmune conditions, and increased risk of infections [10]. Association does not equal causation. Thus, there have been multiple studies to determine the role of vitamin D outside of its effects on bone and mineral metabolism [11].

Measurement of Vitamin D/Epidemiology of Vitamin D Intoxication

Vitamin D insufficiency and deficiency are very common with an estimated one-third of the world population being affected [10, 11], although there are problems of measurement and controversies in defining deficiency. The negative sequelae of deficiency and potential for benefits have led to increased public and provider interest in supplementation [10]. There has been a resultant dramatic increase in both medical prescription and over-the-counter purchases of vitamin D supplements [12].

Serum levels of 25(OH)D remain the most often used marker of vitamin D status and are generally accepted worldwide. However, there is variability among measurements with regard to assay quality and lack of standardization. This has led to difficulty in determining a clear consensus of what qualifies as deficiency as well as excess. In general, multiple medical and scientific societies recommend vitamin D intake of 400 IU to 2000 IU per day depending on age from infancy to the elderly with the goal of a serum 25(OH)D levels of 20–30 ng/mL (50–75 nmol/L) [11]. Vitamin D toxicity (VDT) was generally defined as a level that would result in hypercalcemia, but this has been revised to values >100–150 ng/mL (250–375 nmol/L) due to negative effects of VDT being noted starting at that range even in the absence of hypercalcemia [11, 13].

There appears to be a reverse J-shaped relationship of serum 25(OH)D levels and outcomes such as mortality [14]. Therefore, while deficiency is important to correct, VDT is also of great clinical importance [15]. Although the prevalence is unknown, reports in the literature, lay press, and on the Internet have increased public awareness of real and potential health benefits of vitamin D [7, 13]. VDT is often related to excessive ingestion through use of over-the-counter supplements (most common), manufacturing errors resulting in excess amounts as D preparations or as fortification of foods, and prescribing errors (least common) [7, 16, 17]. Retrospective analysis of data from the National Poison Data System showed that VDT increased from a mean of 196 cases per year from 2000 to 2005 to 4535 exposures per year from 2005 to 2011 [10]. Review of Mayo Clinic data from 2001 to 2011 by Dudenkov et al. [18] showed that the number of individuals with a serum 25(OH)D concentration >50 ng/mL (>75 nmol/l) had increased by 20 fold over that period. Of note, only one patient, with a 25(OH)D concentration of 364 ng/mL (910 nmol/l), was diagnosed with hypercalcemia in the Mayo series. This is consistent with data reported by Pietras et al. [19] and Ekwaru et al. [20] that serum 25(OH)D concentrations of 40–60 ng/mL (100–150 nmol/l) did not result in symptoms of VDT [13].

Due to a wide therapeutic index, the highest daily intake of vitamin D that will result in no adverse effects is not known [15, 17]. Reports show that vitamin D supplementation up to 10,000 IU per day will not result in serum levels at risk for toxicity, but there appears to be no improvement for bone health at doses greater than 4000 IU per day [7, 11]. In the VITAL trial, there were no safety concerns with regard to hypercalcemia, nephrolithiasis, or renal injury with a daily supplementation of 2000 IU, one of the more common supplementation doses available [15].

Though serum 25(OH)D levels are most often used to determine toxicity, patients taking other forms of vitamin D (such as α-hydroxylated vitamin D analogs) may have normal or low 25(OH)D concentration with increased calcitriol levels [13].

Pathophysiology of Hypercalcemia Related to Vitamin D Intoxication

Vitamin D toxicity can result in life-threatening hypercalcemia and therefore must not be overlooked as an etiology in patients presenting with hypercalcemia [17]. There are currently three hypotheses about the mechanism through which vitamin D excess results in toxicity with all proposed mechanisms resulting in increased VDR nuclear activity with resultant increased transcription and gene expression [5, 13].

One hypothesis is that toxicity is mediated by elevated serum calcitriol levels that lead to increased intracellular activity. However, many animal studies and human cases have shown that calcitriol levels were normal or only slightly elevated in some patients with VDT-related hypercalcemia. Therefore, increased concentrations of the active vitamin D hormone calcitriol do not appear to be the sole mechanism of inducing hypercalcemia [5, 13].

A second hypothesis is that marked increases in vitamin D metabolites result in the metabolites saturating VDBP and freeing calcitriol to enter target cells through diffusion and to activate VDRs. However, this is an unlikely mechanism because preclinical studies have shown that mice lacking 1α-hydroxylase (and therefore unable to synthesize calcitriol) still develop VDT at high doses of vitamin D supplementation [5, 13]. This biochemical finding has also been shown in pigs and dairy cows. However, in conflict with the animal data, a report of a family with accidental VDT noted normal total calcitriol levels, but markedly elevated free calcitriol levels. This supports the mechanism of "free" calcitriol being the primary mediator of VDT [5].

The third, and most likely, hypothesis is that increases in metabolites other than calcitriol saturate the binding capacity of VDBP and allow for the various vitamin D metabolites to enter the cell and activate VDRs to stimulate gene expression. 25(OH)D has been shown to have a high affinity for VDBP but also has the strongest affinity for VDRs at high concentrations, thus allowing it to directly exert genomic effects when in excess [6, 12, 13].

Presentation

The diagnosis of VDT can often be determined clinically with a thorough history and review of medications.

Due to the primary effects of vitamin D increasing calcium absorption in the gastrointestinal tract, VDT manifests as symptoms due to hypercalcemia and hypercalciuria. These symptoms can range from nonspecific to lethal: muscle weakness, hypertension, neuropsychiatric disturbances, gastrointestinal upset (vomiting, abdominal pain, peptic ulcer), pancreatitis, polyuria and polydipsia, dehydration, renal calculi, renal failure, irreversible deposition of calcium phosphate crystals in soft tissues, cardiac arrhythmias, coronary vessel calcification, and heart valve calcification [12, 13, 17].

Hypercalciuria precedes hypercalcemia and can be seen with 25(OH)D levels starting at 100–150 ng/mL (250–375 nmol/L), whereas hypercalcemia does not usually occur until serum levels are >150 ng/mL (375 nmol/L) and is rare [11, 15]. Hypercalciuria is due to the increased filtered load of calcium plus parathyroid hormone (PTH) suppression leading to decreased renal tubular calcium reabsorption. Lacking the effect of parathyroid hormone, even with hypercalciuria, the increased calcium load overwhelms renal tubular function, and serum calcium rises [8].

Due to the large storage pool in fatty tissue, vitamin D has a long half-life, and VDT can result for up to 18 months after discontinuation of chronic supplementation. However, in the plasma, the half-lives of 25(OH)D and 1,25(OH)$_2$D are much shorter, and VDT from acute overdose of 25(OH)D may last for weeks and

$1,25(OH)_2D$ for few days [13]. Acute VDT is usually caused by doses of vitamin D >10,000 IU per day resulting in serum 25(OH)D concentrations >150 ng/mL (375 nmol/L). Chronic VDT, though, can occur with doses >4000 IU per day over an extended period (i.e., years) with 25(OH)D concentrations in the 50–150 ng/mL range (125–375 nmol/L) [10, 15].

In contrast VDT cannot result from excess sun exposure. A diversified adult diet (even with fortified foods) does not provide excess amounts of vitamin D, although if it is supplemented by cod liver oil, VDT is possible. VDT is a rare diagnosis and is most often seen in prolonged use of large vitamin D supplementation doses. In adults, patients taking vitamin D for a non-mineral/bone reason may be more likely to take excessive doses. For example, multiple sclerosis is associated with low serum 25 (OH)vitamin D levels [21], and patients may believe that the more vitamin D they ingest, the better their course will be. For example, some studies of vitamin D therapy on multiple sclerosis have utilized very high doses [e.g., 22].

Similarly, in children, parents may provide more vitamin D than needed as an attempt to maximize health. There have also been cases in children related to excessive amounts of vitamin D in fortified foods [23]. Patients prescribed monthly or weekly 50,000 unit doses of ergocalciferol (in the United States) or cholecalciferol (in Europe) may take it daily and thus acutely raise the serum 25(OH)D level. In Europe 25-OH vitamin D preparations are available by prescription [24] and are also potential sources of vitamin D excess. Calcitriol has a much shorter half-life than cholecalciferol. When used in high doses in hypoparathyroidism or end-stage chronic kidney disease (CKD 5), there is at least potential for transient hypercalcemia, particularly if the patient with hypoparathyroidism is transitioning to a parathyroid hormone preparation.

VDT cannot be diagnosed solely based on 25(OH)D serum levels. Biochemically, in addition to 25(OH)D concentrations >150 ng/mL, the patient will have hypercalciuria with or without hypercalcemia, suppressed PTH activity, and hyperphosphatemia. Calcitriol may be low, normal, or mildly increased due to decreased 1α-hydroxylase activity and increased 24-hydroxylase activity as a result of PTH suppression [13]. Vitamin D increases phosphate absorption in the gut, such that the calcium-phosphate product may be very high in VDT patients.

Separate from its effect on calcium, intermittent high-dose supplementation in older individuals over a prolonged period may lead to increased risk of falls with serum levels of 25OHD as low as 45 ng/mL (113 nmol/L) [11, 25]. This surprising finding discouraged the use of large intermittent doses of vitamin D in institutionalized older people at risk for falls and fracture.

Treatment for Vitamin D Intoxication

The first line of treatment is to stabilize the patient and correct hypercalcemia [10]. To stabilize a critical patient, resuscitative measures must be immediately started with protection of the airway, administration of intravenous fluid (IVF), and transfer to a higher level of care if needed. Isotonic sodium chloride is the preferred IVF to correct dehydration and restore renal function. Hemodialysis may also be considered in those with severe/life-threatening hypercalcemia or sequelae of hypercalcemia. Continuous veno-venous hemofiltration (CVVH) can be used in hemodynamically unstable patients [10, 13]. Hypercalcemia of any cause decreases the ability of the kidney to reabsorb water, leading to volume loss, which may be severe. Thus, restoration of volume is the first goal of the treatment protocol.

To correct hypercalcemia, all vitamin D supplementation should be discontinued, and dietary calcium intake should be reduced. Loop diuretics can be used only after volume resuscitation to promote urine calcium loss. Early use of loop diuretics can exacerbate volume contraction and worsen hypercalcemia. Antiresorptive medications such as calcitonin and/or bisphosphonates can be used as well. Intravenous (IV) calcitonin 4 U/kg can be administered with assessment of serial calcium levels and repeated after 6–12 hours. Serum calcium is lowered through calcitonin's effects as an inhibitor of bone resorption. However, calcitonin can cause tachyphylaxis, such that it is often used as a bridge to intravenous bisphosphonate administration, which can take effect in a few days. Intravenous bisphosphonates (such as zoledronic acid) can be administered concurrently with calcitonin, with action then persisting for a prolonged period depending on formulation. Glucocorticoids (hydrocortisone 100 mg per day or equivalent steroid dosing) decrease serum calcium levels through decreased intestinal calcium absorption, increased urinary excretion, and increased synthesis of inactive metabolites with reduced production of calcitriol. Serum calcium levels usually return to normal over several days with steroid initiation, but prolonged use is associated with a wide host of adverse effects [10, 13]. Good hydration must be maintained throughout the treatment period.

A second-line treatment strategy is to reduce vitamin D levels, but these are currently under investigation and are currently not preferred [10, 13]:

- Phenobarbital can decrease 25(OH)D levels via suppression of 25-hydroxylation [26].
- Ketoconazole suppresses1α-hydroxylase activity through nonspecific suppression of the cytochrome P450 CYP27B1 [10, 13].
- Drugs such as rifampin induce enzymatic conversion to inactive vitamin D metabolites.
- Specific inhibitors of CYP27B1 that might block calcitriol production without affecting other cytochrome P450 enzymes [10, 13].

Conclusion

With increasing vitamin D supplementation worldwide, reports of vitamin D toxicity have increased. Though it continues to be an overall rare diagnosis, recognition and treatment are critical due to its potentially fatal consequences. The mechanisms through which toxicity occurs and the maximum tolerated dose of vitamin D are unknown, but the constellation of presenting symptoms and a serum 25(OH)D concentration >100 ng/mL should prompt consideration of vitamin D excess as the cause of hypercalcemia. Fortunately, toxicity is usually self-limited, and well-established treatment options exist with many second-line treatments currently under study. Overall, practitioners should remain vigilant in all patients who are on vitamin D supplementation and help educate the public on the danger of excess ingestion. When it comes to vitamin D intake, more is not necessarily better.

Case

A 47-year-old healthy woman presented to the emergency department with anorexia, nausea, vomiting, and confusion that culminated in a fall. On evaluation in the emergency department, her serum calcium was found to be 16.9 mg/dL (normal 8.5–10.2 mg/dL). She reported a history of wrist fracture 2 years prior. As a result, dual-energy X-ray absorptiometry had been performed about 1 year ago. She was diagnosed with osteopenia at that time. Due to the diagnosis of osteopenia, she had started taking vitamin D 5000 units three times per day about 6 months ago. Recently she also added calcium supplementation 500 mg twice-daily based upon the advice of a friend who was a nutritionist. She had no other relevant medical history and took no other medications. She was a nonsmoker and consumed one glass of wine weekly. Her family history was negative for hypercalcemia, but she has a history of osteoporosis in her mother. On exam, weight was 130 pounds with height 65 inches. She was lethargic and oriented to person, but not place or time. Mucous membranes were dry, she was tachycardic, and bowel sounds were diminished. Her exam was otherwise unremarkable. Lab evaluation revealed PTH 9.5 (normal 15–65 pg/mL) with serum calcium 16.2 mg/dL (normal 8.5–10.2 mg/dL). Serum creatinine was 2.6 mg/dL and bicarbonate was 34 mEq/L. Phosphate was 4.9 mg/dL (normal 2.5–4.5 mg/dL). 25-Hydroxyvitamin D was 320 ng/mL (normal 20–50 ng/mL), and 1,25-dihydroxyvitamin D was 55.5 pg/mL (20–79 pg/mL). Complete blood count, liver and thyroid function tests, serum cortisol, PTHrP, and serum and urine electrophoresis were normal. She was treated with intravenous saline at 250 cc/hour and was given calcitonin 4 IU/kg every 12 hours for four doses. Her supplements were discontinued. Over the next 48 hours, her serum calcium declined to 12.4 mg/dL and subsequently normalized. The patient improved clinically and her serum creatinine improved to 1.3 mg/dL. She was able to begin eating and drinking, and her serum calcium remained normal after intravenous fluids were discontinued. She was seen in endocrinology clinic 2 months later in the outpatient setting. At that time, she was feeling well and had discontinued all of her supplements upon discharge from the hospital. Her serum calcium was 10.1 mg/dL (normal 8.5–10.2 mg/dL), and 25-hydroxyvitamin D was over 150 ng/mL. Her creatinine was 1.0 mg/dL.

The patient in this case had laboratories consistent with vitamin D toxicity, probably accompanied by milk-alkali syndrome (see Chap. 14 for a discussion of milk-alkali syndrome). The presentation is notable for symptomatic and marked hypercalcemia in the setting of prolonged very high-dose vitamin

D intake. Her laboratory evaluation revealed non-PTH-mediated hypercalcemia, and her 25-hydroxyvitamin D level was consistent with levels observed in patients with vitamin D toxicity. Notably, the 1,25-dihydroxyvitamin D level was not elevated, which is not uncommon since the suppression of PTH reduces transcription of the 1-alpha-hydroxylase. Other causes of hypercalcemia were excluded by lab evaluation. Because the half-life of vitamin D is long, this patient's 25-hydroxyvitamin D level was still elevated months after discontinuation of supplements.

References

1. Tripkovic L, Lambert H, Hart K, Smith CP, Bucca G, Penson S, et al. Comparison of vitamin D2 and vitamin D3 supplementation in raising serum 25-hydroxyvitamin D status: a systematic review and meta-analysis. Am J Clin Nutr. 2012;95(6):1357–64.
2. Holick MF. Vitamin D deficiency. N Engl J Med. 2007;357(3):266–81.
3. Nair R, Maseeh A. Vitamin D: the "sunshine" vitamin. J Pharmacol Pharmacother. 2012;3(2):118–26.
4. Shroff R, Knott C, Rees L. The virtues of vitamin D – but how much is too much? Pediatr Nephrol. 2010;25(9):1607–20.
5. Jones G. Pharmacokinetics of vitamin D toxicity. Am J Clin Nutr. 2008;88(2):582S–6S.
6. Bouillon R, Schuit F, Antonio L, Rastinejad F. Vitamin D binding protein: a historic overview. Front Endocrinol (Lausanne). 2020;10:910.
7. Taylor PN, Davies JS. A review of the growing risk of vitamin D toxicity from inappropriate practice. Br J Clin Pharmacol. 2018;84:1121–7.
8. Misgar RA, Sahu D, Bhat MH, Wani AI, Bashir MI. Vitamin D toxicity: a prospective study from a tertiary care centre in Kashmir Valley. Indian J Endocrinol Metab. 2019;23(3):363–6.
9. Prietl B, Treiber G, Pieber TR, Amrein K. Vitamin D and immune function. Nutrients. 2013;5(7):2502–21.
10. Lim K, Thadhani R. Vitamin D toxicity. Br J Nephrol. 2020;42(2):238–44.
11. Giustina A, Bouillon R, Binkley N, Sempos C, Adler RA, Bollerslev J, et al. Controversies in vitamin D: a statement from the third international conference. JBMR Plus. 2020;4(12):e10417.
12. Pérez-Barrios C, Hernández-Álvarez E, Blanco-Navarro I, Pérez-Sacristán B, Granado-Lorencio F. Prevalence of hypercalcemia related to hypervitaminosis D in clinical practice. Clin Nutr. 2016;35(6):1354–8.
13. Marcinowska-Suchowierska E, Kupisz-Urbańska M, Łukaszkiewicz J, Płudowski P, Jones G. Vitamin D toxicity-a clinical perspective. Front Endocrinol (Lausanne). 2018;9:550.
14. Durazo-Arvizu RA, Dawson-Hughes B, Kramer H, et al. The reverse J-shaped association between serum total 25-hydroxyvitamin D concentration and all-cause mortality: the impact of assay standardization. Am J Epidemiol. 2017;185(8):720–6.
15. Pilz S, Zittermann A, Trummer C, Theiler-Schwetz V, Lerchbaum E, Keppel M, et al. Vitamin D testing and treatment: a narrative review of current evidence. Endocr Connect. 2019 Feb;8(2):R27–43.
16. Rahesh J, Chu V, Peiris AN. Hypervitaminosis D without toxicity. Proc (Bayl Univ Med Cent). 2019;33(1):42–3.
17. Galior K, Grebe S, Singh R. Development of vitamin D toxicity from overcorrection of vitamin D deficiency: a review of case reports. Nutrients. 2018;10(8):953.

18. Dudenkov DV, Yawn BP, Oberhelman SS, Fischer PR, Singh RJ, Cha SS, Maxson JA, Quigg SM, Thatcher TD. Changing incidence of serum 25-hydroxyvitamin D values above 50 ng/mL: A 10-year population-based study. Mayo Clin Proc. 2015;90(5):577–86.
19. Pietras SM, Obayan BK, Cai MH, Holick MF. Vitamin D2 treatment for vitamin D deficiency and insufficiency for up to 6 years. Arch Intern Med. 2009;169(19):1806–8.
20. Ekwaru JP, Zwicker JD, Holick MF, Giovannucci E, Veugelers PJ. The importance of body weight for the dose response relationship of oral vitamin D supplementation and serum 25-hydroxyvitamin D in healthy volunteers. PLoS One. 2014;9(11):e11265.
21. Feige J, Moser T, Bieler L, Schwenker K, Hauer L, Sellner J. Vitamin D supplementation in multiple sclerosis: a critical analysis of potentials and threats. Nutrients. 2020;12:783.
22. Dorr J, Backer-Koduah P, Wernecke KD, Becker E, Hoffmann F, Faiss J, Brockmeier B, Hoffmann O, Anvari K, Wuerfel J, et al. High-dose vitamin D supplementation in multiple sclerosis – results from the randomized EVIDIMS (efficacy of vitamin D supplementation in multiple sclerosis) trial. Mult Scler J Exp Transl Clin. 2020;6(1):2055217320903474.
23. Vogiatzi MG, Jacobson-Dickman K, De Boer MD, Drugs and Therapeutic Committee of the Pediatric Endocrine Society. Vitamin D supplementations and risk of toxicity in pediatrics: a review of current literature. J Clin Endocrinol Metab. 2014;99:1132–41.
24. Minisola S, Cianferotti L, Biondi P, Cipriani C, Fossi C, Franceschelli GF, Leoncini G, Pepe J, Bischoff-Ferrari HA, Brandi ML. Correction of vitamin D status by calcidiol: pharmacokinetic profile, safety, and biochemical effects on bone and mineral metabolism of daily and weekly dosage regimens. Osteoporos Int. 2017;28:3239–49.
25. Sanders KM, Stuart AI, Williamson EJ, Simpson JA, Kotowicz MA, Young D, Nicholson GC. Annual high-dose oral vitamin D and falls and fractures in older women: a randomized controlled trial. JAMA. 2010;303(18):1815–22.
26. Hosseinpour F, Ellfolk M, Norlin M, Wikvall K. Phenobarbital suppresses vitamin D3 25-hydroxylase expression: a potential new mechanism for drug-induced osteomalacia. Biochem Biophys Res Commun. 2007;357(3):603–7.

Chapter 13
Benign 1,25-Dihydroxyvitamin D–Mediated Hypercalcemia

Naim M. Maalouf and Li Song

Introduction

Hypercalcemia is encountered in 0.2–4% in the general population [1]. Primary hyperparathyroidism (PHPT) and hypercalcemia of malignancy account for 80–90% of the cases being the most common cause in community dwelling and hospitalized individuals, respectively [2]. Etiologies of hypercalcemia can be divided into parathyroid hormone (PTH)-dependent and PTH-independent conditions. Vitamin D-mediated hypercalcemia is PTH-independent hypercalcemia mediated by elevated 1,25-dihydroxyvitamin D [1,25(OH)$_2$D] with suppressed PTH. There are benign and malignant causes. This chapter focuses on the benign causes of 1,25(OH)$_2$D-mediated hypercalcemia.

Vitamin D Production, Metabolism, and Actions

Endogenous vitamin D production starts with photolysis of 7-dehydrocholesterol by UVB to pre-vitamin D which undergoes thermal isomerization to form vitamin D in skin (Fig. 13.1). Continued UVB exposure converts pre-vitamin D and vitamin D to biologically inactive metabolites which provide a mechanism to prevent vitamin D toxicity from prolonged sunlight exposure [3]. Vitamin D is transported mostly by vitamin D-binding protein (DBP) and albumin to fat and muscle for storage and liver for further metabolism [4–6]. In the liver, vitamin D is metabolized to

N. M. Maalouf (✉) · L. Song
Division of Endocrinology, Department of Internal Medicine and the Charles and Jane Pak Center of Mineral Metabolism and Clinical Research, University of Texas Southwestern Medical Center, Dallas, TX, USA
e-mail: Naim.maalouf@utsouthwestern.edu; Li.Song@UTSouthwestern.edu

© The Author(s), under exclusive license to Springer Nature Switzerland AG 2022
M. D. Walker (ed.), *Hypercalcemia*, Contemporary Endocrinology,
https://doi.org/10.1007/978-3-030-93182-7_13

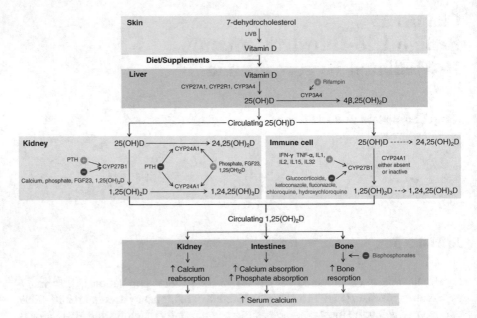

Fig. 13.1 Vitamin D metabolism, classical actions, and regulation relevant to 1,25(OH)$_2$D-mediated hypercalcemia. Medications used in the treatment of 1,25(OH)$_2$D-mediated hypercalcemia are indicated in red. 7-Dehydrocholesterol is transformed to vitamin D by UVB and thermal isomerization in the skin. Endogenous, dietary, and supplemental vitamin D is converted to 25(OH) D by 25-hydroxylases (CYP27A1, CYP2R1, and CYP3A4) in the liver. 25(OH)D is converted to 1,25(OH)$_2$D by 1α-hydroxylase (CYP27B1) in the kidneys and other tissues including immune cells. 1,25(OH)$_2$D is the most active vitamin D metabolite and mediates the classical actions of vitamin D including increased calcium and phosphate intestinal absorption, increased renal calcium reabsorption, and increased bone resorption and mobilization of calcium. In the liver, 25(OH) D is catabolized to an inactive metabolite by CYP3A4, which is induced by rifampin. In the kidneys, 25(OH)D and 1,25(OH)$_2$D are catabolized by CYP24A1. Renal CYP27B1 and CYP24A1 are highly regulated. Renal CYP27B1 is stimulated by PTH and inhibited by calcium, phosphate, FGF23, and 1,25(OH)$_2$D. Renal CYP24A1 is inhibited by PTH and stimulated by phosphate, FGF23, and 1,25(OH)$_2$D. Immune cells also express CYP27B1 which is under a differential regulation. It is stimulated by pro-inflammatory cytokines and inhibited by glucocorticoids, chloroquine, hydroxychloroquine, ketoconazole, and fluconazole

25-hydroxyvitamin D [25(OH)D] by 25-hydroxylases including CYP2R1, CYP27A1, and CYP3A4 [7–9]. 25(OH)D is further metabolized to its most active metabolite 1,25(OH)$_2$D in kidneys, where 1,25(OH)$_2$D production and degradation are tightly controlled mainly by regulation of two enzymes: 1α-hydroxylase (CYP27B1) and 24-hydroxylase (CYP24A1) (Fig. 13.1). CYP27B1 converts 25(OH)D to 1,25(OH)$_2$D. CYP24A1 catabolizes 25(OH)D and 1,25(OH)$_2$D to their respective biologically inactive metabolites, 24,25(OH)$_2$D and 1,24,25(OH)$_3$D, which are eventually catabolized to calcitroic acid. Renal CYP27B1 expression is stimulated by PTH and inhibited by calcium, phosphorus, fibroblast growth factor-23 (FGF23), and 1,25(OH)$_2$D [10, 11]. Renal CYP24A1 expression is stimulated by 1,25(OH)$_2$D, phosphorus, and FGF23 and inhibited by PTH [10]. Disruption in this regulation may result in increased $1,25(OH)_2D$ and hypercalcemia as in CYP24A1 loss-of-function mutations found in idiopathic infantile hypercalcemia and some adults with the syndrome of hypercalcemia, hypercalciuria, nephrolithiasis, and nephrocalcinosis [12, 13]. CYP27B1 is also expressed in other tissues including immune cells, keratinocytes, parathyroid glands, placenta, testes, intestines, lungs, breasts, chondrocytes, and osteoblasts. In immune cells, CYP27B1 activity is primarily regulated by the availability of its substrate 25(OH)D and cytokines, but not by PTH, calcium, phosphate, or FGF23 [10, 14–16]. In addition, CYP24A1 is either absent or defective in macrophages [10, 14]. In granulomatous diseases, activated macrophages and lymphocytes may produce excessive amount of $1,25(OH)_2D$ that overspills to systemic circulation and exerts its endocrine effects leading to hypercalcemia [17].

The biological actions of vitamin D are primarily mediated by $1,25(OH)_2D$ on the vitamin D receptor (VDR) that forms a heterodimer with retinoid X receptor. This complex interacts with vitamin D response elements to regulate transcription of target genes. The classical actions of vitamin D are to mediate calcium and phosphate homeostasis (Fig. 13.1). In the presence of a calcium deficit, $1,25(OH)_2D$ increases calcium absorption in the duodenum by inducing expression of proteins that facilitate transcellular calcium transport including TRPV6 (a calcium channel on the brush border), calbindin-D9k (an intracellular calcium-binding protein), and PMCA1b (a basolateral membrane calcium ATPase) [18]. $1,25(OH)_2D$ also increases the expression of NaPi-IIb (a sodium phosphate cotransporter) which enhances intestinal phosphate absorption [19]. In the kidneys, 10–15% of calcium is reabsorbed in the distal tubule through a mechanism similar to that in the duodenum involving TRPV5, calbindin-D28k, and PMCA1b which are induced by $1,25(OH)_2D$ [20]. $1,25(OH)_2D$ also stimulates the expression of the PTH receptor in the kidneys which in turn enhances PTH's effect and reabsorption of calcium [21]. In bone, $1,25(OH)_2D$ stimulates bone mineralization indirectly by increasing intestinal calcium and phosphate absorption [22, 23]. In vitro, $1,25(OH)_2D$ directly stimulates osteoblast differentiation, upregulates receptor activator of nuclear factor-κB ligand, reduces osteoprotegerin, and thus, in turn, promotes osteoclastogenesis. In vivo, supraphysiologic doses of $1,25(OH)_2D$ induce bone resorption and calcium mobilization [24, 25].

Vitamin D has many non-classical actions. In the parathyroid glands, $1,25(OH)_2D$ decreases PTH synthesis and secretion, decreases proliferation of PTH-producing cells, and increases the calcium-sensing receptor making parathyroid glands more sensitive to the regulation by calcium [26, 27]. Vitamin D also modulates the immune response by promoting the innate immune response and microbial killing but suppressing the adaptive immune response to prevent overzealous inflammatory response [28–30].

Signs and Symptoms

Signs and symptoms of 1,25(OH)$_2$D-mediated hypercalcemia are similar to those of hypercalcemia of other causes. They vary based on the onset and severity of hypercalcemia. In acute and/or severe hypercalcemia (serum calcium >12 mg/dL), patients may present with overt symptoms of altered mentation, anorexia, nausea, vomiting, polyuria, dehydration, acute kidney injury (AKI), ectopy, shortened QT interval, broadened T wave, bradycardia, or first-degree heart block [31]. In chronic and mild hypercalcemia, patients may present with depression, constipation, dyspepsia, pancreatitis, nephrolithiasis, nephrocalcinosis, or no symptoms [31]. 1,25(OH)$_2$D-mediated hypercalcemia may be exacerbated in summer months, increased sunlight exposure, and vitamin D supplementation [32–34].

Causes of 1,25(OH)$_2$D-Mediated Hypercalcemia

Several disorders are associated with 1,25(OH)$_2$D-mediated hypercalcemia (Table 13.1). These can be categorized into congenital vs. acquired disorders that lead to overproduction or under-metabolism of 1,25(OH)$_2$D. Acquired ectopic overproduction of 1,25(OH)$_2$D can be subdivided into malignant vs. nonmalignant diseases. Nonmalignant disorders can be further classified into infectious vs. noninfectious granulomatous conditions (Table 13.1).

Congenital Conditions

Congenital disorders associated with 1,25(OH)$_2$D-mediated hypercalcemia include idiopathic infantile hypercalcemia (IIH) and hypercalcemia associated with Williams syndrome.

Idiopathic infantile hypercalcemia, also known as infantile hypercalcemia, is characterized by severe hypercalcemia, failure to thrive, vomiting, dehydration, and nephrocalcinosis. The term IIH was coined after an epidemic of hypercalcemia in the United Kingdom in the 1950s following the implementation of higher prophylactic doses of vitamin D supplementation [35]. Since most infants receiving the prophylaxis remained normocalcemic, intrinsic hypersensitivity to vitamin D was proposed as the pathogenetic factor.

The familial occurrence of IIH led to the suspicion of a genetic basis for this disorder. In 2011, Schlingmann and colleagues identified inactivating recessive mutations in the *CYP24A1* gene in six patients from four families with IIH and in a second cohort of infants in whom severe hypercalcemia had developed after bolus prophylaxis with vitamin D [13]. These loss-of-function mutations led to a variable degree of elevation in serum 1,25(OH)$_2$D, hypercalcemia and hypercalciuria and

Table 13.1 Etiology of 1,25(OH)$_2$D-mediated hypercalcemia

1. Congenital
(a) Idiopathic infantile hypercalcemia
(i) Inactivating mutations of the *CYP24A1* gene
(ii) Inactivating mutations of the *SLC34A1* gene
(b) Other
(i) Williams syndrome
2. Acquired ectopic 1,25(OH)$_2$D production
(a) Nonmalignant granulomatous diseases
(i) Noninfectious
1. Sarcoidosis
2. Crohn's disease
3. Granulomatosis with polyangiitis
4. Langerhans cell histiocytosis
5. Subcutaneous fat necrosis of the newborn
6. Foreign body granulomatosis
(a) Silicosis
(b) Cosmetic injection-induced: paraffin and polymethylmethacrylate
(c) Chronic beryllium disease
(d) Talc granulomatosis
(e) Textiloma
7. Other
(ii) Infectious
1. Mycobacterial
(a) Tuberculosis
(b) Leprosy
(c) *Mycobacterium avium* complex
2. Fungal
(a) Histoplasmosis
(b) Paracoccidioidomycosis
(c) Candidiasis
(d) *Pneumocystis jiroveci* pneumonia
(e) Cryptococcosis
3. Bacterial
(a) Cat scratch disease
(b) Malignant disorders

low to undetectable plasma PTH. Discontinuation of vitamin D supplementation resulted in improvement in some, but not all patients. Since that original report, different clinical scenarios have been described in patients with inactivating recessive *CYP24A1* mutations, ranging from severe forms characterized by early diagnosis in infancy, severe hypercalcemia, dehydration, and vomiting to milder forms, often diagnosed in the adulthood during workup for recurrent hypercalciuric nephrolithiasis [36]. Thus, IIH is now considered a misnomer since the diagnosis may also be made in adults. While IIH is reported in carriers of biallelic mutations (homozygotes), heterozygous carriers of *CYP24A1* mutations may display milder elevation in serum calcium than non-carriers (wild type) [37]. Currently, the prevalence of *CYP24A1* mutations in the general population and among patients with hypercalciuric nephrolithiasis remains unknown [36].

Genetic heterogeneity in IIH was recognized after mutations in *CYP24A1* were excluded in several patients presenting with symptomatic $1,25(OH)_2D$-mediated hypercalcemia in early infancy [38]. These patients also exhibited hypophosphatemia due to renal phosphate wasting and were eventually found to harbor autosomal recessive mutations in the *SLC34A1* gene encoding renal sodium phosphate cotransporter 2A (NaPi-IIa) [38]. In one affected patient with persistent hypercalcemia despite discontinuation of vitamin D supplementation, oral phosphate supplementation corrected hypophosphatemia and normalized calcium metabolism [38]. This clinical finding, coupled with experiments in Slc34a1 knockout mice, an animal model of this condition, suggested that hypophosphatemia-induced CYP27B1 activation and CYP24A1 inactivation (Fig. 13.1) was the driver of $1,25(OH)_2D$-mediated hypercalcemia.

Williams syndrome is a relatively common multisystem syndrome caused by deletion of 1.5–1.8 Mb on chromosome 7q11.23, with an estimated incidence of 1:7500 live births [39]. It presents with variable expression of the clinical manifestations including dysmorphic facial features ("Elfin facies"), cardiovascular anomalies (supravalvar aortic stenosis and peripheral pulmonary artery stenosis), hypertension, and endocrine abnormalities including hypercalcemia and hypothyroidism [39]. Patients with Williams syndrome occasionally present with symptomatic hypercalcemia in the first 2 years of life complicated by dehydration, hypercalciuria, and nephrocalcinosis. Although hypercalcemia tends to resolve spontaneously during childhood, some patients continue to experience calcium disorders in adulthood [40]. Some studies have identified elevated $1,25(OH)_2D$ as the cause of hypercalcemia in this syndrome [41], although other proposed mechanisms include increased sensitivity to vitamin D and defective calcitonin synthesis and release [42].

Granulomatous Diseases

Granulomas are organized aggregations of macrophages and other immune cells formed in response to intracellular pathogens, foreign bodies, or unknown stimuli (e.g., sarcoidosis, Crohn's disease, and granulomatosis with polyangiitis) [43, 44]. Both noninfectious and infectious granulomatous diseases may cause $1,25(OH)_2D$-mediated hypercalcemia. Among these, sarcoidosis and tuberculosis are the most common and best studied.

Sarcoidosis is an inflammatory condition characterized by granuloma formation in involved organs, mainly the lungs. Hypercalcemia occurs in 5.2–7.7% of sarcoidosis patients and hypercalciuria in up to 50% [45]. Sarcoidosis-associated hypercalcemia was first described in the 1930s [46]. The possible role of dysregulated vitamin D metabolism was speculated from calcium balance studies showing increased intestinal calcium absorption, negative calcium balance attributed to increased bone resorption, and increased sensitivity to vitamin D supplementation and UV light in sarcoidosis patients [47, 48]. In 1979, increased serum $1,25(OH)_2D$ was first described as the cause of hypercalcemia in sarcoidosis [49, 50]. Subsequently, observation of hypercalcemia and increased $1,25(OH)_2D$ in sarcoidosis patients with end-stage renal disease (ESRD) and after bilateral nephrectomy suggested *extrarenal* production of $1,25(OH)_2D$ [51, 52]. This was supported by in vitro studies demonstrating $1,25(OH)_2D$ production in cultured pulmonary alveolar macrophages (PAM) and lymph node homogenate from sarcoidosis patients [53–55] and detection of CYP27B1 mRNA in PAM [56]. The excessive production of $1,25(OH)_2D$ despite hypercalcemia and low PTH (which normally suppress CYP27B1 and induce CYP24A1 in kidneys) suggests differential regulation of these enzymes in macrophages. In macrophages, CYP27B1 activity is not regulated by PTH, calcium, or phosphate [17, 57]. Rather, it is highly substrate-dependent, stimulated by pro-inflammatory cytokines including IFN-γ, TNF-α, IL-1, IL-2, IL-15, and IL-32, and inhibited by dexamethasone, chloroquine, and ketoconazole [15–17, 57–60]. IFN-γ also inhibits CYP24A1 mRNA expression in macrophages in vitro [61, 62]. There is also alternative splicing of CYP24A1 that results in a peptide lacking the metabolic activity of 24-hydroxylase [63]. The combination of increased CYP27B1 activity and lack of CYP24A activity creates an environment for excessive and dysregulated $1,25(OH)_2D$ production in macrophages which may overspill to the systemic circulation and result in hypercalcemia [14]. Although sarcoidosis-associated hypercalcemia is mainly mediated by $1,25(OH)_2D$, PTH-related peptide (PTHrP) may also contribute in some patients [64].

$1,25(OH)_2D$-mediated hypercalcemia has been reported in other noninfectious granulomatous conditions including Crohn's disease [65–69], granulomatosis with polyangiitis [70–72], Langerhans cell histiocytosis [73, 74], subcutaneous fat necrosis of the newborn [75–79], foreign body granulomatosis [80–94], rheumatoid arthritis [95], hepatic granulomatosis in chronic dialysis [96], disseminated giant cell myositis [97], and chronic granulomatous prostatitis [98].

In Crohn's disease (CD), granulomatous inflammation is seen in up to 33% of patients, elevated $1,25(OH)_2D$ is found in 42% of patients without hypercalcemia [99, 100], and $1,25(OH)_2D$-mediated hypercalcemia has been reported [65–69]. 1α-Hydroxylase expression was found in macrophages and giant cells in the lamina propria [99] and is increased in colonic biopsies from patients with active CD compared to normal colon, quiescent CD, and ulcerative colitis [99].

Granulomatosis with polyangiitis (GPA) is an antineutrophil cytoplasmic autoantibody-associated vasculitis characterized by granulomatous inflammation of the respiratory tract and systemic small vessel vasculitis [44]. There are a few cases of hypercalcemia associated with GPA with some mediated by $1,25(OH)_2D$ [70–72] and one by immobilization due to severe GPA-associated neuropathy [101].

Langerhans cell histiocytosis (LCH) is a histiocytic disorder with granulomas comprising langerin-positive histocytes and other inflammatory infiltrate that can affect virtually any organ most commonly the bone, skin, lungs, and pituitary [102, 103]. Hypercalcemia was reported in five cases [73, 74, 104–106]. The mechanism has been attributed to $1,25(OH)_2D$ [73, 74], bone-resorbing cytokines such IL-1 and prostaglandin [106] and treatment with vinblastine without concurrent use of glucocorticoid [104].

Subcutaneous fat necrosis (SCFN) of the newborn is a rare disorder characterized by subcutaneous nodules and plaques infiltrated with fat necrosis and granulomatous inflammation that primary affects full- and post-term infants within the first few weeks of life most commonly precipitated by asphyxia and hypothermia [107–109]. Hypercalcemia occurs in 25–69% newborns with SCFN [107, 109]. The mechanism has been attributed to $1,25(OH)_2D$ and prostaglandin [75–79, 110]. 1α-Hydroxylase expression was found in the inflammatory infiltrate in SCFN skin lesions [78].

Foreign body granulomatosis is a rare cause of hypercalcemia. $1,25(OH)_2D$-mediated hypercalcemia has been reported in chronic beryllium disease [93], talc granulomatosis [92], textiloma [111], and granuloma induced by foreign particles produced by artificial joint replacement [112]. There has also been an increased incidence of hypercalcemia associated with cosmetic injections and fillers. Among these, silicone was the most commonly used, followed by polymethylmethacrylate and paraffin oil [91]. Hypercalcemia occurred in a few months to 28 years after the first injection [91]. Elevated $1,25(OH)_2D$ was found in majority of the cases [91]. Immunohistochemistry in biopsies of the skin lesions showed a strong CYP27B1 expression [83, 84, 86, 94] and a trend to a decreased CYP24A1 expression [83].

$1,25(OH)_2D$-mediated hypercalcemia has also been reported in infectious granulomatous diseases including tuberculosis [113–118], leprosy [119–121], *Mycobacterium avium* complex [122, 123], histoplasmosis [124–127], paracoccidioidomycosis [128], disseminated Candidiasis [129], *Pneumocystis jirovecii* pneumonia [130–138], cryptococcosis [139–142], and cat scratch disease [143].

The frequency of hypercalcemia in tuberculosis varies between 2.3% and 50.6% which may be attributed to regional difference in calcium intake and vitamin D levels [115, 144]. The mechanism of hypercalcemia is thought to be extrarenal production of $1,25(OH)_2D$. In the 1980s, $1,25(OH)_2D$-mediated hypercalcemia was found in tuberculosis patients with ESRD providing evidence for extrarenal 1,25(OH)$_2$D production [113, 114]. Subsequently, pleural fluid from tuberculosis patients rich in IFN-γ was found to potentiate 1,25(OH)$_2$D synthesis by PAM [145]. CD8+ T lymphocytes in bronchial alveolar lavage from tuberculosis patients also appeared to be an important source of 1,25(OH)$_2$D [146]. 1,25(OH)$_2$D exerts an autocrine/paracrine effect to modulate the immune response to *Mycobacterium tuberculosis (Mtb)*. Activation of toll-like receptor 2/1 (TLR2/TLR1) heterodimers on macrophages by *Mtb* increases the expression of CYP27B1 and VDR [147]. When provided 25(OH)D or 1,25(OH)$_2$D, the substrate for CYP27B1 or the ligand for VDR, respectively, there was an increased expression of cathelicidin which enhances microbial killing in activated macrophages [147]. 1,25(OH)$_2$D inhibits proliferation of T-cell helper type 1 (TH1) (pro-inflammatory) over TH2 cells (anti-inflammatory) leading to a relative increase of TH2 cell-derived cytokines which decrease the 1,25(OH)$_2$D production and prevent an overzealous innate immune response to *Mtb* [14]. If 1,25(OH)$_2$D is produced in sufficient quantity, it can over-spill to the systemic circulation and cause hypercalcemia [14].

1,25(OH)$_2$D-mediated hypercalcemia was found in lepromatous and borderline lepromatous leprosy [119–121], but not in tuberculoid leprosy [148]. In the latter case, 1,25(OH)$_2$D was low, and hypercalcemia was attributed to increased bone resorption [148]. Hypercalcemia in histoplasmosis mostly occurs in disseminated disease and can be attributed to at least two potential mechanisms: extrarenal production of 1,25(OH)$_2$D [124–127] and adrenal insufficiency due to infection of the adrenal glands [149, 150]. Paracoccidioidomycosis-associated hypercalcemia is very rare and may be mediated by 1,25(OH)$_2$D [128] or osteolytic lesions [151]. Hypercalcemia in *Pneumocystis jirovecii* pneumonia (PJP) was first reported in 1993 in a patient with HIV/AIDS [130]. Since year 2002, there has been an increase in reports of 1,25(OH)$_2$D-mediated hypercalcemia mostly in renal transplant recipients with PJP [131, 132, 135, 136, 138]. 1,25(OH)$_2$D-mediated hypercalcemia in pulmonary cryptococcosis was described in patients with HIV/AIDS [139, 152] and non-HIV-infected patients including a patient with ESRD suggesting extrarenal production of 1,25(OH)$_2$D [141, 142].

Evaluation

Evaluation of patients with suspected 1,25(OH)$_2$D-mediated hypercalcemia requires a detailed history to uncover the underlying etiology and/or exacerbating factors, laboratory studies to establish the diagnosis, and occasionally imaging studies, genetic testing, or a biopsy for definitive diagnosis.

In addition to eliciting symptoms of hypercalcemia (neuropsychiatric, gastrointestinal, musculoskeletal, and renal manifestations), symptoms that could guide to a specific underlying condition should be sought. Young age at diagnosis and/or family history of hypercalcemia or hypercalciuric nephrolithiasis are more suggestive of a congenital condition. History of immunodeficiency and constitutional symptoms including fever and night sweats suggest an infectious etiology. Pulmonary symptoms (cough, dyspnea) occur with respiratory infections or sarcoidosis, while gastrointestinal symptoms (diarrhea, hematochezia) may be from Crohn's disease. Specific foreign body exposure (cosmetic injections) or other unusual exposure (silica, beryllium, talc) can be assessed by history. Finally, exposure to sunlight and/or intake of vitamin D supplements should be elicited to identify factors that potentially worsen $1,25(OH)_2D$-mediated hypercalcemia by greater provision of substrate [45].

On laboratory evaluation, hyperphosphatemia concomitant with hypercalcemia can be a clue to the presence of $1,25(OH)_2D$ excess. Serum $1,25(OH)_2D$ can be elevated in some patients with PHPT, but a suppressed serum PTH differentiates $1,25(OH)_2D$-mediated hypercalcemia from PHPT. Hypercalciuria is common in patients with $1,25(OH)_2D$ excess and frequently precedes hypercalcemia.

The ratio of circulating $25(OH)D$ to $24,25(OH)_2D$ is a helpful screening test to identify patients with IIH due to inactivating mutations in *CYP24A1*: The synthesis of $24,25(OH)_2D$ by the CYP24A1 enzyme is dependent on both the concentration of the substrate $25(OH)D$ and CYP24A1 enzymatic activity (Fig. 13.1). Therefore, the ratio of $25(OH)D$ to $24,25(OH)_2D$ provides the most reliable estimation of CYP24A1 activity, superseding the isolated measurement of $24,25(OH)_2D$ concentration [153]. In healthy individuals, this ratio is typically under 25, whereas carriers of biallelic *CYP24A1* mutation or deletion exhibit a ratio over 80, and heterozygous carriers exhibit a ratio between 25 and 80 [1]. Because of the substrate dependency of the $25(OH)D$ to $24,25(OH)_2D$ ratio, it is essential that both $25(OH)D$ and $24,25(OH)_2D$ are measured in the same draw and assessed using the same methodology used for establishing the reference range for the ratio [153]. Furthermore, in cases of vitamin D deficiency [$25(OH)D < 20$ ng/mL], the ratio of $25(OH)D$ to $24,25(OH)_2D$ can be falsely elevated since there is no inactivation of $25(OH)D$ to $24,25(OH)_2D$.

The diagnosis of sarcoidosis is not standardized, but is based on three major criteria: a compatible clinical presentation, the finding of non-necrotizing granulomatous inflammation in one or more tissue samples, and the exclusion of alternative causes of granulomatous disease [154]. Serum angiotensin-converting enzyme (ACE) is helpful in the evaluation of patients with suspected sarcoidosis, with greater disease activity associated with higher ACE levels. In the proper clinical context (radiographic evidence of infiltrates or adenopathy and organ biopsies showing noncaseating granulomas), ACE elevation is highly suggestive of a diagnosis of sarcoidosis. However, other diseases such as untreated hyperthyroidism, amyloidosis, or even conditions associated with $1,25(OH)_2D$-mediated hypercalcemia such as leprosy and histoplasmosis have been associated with increased serum ACE activity [155].

Acute mycobacterium tuberculosis (TB) and atypical mycobacterial infections can be screened for by staining biopsies for acid-fast bacilli. On the other hand, latent TB infection can be detected by performing IFN-γ release assay testing (QuantiFERON gold) or by delayed-type hypersensitivity skin testing to TB antigens (PPD). False-negative IFN-γ release or skin test results may occur in the setting of acute active forms of TB due to concurrent T-cell anergy.

Concern for fungal infection and type of fungal testing are dependent on several factors including the patient's geographic exposure, immune status, and whether there is suspicion for disseminated disease or localized pulmonary disease: For isolated pulmonary disease or in an immunocompetent patients, serology (complement fixation and immunodiffusion) is the preferred test for diagnosing histoplasmosis, whereas antigen testing is recommended in immunocompromised patients (transplant recipients or patients with AIDS).

Management

Treatment of 1,25(OH)$_2$D-mediated hypercalcemia is aimed at treating the underlying disease. Supraphysiologic 1,25(OH)$_2$D causes hypercalcemia through increased intestinal calcium absorption, increased renal calcium reabsorption, and increased bone resorption which can be targets for dietary and pharmacological therapies. Limiting calcium intake, eliminating vitamin D supplementation, and avoiding sunlight exposure may help reduce 1,25(OH)$_2$D production and intestinal absorption of calcium. A restricted calcium intake increases the availability of oxalate in the intestines for absorption and results in hyperoxaluria which increases the risk of nephrolithiasis; therefore, it is important to also restrict dietary oxalate intake [156].

Acute therapies for 1,25(OH)$_2$D-mediated hypercalcemia are similar to those for treatment of hypercalcemia of other causes. Volume expansion with isotonic saline restores renal perfusion and enhances calciuresis. Furosemide increases calciuresis and can be used with caution to avoid volume overload from intravenous (IV) fluids, although only after intravascular volume repletion is achieved. Intramuscular or subcutaneous calcitonin primarily inhibits bone resorption but also decreases renal calcium reabsorption, which in turn improves hypercalcemia quickly but is limited by tachyphylaxis after 48 hours. IV bisphosphonate reduces serum calcium by inhibiting bone resorption. IV pamidronate and zoledronic acid have been shown to reduce serum calcium in sarcoidosis patients with hypercalcemia [157, 158].

For more specific pharmacological therapies to 1,25(OH)$_2$D-mediated hypercalcemia, glucocorticoid therapy is the most commonly used, particularly in sarcoidosis. Glucocorticoids suppress the expression of IFN-γ and TNF-α which are important in the development of granulomas and reduce disease activity in sarcoidosis [159–161]. Glucocorticoids also inhibit extrarenal 1α-hydroxylase resulting in decreased 1,25(OH)$_2$D [58, 60, 162]. Independent from its action on 1,25(OH)$_2$D, glucocorticoid therapy directly inhibits the transcription of TRPV6 and calbindin-D9k and reduces intestinal calcium absorption [163] and decreases renal tubular reabsorption of calcium [164, 165]. There is no clear guide on the optimal dose, duration, or tapering of glucocorticoids in sarcoidosis. Prednisone 20–40 mg per day is typically recommended as the initial dose for pulmonary sarcoidosis [166].

After 1–3 months on initial therapy, the dose is tapered over several months down to 5–10 mg per day as a maintenance dose for 1 year before discontinuation in patients with adequate response [166]. Serum calcium starts to fall within 2 days of glucocorticoid initiation and tends to fully normalize within 7–10 days [45]. A lack of response to glucocorticoids after 2 weeks should prompt consideration of potential alternative causes of hypercalcemia. In patients with 1,25(OH)₂D-mediated hypercalcemia who do not respond to glucocorticoids, glucocorticoid-sparing therapies can be considered.

Antimalarial medications chloroquine 500 mg per day and the less toxic hydroxychloroquine 400 mg per day have been used with some success in sarcoidosis with cutaneous [167] and neurological involvement [168] and hypercalcemia [169–171]. They were used either as monotherapy or in addition to glucocorticoid therapy in patients intolerant to glucocorticoids at the doses required to maintain normocalcemia [169–171]. Chloroquine inhibits extrarenal 1α-hydroxylase and stimulates 24-hydroxylase in vitro in sarcoid PAM, which in turn decreases 1,25(OH)₂D [58, 60].

Ketoconazole is an antifungal medication that has been shown to reduce 1,25(OH)₂D in normal patients and patients with PHPT [172, 173], sarcoidosis [174, 175], tuberculosis [117], and inactivating mutations in *CYP24A1* [12, 176–178]. It induces a dose-dependent reduction in 1,25(OH)₂D production in vitro in sarcoid PAM due to presumed inhibition on cytochrome P450-linked 1α-hydroxylase [174] Fluconazole, a less toxic but less potent inhibitor of 1α-hydroxylase, has been shown to be effective in treatment of a patient with inactivation mutations in *CYP24A1* [179].

Rifampin is an antibiotic medication typically used in combination with other antimicrobials in the treatment of tuberculosis and leprosy which are granulomatous infections that can cause 1,25(OH)₂D-mediated hypercalcemia. In addition to its microbial activity, rifampin has been shown to induce the expression of 25(OH)D degradative enzymes including CYP24A1, CYP3A4, UGT1A4, and UGT1A3 and to lower 1,25(OH)₂D concentration by reducing the substrate (i.e., 25(OH)D) to 1α-hydroxylase [180–183]. Rifampin at doses of 300–600 mg/day normalized serum 1,25(OH)₂D and serum and urine calcium in two patients with IIH from inactivating mutations in *CYP24A1* [183]. This suggests that rifampin-induced overexpression of CYP3A4 provides an alternative pathway for inactivation of vitamin D metabolites in patients who lack CYP24A1 function.

Case
A 69-year-old woman presented to the emergency department for hypercalcemia and AKI noted on outpatient laboratory studies. She had a 2-week history of fatigue, nausea, vomiting, and anorexia. She had no known medical history and did not take any medications. She never smoked. Physical exam was unremarkable except tachycardia. Laboratory studies showed serum calcium 14.4 mg/dL (reference 8.4–10.2), albumin 3.4 g/dL (reference 3.5–5.2), and creatinine 9.47 mg/dL (reference 0.51–0.95).

Further evaluation for the hypercalcemia showed phosphorus 6.2 mg/dL (reference 2.4–4.5), PTH 10.4 pg/mL (reference 15–65), PTHrP 0.5 pmol/L (reference <2.0), 25(OH)D 33.4 ng/mL (reference 20–100), and 1,25(OH)$_2$D 114 pg/mL (reference 18–78). These suggest 1,25(OH)$_2$D-mediated hypercalcemia. Additional studies showed elevated serum ACE 147 U/L (reference 8–53) and negative QuantiFERON Gold and sputum fungal culture. CT chest showed a 3.2-cm pulmonary mass, multiple smaller nodules, and mediastinal, hilar, and supraclavicular lymphadenopathy. Biopsy of the lung mass showed fibrosis with chronic inflammation and non-necrotizing granuloma. There was no evidence of malignancy. Tissue cultures were negative for aerobic, anaerobic, acid-fast bacterial, or fungal infections. A diagnosis of sarcoidosis was made.

The patient presented with symptomatic severe hypercalcemia and AKI. She was given bolus normal saline (NS) followed by continuous NS infusion and intravenous (IV) furosemide 80 mg once after volume expansion. She also received subcutaneous calcitonin. IV bisphosphonate was not given because of the degree of AKI. Over the following 4 days, serum calcium and creatinine improved from 14.4 mg/dL and 9.47 mg/dL to 11.2 mg/dL and 5.59 mg/dL, respectively. After the diagnosis of 1,25(OH)$_2$D-mediated hypercalcemia associated with sarcoidosis was made, prednisone 40 mg daily was initiated and tapered to 20 mg daily by 3 months. Serum calcium and creatinine improved to 10.4 mg/dL and 1.60 mg/dL, respectively. 1,25(OH)$_2$D and ACE both improved to normal. Hydroxychloroquine was added and increased to 200 mg twice daily as prednisone was further tapered off over the next 9 months. Serum calcium normalized and serum creatinine improved to baseline 1.35–1.55 mg/dL. She continued a diet limited in calcium, oxalate, and vitamin D.

References

1. Tebben PJ, Singh RJ, Kumar R. Vitamin D-mediated hypercalcemia: mechanisms, diagnosis, and treatment. Endocr Rev. 2016;37(5):521–47.
2. Lafferty FW. Differential diagnosis of hypercalcemia. J Bone Miner Res. 1991;6 Suppl 2:S51–9; discussion S61.
3. Webb AR, DeCosta BR, Holick MF. Sunlight regulates the cutaneous production of vitamin D3 by causing its photodegradation. J Clin Endocrinol Metab. 1989;68(5):882–7.
4. Cooke NE, Haddad JG. Vitamin D binding protein (Gc-globulin). Endocr Rev. 1989;10(3):294–307.
5. Mawer EB, Backhouse J, Holman CA, Lumb GA, Stanbury SW. The distribution and storage of vitamin D and its metabolites in human tissues. Clin Sci. 1972;43(3):413–31.
6. Heaney RP, Horst RL, Cullen DM, Armas LA. Vitamin D3 distribution and status in the body. J Am Coll Nutr. 2009;28(3):252–6.
7. Zhu JG, Ochalek JT, Kaufmann M, Jones G, Deluca HF. CYP2R1 is a major, but not exclusive, contributor to 25-hydroxyvitamin D production in vivo. Proc Natl Acad Sci U S A. 2013;110(39):15650–5.

8. Cheng JB, Levine MA, Bell NH, Mangelsdorf DJ, Russell DW. Genetic evidence that the human CYP2R1 enzyme is a key vitamin D 25-hydroxylase. Proc Natl Acad Sci U S A. 2004;101(20):7711–5.

9. Gupta RP, Hollis BW, Patel SB, Patrick KS, Bell NH. CYP3A4 is a human microsomal vitamin D 25-hydroxylase. J Bone Miner Res. 2004;19(4):680–8.

10. Meyer MB, Pike JW. Mechanistic homeostasis of vitamin D metabolism in the kidney through reciprocal modulation of Cyp27b1 and Cyp24a1 expression. J Steroid Biochem Mol Biol. 2020;196:105500.

11. Jones G, Prosser DE, Kaufmann M. Cytochrome P450-mediated metabolism of vitamin D. J Lipid Res. 2014;55(1):13–31.

12. Jacobs TP, Kaufman M, Jones G, Kumar R, Schlingmann KP, Shapses S, et al. A lifetime of hypercalcemia and hypercalciuria, finally explained. J Clin Endocrinol Metab. 2014;99(3):708–12.

13. Schlingmann KP, Kaufmann M, Weber S, Irwin A, Goos C, John U, et al. Mutations in CYP24A1 and idiopathic infantile hypercalcemia. N Engl J Med. 2011;365(5):410–21.

14. Adams JS, Rafison B, Witzel S, Reyes RE, Shieh A, Chun R, et al. Regulation of the extrarenal CYP27B1-hydroxylase. J Steroid Biochem Mol Biol. 2014;144 Pt A:22–7.

15. Krutzik SR, Hewison M, Liu PT, Robles JA, Stenger S, Adams JS, et al. IL-15 links TLR2/1-induced macrophage differentiation to the vitamin D-dependent antimicrobial pathway. J Immunol. 2008;181(10):7115–20.

16. Montoya D, Inkeles MS, Liu PT, Realegeno S, Teles RM, Vaidya P, et al. IL-32 is a molecular marker of a host defense network in human tuberculosis. Sci Transl Med. 2014;6(250):250ra114.

17. Adams JS, Hewison M. Extrarenal expression of the 25-hydroxyvitamin D-1-hydroxylase. Arch Biochem Biophys. 2012;523(1):95–102.

18. Fleet JC, Schoch RD. Molecular mechanisms for regulation of intestinal calcium absorption by vitamin D and other factors. Crit Rev Clin Lab Sci. 2010;47(4):181–95.

19. Hernando N, Pastor-Arroyo EM, Marks J, Schnitzbauer U, Knopfel T, Burki M, et al. 1,25(OH)2 vitamin D3 stimulates active phosphate transport but not paracellular phosphate absorption in mouse intestine. J Physiol. 2021;599:1131–50.

20. Kumar R, Tebben PJ, Thompson JR. Vitamin D and the kidney. Arch Biochem Biophys. 2012;523(1):77–86.

21. Sneddon WB, Barry EL, Coutermarsh BA, Gesek FA, Liu F, Friedman PA. Regulation of renal parathyroid hormone receptor expression by 1, 25-dihydroxyvitamin D3 and retinoic acid. Cell Physiol Biochem. 1998;8(5):261–77.

22. Amling M, Priemel M, Holzmann T, Chapin K, Rueger JM, Baron R, et al. Rescue of the skeletal phenotype of vitamin D receptor-ablated mice in the setting of normal mineral ion homeostasis: formal histomorphometric and biomechanical analyses. Endocrinology. 1999;140(11):4982–7.

23. Bikle DD. Vitamin D and bone. Curr Osteoporos Rep. 2012;10(2):151–9.

24. DeLuca HF. Overview of general physiologic features and functions of vitamin D. Am J Clin Nutr. 2004;80(6 Suppl):1689S–96S.

25. Suda T, Ueno Y, Fujii K, Shinki T. Vitamin D and bone. J Cell Biochem. 2003;88(2):259–66.

26. Beckerman P, Silver J. Vitamin D and the parathyroid. Am J Med Sci. 1999;317(6):363–9.

27. Canaff L, Hendy GN. Human calcium-sensing receptor gene. Vitamin D response elements in promoters P1 and P2 confer transcriptional responsiveness to 1,25-dihydroxyvitamin D. J Biol Chem. 2002;277(33):30337–50.

28. Hewison M. Antibacterial effects of vitamin D. Nat Rev Endocrinol. 2011;7(6):337–45.

29. Adams JS, Hewison M. Unexpected actions of vitamin D: new perspectives on the regulation of innate and adaptive immunity. Nat Clin Pract Endocrinol Metab. 2008;4(2):80–90.

30. Bishop E, Ismailova A, Dimeloe SK, Hewison M, White JH. Vitamin D and immune regulation: antibacterial, antiviral, anti-inflammatory. JBMR Plus. 2020;5:e10405.

31. Goltzman D. In: Feingold KR, Anawalt B, Boyce A, Chrousos G, de Herder WW, Dungan K, et al., editors. Approach to hypercalcemia. South Dartmouth: Endotext; 2000.
32. Taylor RL, Lynch HJ Jr, Wysor WG Jr. Seasonal influence of sunlight on the hypercalcemia of sarcoidosis. Am J Med. 1963;34:221–7.
33. Sodhi A, Aldrich T. Vitamin D supplementation: not so simple in sarcoidosis. Am J Med Sci. 2016;352(3):252–7.
34. Sarathi V, Karethimmaiah H, Goel A. High-dose vitamin D supplementation precipitating hypercalcemic crisis in granulomatous disorders. Indian J Endocrinol Metab. 2017;21(6):815–9.
35. Hypercalcaemia in infants and vitamin D. Br Med J. 1956;2(4985):149.
36. Carpenter TO. CYP24A1 loss of function: clinical phenotype of monoallelic and biallelic mutations. J Steroid Biochem Mol Biol. 2017;173:337–40.
37. Brancatella A, Cappellani D, Kaufmann M, Borsari S, Piaggi P, Baldinotti F, et al. Do the heterozygous carriers of a CYP24A1 mutation display a different biochemical phenotype than wild types? J Clin Endocrinol Metab. 2021;106:708–17.
38. Schlingmann KP, Ruminska J, Kaufmann M, Dursun I, Patti M, Kranz B, et al. Autosomal-recessive mutations in SLC34A1 encoding sodium-phosphate cotransporter 2A cause idiopathic infantile hypercalcemia. J Am Soc Nephrol. 2016;27(2):604–14.
39. Morris CA, Braddock SR. Health care supervision for children with Williams syndrome. Pediatrics. 2020;145(2):e20193761.
40. Sindhar S, Lugo M, Levin MD, Danback JR, Brink BD, Yu E, et al. Hypercalcemia in patients with Williams-Beuren syndrome. J Pediatr. 2016;178:254–60.e4.
41. Garabédian M, Jacqz E, Guillozo H, Grimberg R, Guillot M, Gagnadoux MF, et al. Elevated plasma 1,25-dihydroxyvitamin D concentrations in infants with hypercalcemia and an elfin facies. N Engl J Med. 1985;312(15):948–52.
42. Culler FL, Jones KL, Deftos LJ. Impaired calcitonin secretion in patients with Williams syndrome. J Pediatr. 1985;107(5):720–3.
43. Pagan AJ, Ramakrishnan L. The formation and function of granulomas. Annu Rev Immunol. 2018;36:639–65.
44. Schilder AM. Wegener's Granulomatosis vasculitis and granuloma. Autoimmun Rev. 2010;9(7):483–7.
45. Gianella F, Hsia C, Sakhaee K, editors. The role of vitamin D in sarcoidosis; 2020.
46. Harrell GT, Fisher S. Blood chemical changes in Boeck's sarcoid with particular reference to protein, calcium and phosphatase values. J Clin Invest. 1939;18(6):687–93.
47. Bell NH, Gill JR Jr, Bartter FC. On the abnormal calcium absorption in sarcoidosis. Evidence for increased sensitivity to vitamin D. Am J Med. 1964;36:500–13.
48. Albright F, Carroll EL, Dempsey EF, Henneman PH. The cause of hypercalcuria in sarcoid and its treatment with cortisone and sodium phytate. J Clin Invest. 1956;35(11):1229–42.
49. Bell NH, Stern PH, Pantzer E, Sinha TK, DeLuca HF. Evidence that increased circulating 1 alpha, 25-dihydroxyvitamin D is the probable cause for abnormal calcium metabolism in sarcoidosis. J Clin Invest. 1979;64(1):218–25.
50. Papapoulos SE, Clemens TL, Fraher LJ, Lewin IG, Sandler LM, O'Riordan JL. 1, 25-dihydroxycholecalciferol in the pathogenesis of the hypercalcaemia of sarcoidosis. Lancet. 1979;1(8117):627–30.
51. Barbour GL, Coburn JW, Slatopolsky E, Norman AW, Horst RL. Hypercalcemia in an anephric patient with sarcoidosis: evidence for extrarenal generation of 1,25-dihydroxyvitamin D. N Engl J Med. 1981;305(8):440–3.
52. Maesaka JK, Batuman V, Pablo NC, Shakamuri S. Elevated 1,25-dihydroxyvitamin D levels: occurrence with sarcoidosis with end-stage renal disease. Arch Intern Med. 1982;142(6):1206–7.
53. Adams JS, Sharma OP, Gacad MA, Singer FR. Metabolism of 25-hydroxyvitamin D3 by cultured pulmonary alveolar macrophages in sarcoidosis. J Clin Invest. 1983;72(5):1856–60.

54. Adams JS, Singer FR, Gacad MA, Sharma OP, Hayes MJ, Vouros P, et al. Isolation and structural identification of 1,25-dihydroxyvitamin D3 produced by cultured alveolar macrophages in sarcoidosis. J Clin Endocrinol Metab. 1985;60(5):960–6.
55. Mason RS, Frankel T, Chan YL, Lissner D, Posen S. Vitamin D conversion by sarcoid lymph node homogenate. Ann Intern Med. 1984;100(1):59–61.
56. Inui N, Murayama A, Sasaki S, Suda T, Chida K, Kato S, et al. Correlation between 25-hydroxyvitamin D3 1 alpha-hydroxylase gene expression in alveolar macrophages and the activity of sarcoidosis. Am J Med. 2001;110(9):687–93.
57. Adams JS, Ren SY, Arbelle JE, Horiuchi N, Gray RW, Clemens TL, et al. Regulated production and intracrine action of 1,25-dihydroxyvitamin D3 in the chick myelomonocytic cell line HD-11. Endocrinology. 1994;134(6):2567–73.
58. Adams JS, Gacad MA. Characterization of 1 alpha-hydroxylation of vitamin D3 sterols by cultured alveolar macrophages from patients with sarcoidosis. J Exp Med. 1985;161(4):755–65.
59. Adams JS, Gacad MA, Diz MM, Nadler JL. A role for endogenous arachidonate metabolites in the regulated expression of the 25-hydroxyvitamin D-1-hydroxylation reaction in cultured alveolar macrophages from patients with sarcoidosis. J Clin Endocrinol Metab. 1990;70(3):595–600.
60. Reichel H, Koeffler HP, Barbers R, Norman AW. Regulation of 1,25-dihydroxyvitamin D3 production by cultured alveolar macrophages from normal human donors and from patients with pulmonary sarcoidosis. J Clin Endocrinol Metab. 1987;65(6):1201–9.
61. Monkawa T, Yoshida T, Hayashi M, Saruta T. Identification of 25-hydroxyvitamin D3 1alpha-hydroxylase gene expression in macrophages. Kidney Int. 2000;58(2):559–68.
62. Dusso AS, Kamimura S, Gallieni M, Zhong M, Negrea L, Shapiro S, et al. gamma-Interferon-induced resistance to 1,25-(OH)2 D3 in human monocytes and macrophages: a mechanism for the hypercalcemia of various granulomatoses. J Clin Endocrinol Metab. 1997;82(7):2222–32.
63. Ren S, Nguyen L, Wu S, Encinas C, Adams JS, Hewison M. Alternative splicing of vitamin D-24-hydroxylase: a novel mechanism for the regulation of extrarenal 1,25-dihydroxyvitamin D synthesis. J Biol Chem. 2005;280(21):20604–11.
64. Zeimer HJ, Greenaway TM, Slavin J, Hards DK, Zhou H, Doery JC, et al. Parathyroid-hormone-related protein in sarcoidosis. Am J Pathol. 1998;152(1):17–21.
65. Bosch X. Hypercalcemia due to endogenous overproduction of 1,25-dihydroxyvitamin D in Crohn's disease. Gastroenterology. 1998;114(5):1061–5.
66. Inayat F, Saleem S, Mohyudin A, Khan Z. Hypercalcaemia due to isolated elevation of 1,25-dihydroxyvitamin D in patients with Crohn's disease. BMJ Case Rep. 2019;12(9):e230099.
67. Ioachimescu AG, Bauer TW, Licata A. Active crohn disease and hypercalcemia treated with infliximab: case report and literature review. Endocr Pract. 2008;14(1):87–92.
68. Tuohy KA, Steinman TI. Hypercalcemia due to excess 1,25-dihydroxyvitamin D in Crohn's disease. Am J Kidney Dis. 2005;45(1):e3–6.
69. Zemrak F, McNeil L, Peden N. Rennies, Crohn's disease and severe hypercalcaemia. BMJ Case Rep. 2010;2010:bcr0720103138.
70. Edelson GW, Talpos GB, Bone HG 3rd. Hypercalcemia associated with Wegener's granulomatosis and hyperparathyroidism: etiology and management. Am J Nephrol. 1993;13(4):275–7.
71. Bosch X, Lopez-Soto A, Morello A, Olmo A, Urbano-Marquez A. Vitamin D metabolite-mediated hypercalcemia in Wegener's granulomatosis. Mayo Clin Proc. 1997;72(5):440–4.
72. Shaker JL, Redlin KC, Warren GV, Findling JW. Case report: hypercalcemia with inappropriate 1,25-dihydroxyvitamin D in Wegener's granulomatosis. Am J Med Sci. 1994;308(2):115–8.
73. Al-Ali H, Yabis AA, Issa E, Salem Z, Tawil A, Khoury N, et al. Hypercalcemia in Langerhans' cell granulomatosis with elevated 1,25 dihydroxyvitamin D (calcitriol) level. Bone. 2002;30(1):331–4.
74. Zornitzki T, Schattner A, Knobler H. Hypercalcemia in isolated hypothalamic-pituitary Langerhans cell histiocytosis with no bone lesions. Am J Med. 2004;117(7):533–4.

75. Burden AD, Krafchik BR. Subcutaneous fat necrosis of the newborn: a review of 11 cases. Pediatr Dermatol. 1999;16(5):384–7.
76. Cook JS, Stone MS, Hansen JR. Hypercalcemia in association with subcutaneous fat necrosis of the newborn: studies of calcium-regulating hormones. Pediatrics. 1992;90(1 Pt 1):93–6.
77. Finne PH, Sanderud J, Aksnes L, Bratlid D, Aarskog D. Hypercalcemia with increased and unregulated 1,25-dihydroxyvitamin D production in a neonate with subcutaneous fat necrosis. J Pediatr. 1988;112(5):792–4.
78. Farooque A, Moss C, Zehnder D, Hewison M, Shaw NJ. Expression of 25-hydroxyvitamin D3-1alpha-hydroxylase in subcutaneous fat necrosis. Br J Dermatol. 2009;160(2):423–5.
79. Kruse K, Irle U, Uhlig R. Elevated 1,25-dihydroxyvitamin D serum concentrations in infants with subcutaneous fat necrosis. J Pediatr. 1993;122(3):460–3.
80. Agrawal N, Altiner S, Mezitis NH, Helbig S. Silicone-induced granuloma after injection for cosmetic purposes: a rare entity of calcitriol-mediated hypercalcemia. Case Rep Med. 2013;2013:807292.
81. Camuzard O, Dumas P, Foissac R, Fernandez J, David S, Balaguer T, et al. Severe granulomatous reaction associated with hypercalcemia occurring after silicone soft tissue augmentation of the buttocks: a case report. Aesthetic Plast Surg. 2014;38(1):95–9.
82. Dangol GMS, Negrete H. Silicone-induced granulomatous reaction causing severe hypercalcemia: case report and literature review. Case Rep Nephrol. 2019;2019:9126172.
83. Eldrup E, Theilade S, Lorenzen M, Andreassen CH, Poulsen KH, Nielsen JE, et al. Hypercalcemia after cosmetic oil injections: unraveling etiology, pathogenesis, and severity. J Bone Miner Res. 2021;36:322–33.
84. Gyldenlove M, Rorvig S, Skov L, Hansen D. Severe hypercalcaemia, nephrocalcinosis, and multiple paraffinomas caused by paraffin oil injections in a young bodybuilder. Lancet. 2014;383(9934):2098.
85. Melnick S, Abaroa-Salvatierra A, Deshmukh M, Patel A. Calcitriol mediated hypercalcaemia with silicone granulomas due to cosmetic injection. BMJ Case Rep. 2016;2016:bcr2016217269.
86. Hindi SM, Wang Y, Jones KD, Nussbaum JC, Chang Y, Masharani U, et al. A case of hypercalcemia and overexpression of CYP27B1 in skeletal muscle lesions in a patient with HIV infection after cosmetic injections with polymethylmethacrylate (PMMA) for wasting. Calcif Tissue Int. 2015;97(6):634–9.
87. Khanna P, Khatami A, Swiha M, Rachinsky I, Kassam Z, Berberich AJ. Severe hypercalcemia secondary to paraffin oil injections in a bodybuilder with significant findings on scintigraphy. AACE Clin Case Rep. 2020;6(5):e234–e8.
88. Manfro AG, Lutzky M, Dora JM, Kalil MAS, Manfro RC. Case reports of hypercalcemia and chronic renal disease due to cosmetic injections of polymethylmethacrylate (PMMA). J Bras Nefrol. 2021;43:288–92.
89. Negri AL, Rosa Diez G, Del Valle E, Piulats E, Greloni G, Quevedo A, et al. Hypercalcemia secondary to granulomatous disease caused by the injection of methacrylate: a case series. Clin Cases Miner Bone Metab. 2014;11(1):44–8.
90. Solling ASK, Tougaard BG, Harslof T, Langdahl B, Brockstedt HK, Byg KE, et al. Non-parathyroid hypercalcemia associated with paraffin oil injection in 12 younger male bodybuilders: a case series. Eur J Endocrinol. 2018;178(6):K29–37.
91. Tachamo N, Donato A, Timilsina B, Nazir S, Lohani S, Dhital R, et al. Hypercalcemia associated with cosmetic injections: a systematic review. Eur J Endocrinol. 2018;178(4):425–30.
92. Woywodt A, Schneider W, Goebel U, Luft FC. Hypercalcemia due to talc granulomatosis. Chest. 2000;117(4):1195–6.
93. Stoeckle JD, Hardy HL, Weber AL. Chronic beryllium disease. Long-term follow-up of sixty cases and selective review of the literature. Am J Med. 1969;46(4):545–61.
94. Moraitis AG, Hewison M, Collins M, Anaya C, Holick MF. Hypercalcemia associated with mineral oil-induced sclerosing paraffinomas. Endocr Pract. 2013;19(2):e50–6.
95. Gates S, Shary J, Turner RT, Wallach S, Bell NH. Abnormal calcium metabolism caused by increased circulating 1,25-dihydroxyvitamin D in a patient with rheumatoid arthritis. J Bone Miner Res. 1986;1(2):221–6.

96. Hardy P, Moriniere PH, Tribout B, Hamdini N, Marie A, Bouffandeau B, et al. Liver granulomatosis is not an exceptional cause of hypercalcemia with hypoparathyroidism in dialysis patients. J Nephrol. 1999;12(6):398–403.

97. Kallas M, Green F, Hewison M, White C, Kline G. Rare causes of calcitriol-mediated hypercalcemia: a case report and literature review. J Clin Endocrinol Metab. 2010;95(7):3111–7.

98. Zouras S, Surya A, Abusahmin H, Hassan M, Humphreys E, Nagaraja P, et al. Granulomatous disease of unusual sites causing hypercalcemia: two case reports. AACE Clin Case Rep. 2019;5(1):e44–e9.

99. Abreu MT, Kantorovich V, Vasiliauskas EA, Gruntmanis U, Matuk R, Daigle K, et al. Measurement of vitamin D levels in inflammatory bowel disease patients reveals a subset of Crohn's disease patients with elevated 1,25-dihydroxyvitamin D and low bone mineral density. Gut. 2004;53(8):1129–36.

100. Lichtenstein GR, Loftus EV, Isaacs KL, Regueiro MD, Gerson LB, Sands BE. ACG clinical guideline: management of Crohn's disease in adults. Am J Gastroenterol. 2018;113(4):481–517.

101. Helvaci O, Erdogan Yon ME, Kucuk H, Tufan A, Guz G. Hypercalcemia in a patient with granulomatosis with polyangiitis. Am J Kidney Dis. 2020;76(5):A18–20.

102. Allen CE, Beverley PCL, Collin M, Diamond EL, Egeler RM, Ginhoux F, et al. The coming of age of Langerhans cell histiocytosis. Nat Immunol. 2020;21(1):1–7.

103. Allen CE, Merad M, McClain KL. Langerhans-cell histiocytosis. N Engl J Med. 2018;379(9):856–68.

104. Jubinsky PT. Hypercalcemia in Langerhans cell histiocytosis: is it therapy-related? J Pediatr Hematol Oncol. 2003;25(2):176–9.

105. Jurney TH. Hypercalcemia in a patient with eosinophilic granuloma. Am J Med. 1984;76(3):527–8.

106. McLean TW, Pritchard J. Langerhans cell histiocytosis and hypercalcemia: clinical response to indomethacin. J Pediatr Hematol Oncol. 1996;18(3):318–20.

107. Stefanko NS, Drolet BA. Subcutaneous fat necrosis of the newborn and associated hypercalcemia: a systematic review of the literature. Pediatr Dermatol. 2019;36(1):24–30.

108. Schofield R, McMaster D, Cotterill A, Musthaffa Y. Lessons learnt in the management of hypercalcaemia secondary to subcutaneous fat necrosis of the newborn. J Paediatr Child Health. 2021;57:947–9.

109. Del Pozzo-Magana BR, Ho N. Subcutaneous fat necrosis of the newborn: a 20-year retrospective study. Pediatr Dermatol. 2016;33(6):e353–e5.

110. Sharata H, Postellon DC, Hashimoto K. Subcutaneous fat necrosis, hypercalcemia, and prostaglandin E. Pediatr Dermatol. 1995;12(1):43–7.

111. de Bellefroid J, Vandecasteele S, Van Cauwenberge S, Bouillon R, Van den Bruel A. Textiloma-induced 1,25-dihydroxyvitamin D-mediated hypercalcemia: a case report and literature study. J Endocr Soc. 2019;3(11):2158–64.

112. Zhang J, Sellmeyer DE. Particle disease: a unique cause of hypercalcemia. Osteoporos Int. 2020;31(12):2481–4.

113. Gkonos PJ, London R, Hendler ED. Hypercalcemia and elevated 1,25-dihydroxyvitamin D levels in a patient with end-stage renal disease and active tuberculosis. N Engl J Med. 1984;311(26):1683–5.

114. Felsenfeld AJ, Drezner MK, Llach F. Hypercalcemia and elevated calcitriol in a maintenance dialysis patient with tuberculosis. Arch Intern Med. 1986;146(10):1941–5.

115. Wada T, Hanibuchi M, Saijo A. Acute hypercalcemia and hypervitaminosis D associated with pulmonary tuberculosis in an elderly patient : a case report and review of the literature. J Med Invest. 2019;66(3.4):351–4.

116. Rajendra A, Mishra AK, Francis NR, Carey RA. Severe hypercalcemia in a patient with pulmonary tuberculosis. J Family Med Prim Care. 2016;5(2):509–11.

117. Saggese G, Bertelloni S, Baroncelli GI, Di Nero G. Ketoconazole decreases the serum ionized calcium and 1,25-dihydroxyvitamin D levels in tuberculosis-associated hypercalcemia. Am J Dis Child. 1993;147(3):270–3.

118. Rizwan A, Islam N. Middle aged male with pulmonary tuberculosis and refractory hypercalcemia at a tertiary care centre in South East Asia: a case report. Cases J. 2009;2:6316.
119. Ryzen E, Rea TH, Singer FR. Hypercalcemia and abnormal 1,25-dihydroxyvitamin D concentrations in leprosy. Am J Med. 1988;84(2):325–9.
120. Couri CE, Foss NT, Dos Santos CS, de Paula FJ. Hypercalcemia secondary to leprosy. Am J Med Sci. 2004;328(6):357–9.
121. Hoffman VN, Korzeniowski OM. Leprosy, hypercalcemia, and elevated serum calcitriol levels. Ann Intern Med. 1986;105(6):890–1.
122. Delahunt JW, Romeril KE. Hypercalcemia in a patient with the acquired immunodeficiency syndrome and Mycobacterium avium intracellulare infection. J Acquir Immune Defic Syndr (1988). 1994;7(8):871–2.
123. Tsao YT, Lee SW, Hsu JC, Ho FM, Wang WJ. Surviving a crisis of HIV-associated immune reconstitution syndrome. Am J Emerg Med. 2012;30(8):1661 e5–7.
124. Liang KV, Ryu JH, Matteson EL. Histoplasmosis with tenosynovitis of the hand and hypercalcemia mimicking sarcoidosis. J Clin Rheumatol. 2004;10(3):138–42.
125. Sonawalla A, Tas V, Raisingani M, Tas E. A rare and potentially fatal etiology of hypercalcemia in an infant. Case Rep Endocrinol. 2019;2019:4270852.
126. Gurram PR, Castillo NE, Esquer Garrigos Z, Vijayvargiya P, Abu Saleh OM. A dimorphic diagnosis of a pleomorphic disease: an unusual cause of hypercalcemia. Am J Med. 2020;133(11):e659–e62.
127. Lopez J, Raval M, Mohan M. Intractable hypercalcemia in a patient with multiple myeloma: an infectious etiology. Transpl Infect Dis. 2020;22(5):e13354.
128. Almeida RM, Cezana L, Tsukumo DM, de Carvalho-Filho MA, Saad MJ. Hypercalcemia in a patient with disseminated paracoccidioidomycosis: a case report. J Med Case Reports. 2008;2:262.
129. Kantarjian HM, Saad MF, Estey EH, Sellin RV, Samaan NA. Hypercalcemia in disseminated candidiasis. Am J Med. 1983;74(4):721–4.
130. Ahmed B, Jaspan JB. Case report: hypercalcemia in a patient with AIDS and Pneumocystis carinii pneumonia. Am J Med Sci. 1993;306(5):313–6.
131. Chen WC, Chang SC, Wu TH, Yang WC, Tarng DC. Hypercalcemia in a renal transplant recipient suffering with Pneumocystis carinii pneumonia. Am J Kidney Dis. 2002;39(2):E8.
132. Taylor LN, Aesif SW, Matson KM. A case of Pneumocystis pneumonia, with a granulomatous response and vitamin D-mediated hypercalcemia, presenting 13 years after renal transplantation. Transpl Infect Dis. 2019;21(3):e13081.
133. Binet Q, Mairesse J, Vanthuyne M, Marot JC, Wieers G. Hypercalcemia heralding pneumocystis jirovecii pneumonia in an HIV-seronegative patient with diffuse cutaneous systemic sclerosis. Mycopathologia. 2019;184(6):787–93.
134. Hajji K, Dalle F, Harzallah A, Tanter Y, Rifle G, Mousson C. Vitamin D metabolite-mediated hypercalcemia with suppressed parathormone concentration in Pneumocystis jiroveci pneumonia after kidney transplantation. Transplant Proc. 2009;41(8):3320–2.
135. Yau AA, Farouk SS. Severe hypercalcemia preceding a diagnosis of Pneumocystis jirovecii pneumonia in a liver transplant recipient. BMC Infect Dis. 2019;19(1):739.
136. Chatzikyrkou C, Clajus C, Haubitz M, Hafer C. Hypercalcemia and pneumocystis Pneumonia after kidney transplantation: report of an exceptional case and literature review. Transpl Infect Dis. 2011;13(5):496–500.
137. VanSickle JS, Srivastava T, Alon US. Life-threatening hypercalcemia during prodrome of pneumocystis jiroveci pneumonia in an immunocompetent infant. Glob Pediatr Health. 2017;4:2333794X17705955.
138. Hamroun A, Lenain R, Bui Nguyen L, Chamley P, Loridant S, Neugebauer Y, et al. Hypercalcemia is common during pneumocystis pneumonia in kidney transplant recipients. Sci Rep. 2019;9(1):12508.
139. Spindel SJ, Hamill RJ, Georghiou PR, Lacke CE, Green LK, Mallette LE. Case report: vitamin D-mediated hypercalcemia in fungal infections. Am J Med Sci. 1995;310(2):71–6.

140. Ali MY, Gopal KV, Llerena LA, Taylor HC. Hypercalcemia associated with infection by Cryptococcus neoformans and Coccidioides immitis. Am J Med Sci. 1999;318(6):419–23.
141. Wang IK, Shen TY, Lee KF, Chang HY, Lin CL, Chuang FR. Hypercalcemia and elevated serum 1.25-dihydroxyvitamin D in an end-stage renal disease patient with pulmonary cryptococcosis. Ren Fail. 2004;26(3):333–8.
142. Huang JC, Kuo MC, Hwang SJ, Hwang DY, Chen HC. Vitamin D-mediated hypercalcemia as the initial manifestation of pulmonary cryptococcosis in an HIV-uninfected patient. Intern Med. 2012;51(13):1793–6.
143. Bosch X. Hypercalcemia due to endogenous overproduction of active vitamin D in identical twins with cat-scratch disease. JAMA. 1998;279(7):532–4.
144. Chan TY. Differences in vitamin D status and calcium intake: possible explanations for the regional variations in the prevalence of hypercalcemia in tuberculosis. Calcif Tissue Int. 1997;60(1):91–3.
145. Adams JS, Modlin RL, Diz MM, Barnes PF. Potentiation of the macrophage 25-hydroxyvitamin D-1-hydroxylation reaction by human tuberculous pleural effusion fluid. J Clin Endocrinol Metab. 1989;69(2):457–60.
146. Cadranel J, Garabedian M, Milleron B, Guillozo H, Akoun G, Hance AJ. 1,25(OH)2D2 production by T lymphocytes and alveolar macrophages recovered by lavage from normocalcemic patients with tuberculosis. J Clin Invest. 1990;85(5):1588–93.
147. Liu PT, Stenger S, Li H, Wenzel L, Tan BH, Krutzik SR, et al. Toll-like receptor triggering of a vitamin D-mediated human antimicrobial response. Science. 2006;311(5768):1770–3.
148. Ryzen E, Singer FR. Hypercalcemia in leprosy. Arch Intern Med. 1985;145(7):1305–6.
149. Agrawal S, Goyal A, Agarwal S, Khadgawat R. Hypercalcaemia, adrenal insufficiency and bilateral adrenal histoplasmosis in a middle-aged man: a diagnostic dilemma. BMJ Case Rep. 2019;12(8):e231142.
150. Agrawal J, Bansal N, Arora A. Disseminated histoplasmosis in India presenting as addisonian crisis with epiglottis involvement. IDCases. 2020;21:e00844.
151. Tresoldi AT, Pereira RM, Castro LC, Rigatto SZ, Belangero VM. Hypercalcemia and multiple osteolytic lesions in a child with disseminated paracoccidioidomycosis and pulmonary tuberculosis. J Pediatr. 2005;81(4):349–52.
152. Bansal N, Shah R, Patel A, Vaidya G, Pantangi P, Manocha D. Hypercalcemia as a primary manifestation of cryptococcal immune reconstitution syndrome-a rare presentation. Am J Emerg Med. 2015;33(4):598 e3–4.
153. Kaufmann M, Gallagher JC, Peacock M, Schlingmann KP, Konrad M, DeLuca HF, et al. Clinical utility of simultaneous quantitation of 25-hydroxyvitamin D and 24,25-dihydroxyvitamin D by LC-MS/MS involving derivatization with DMEQ-TAD. J Clin Endocrinol Metab. 2014;99(7):2567–74.
154. Crouser ED, Maier LA, Wilson KC, Bonham CA, Morgenthau AS, Patterson KC, et al. Diagnosis and detection of sarcoidosis. An official American Thoracic Society clinical practice guideline. Am J Respir Crit Care Med. 2020;201(8):e26–51.
155. Lopez-Sublet M, Caratti di Lanzacco L, Danser AHJ, Lambert M, Elourimi G, Persu A. Focus on increased serum angiotensin-converting enzyme level: from granulomatous diseases to genetic mutations. Clin Biochem. 2018;59:1–8.
156. von Unruh GE, Voss S, Sauerbruch T, Hesse A. Dependence of oxalate absorption on the daily calcium intake. J Am Soc Nephrol. 2004;15(6):1567–73.
157. Gibbs CJ, Peacock M. Hypercalcaemia due to sarcoidosis corrects with bisphosphonate treatment. Postgrad Med J. 1986;62(732):937–8.
158. Kuchay MS, Mishra SK, Bansal B, Farooqui KJ, Sekhar L, Mithal A. Glucocorticoid sparing effect of zoledronic acid in sarcoid hypercalcemia. Arch Osteoporos. 2017;12(1):68.
159. Conron M, Young C, Beynon HL. Calcium metabolism in sarcoidosis and its clinical implications. Rheumatology (Oxford). 2000;39(7):707–13.
160. Siltzbach LE. Effects of cortisone in sarcoidosis; a study of thirteen patients. Am J Med. 1952;12(2):139–60.

161. Paramothayan NS, Lasserson TJ, Jones PW. Corticosteroids for pulmonary sarcoidosis. Cochrane Database Syst Rev. 2005;(2):CD001114.

162. Sandler LM, Winearls CG, Fraher LJ, Clemens TL, Smith R, O'Riordan JL. Studies of the hypercalcaemia of sarcoidosis: effect of steroids and exogenous vitamin D3 on the circulating concentrations of 1,25-dihydroxy vitamin D3. Q J Med. 1984;53(210):165–80.

163. Huybers S, Naber TH, Bindels RJ, Hoenderop JG. Prednisolone-induced Ca2+ malabsorption is caused by diminished expression of the epithelial Ca2+ channel TRPV6. Am J Physiol Gastrointest Liver Physiol. 2007;292(1):G92–7.

164. Reid IR, Ibbertson HK. Evidence for decreased tubular reabsorption of calcium in glucocorticoid-treated asthmatics. Horm Res. 1987;27(4):200–4.

165. Suzuki Y, Ichikawa Y, Saito E, Homma M. Importance of increased urinary calcium excretion in the development of secondary hyperparathyroidism of patients under glucocorticoid therapy. Metabolism. 1983;32(2):151–6.

166. Statement on sarcoidosis. Joint Statement of the American Thoracic Society (ATS), the European Respiratory Society (ERS) and the World Association of Sarcoidosis and Other Granulomatous Disorders (WASOG) adopted by the ATS Board of Directors and by the ERS Executive Committee, February 1999. Am J Respir Crit Care Med. 1999;160(2):736–55.

167. Siltzbach LE, Teirstein AS. Chloroquine therapy in 43 patients with intrathoracic and cutaneous sarcoidosis. Acta Med Scand Suppl. 1964;425:302–8.

168. Sharma OP. Effectiveness of chloroquine and hydroxychloroquine in treating selected patients with sarcoidosis with neurological involvement. Arch Neurol. 1998;55(9):1248–54.

169. Adams JS, Diz MM, Sharma OP. Effective reduction in the serum 1,25-dihydroxyvitamin D and calcium concentration in sarcoidosis-associated hypercalcemia with short-course chloroquine therapy. Ann Intern Med. 1989;111(5):437–8.

170. Barre PE, Gascon-Barre M, Meakins JL, Goltzman D. Hydroxychloroquine treatment of hypercalcemia in a patient with sarcoidosis undergoing hemodialysis. Am J Med. 1987;82(6):1259–62.

171. O'Leary TJ, Jones G, Yip A, Lohnes D, Cohanim M, Yendt ER. The effects of chloroquine on serum 1,25-dihydroxyvitamin D and calcium metabolism in sarcoidosis. N Engl J Med. 1986;315(12):727–30.

172. Glass AR, Eil C. Ketoconazole-induced reduction in serum 1,25-dihydroxyvitamin D. J Clin Endocrinol Metab. 1986;63(3):766–9.

173. Glass AR, Eil C. Ketoconazole-induced reduction in serum 1,25-dihydroxyvitamin D and total serum calcium in hypercalcemic patients. J Clin Endocrinol Metab. 1988;66(5):934–8.

174. Adams JS, Sharma OP, Diz MM, Endres DB. Ketoconazole decreases the serum 1,25-dihydroxyvitamin D and calcium concentration in sarcoidosis-associated hypercalcemia. J Clin Endocrinol Metab. 1990;70(4):1090–5.

175. Young C, Burrows R, Katz J, Beynon H. Hypercalcaemia in sarcoidosis. Lancet. 1999;353(9150):374.

176. Tebben PJ, Milliner DS, Horst RL, Harris PC, Singh RJ, Wu Y, et al. Hypercalcemia, hypercalciuria, and elevated calcitriol concentrations with autosomal dominant transmission due to CYP24A1 mutations: effects of ketoconazole therapy. J Clin Endocrinol Metab. 2012;97(3):E423–7.

177. Dinour D, Beckerman P, Ganon L, Tordjman K, Eisenstein Z, Holtzman EJ. Loss-of-function mutations of CYP24A1, the vitamin D 24-hydroxylase gene, cause long-standing hypercalciuric nephrolithiasis and nephrocalcinosis. J Urol. 2013;190(2):552–7.

178. Nesterova G, Malicdan MC, Yasuda K, Sakaki T, Vilboux T, Ciccone C, et al. 1,25-(OH)2D-24 hydroxylase (CYP24A1) deficiency as a cause of nephrolithiasis. Clin J Am Soc Nephrol. 2013;8(4):649–57.

179. Sayers J, Hynes AM, Srivastava S, Dowen F, Quinton R, Datta HK, et al. Successful treatment of hypercalcaemia associated with a CYP24A1 mutation with fluconazole. Clin Kidney J. 2015;8(4):453–5.

180. Wang Z, Lin YS, Zheng XE, Senn T, Hashizume T, Scian M, et al. An inducible cytochrome P450 3A4-dependent vitamin D catabolic pathway. Mol Pharmacol. 2012;81(4):498–509.
181. Wang Z, Wong T, Hashizume T, Dickmann LZ, Scian M, Koszewski NJ, et al. Human UGT1A4 and UGT1A3 conjugate 25-hydroxyvitamin D3: metabolite structure, kinetics, inducibility, and interindividual variability. Endocrinology. 2014;155(6):2052–63.
182. Pascussi JM, Robert A, Nguyen M, Walrant-Debray O, Garabedian M, Martin P, et al. Possible involvement of pregnane X receptor-enhanced CYP24 expression in drug-induced osteomalacia. J Clin Invest. 2005;115(1):177–86.
183. Hawkes CP, Li D, Hakonarson H, Meyers KE, Thummel KE, Levine MA. CYP3A4 induction by rifampin: an alternative pathway for vitamin D inactivation in patients with CYP24A1 mutations. J Clin Endocrinol Metab. 2017;102(5):1440–6.

Chapter 14
Medication-Induced Hypercalcemia

Robert A. Wermers and Ejigayehu G. Abate

Introduction

There are many medications that can have adverse effects on the skeleton [1] (Table 14.1) and physiologically influence common skeletal biomarker measurements such as serum calcium, phosphorus, and PTH (Table 14.2) [2, 3]. In addition, many endocrine assays use biotin-streptavidin binding to capture antibody onto a solid support before signal read-out from the detection antibody. Excess biotin, as may be seen in patients taking biotin supplements, in a patient sample may prevent this reaction, leading to false low interference in assays using biotin-streptavidin capture such as PTH [4]. Patients should be instructed to hold biotin at least 12 hours prior to blood collection. Thus, a careful medication history, including prescription medications, over-the-counter medications/supplements, and those administered in the office- or hospital-based setting, is a critical part of the evaluation of bone and calcium disorders, including hypercalcemia. In addition, evaluation of the timing of medication initiation in relationship to development of the abnormality in calcium metabolism as well as their influence on the measurement of skeletal biomarkers is important to understanding its contribution to the observed findings. There are several medications that have been specifically linked to the development of hypercalcemia (Table 14.3). In addition, many of the medications one must consider that can

R. A. Wermers (✉)
Department of Internal Medicine and the Division of Endocrinology, Diabetes, Nutrition, and Metabolism, Mayo Clinic, Rochester, MN, USA

Mayo College of Medicine, Rochester, MN, USA
e-mail: wermers.robert@mayo.edu

E. G. Abate
Department of Internal Medicine and the Division of Endocrinology, Mayo Clinic, Jacksonville, FL, USA
e-mail: Abate.Ejigayehu@mayo.edu

Table 14.1 Examples of medication adversely impacting the skeleton

Medication	Predominant mechanism
Glucocorticoids	↓ bone formation > ↑ bone resorption
Unfractionated heparin	↓ bone formation and ↑ bone resorption
Aromatase inhibitors	Reduced estrogen
GnRH agonists/antagonists	Reduced sex steroids
Thyroid hormone (excess)	↑ bone resorption
Thiazolidinediones	↓ bone formation
Canagliflozin	Unknown
Proton pump inhibitors	Unknown
Serotonin selective reuptake inhibitors	Inhibition of serotonin transporter
Antiepileptics (Dilantin/phenobarbital)	Increased 25-hydroxyvitamin D catabolism
Calcineurin inhibitors	↑ bone resorption
Antiretroviral therapy for HIV	↑ bone resorption
Warfarin	Inhibition of γ-carboxylation
Ferric carboxymaltose and polymaltose	Increased intact FGF23
Voriconazole	Fluoride excess
Retinoids	↑ bone resorption

Table 14.2 Medication with physiologic effects on calcium and parathyroid hormone (PTH) measurements

Lowers serum calcium	Lowers PTH	Increases serum calcium	Increases PTH
Denosumab[a]	Calcium	Lithium	Estrogen replacement
Potent IV bisphosphonates	Vitamin D	PTH analogues	Potent IV bisphosphonates
Ferric carboxymaltose	Aromatase inhibitors	Thiazide diuretics	Loop diuretics
Estrogen replacement (in primary hyperparathyroidism)	Renin-angiotensin-aldosterone inhibitors		Calcium channel blockers
Raloxifene (in primary hyperparathyroidism)	Cinacalcet		Ferric carboxymaltose
Romosozumab			Tenofovir
Cinacalcet			Denosumab
Calcitonin			Romosozumab
Glucocorticoids (with concomitant hypovitaminosis D)			Calcitonin

[a]Hypercalcemia has also been reported with denosumab discontinuation

contribute to calcium disorders are over the counter, readily available, and affordable, thereby necessitating a complete medication history when evaluating such patients.

Table 14.3 Medications associated with hypercalcemia

Medication class	Example medications	Predominant mechanism(s)
Calcium	Calcium carbonate	Increased intestinal calcium absorption Reduced renal calcium excretion (due to alkalosis and renal insufficiency)
Vitamin D_3 Vitamin D_2		Increased intestinal calcium absorption
Calcitriol		Increased intestinal calcium absorption
Calcipotriene		Increased intestinal calcium absorption
Vitamin A		Increased bone resorption
Thiazide/thiazide-like	Hydrochlorothiazide Chlorthalidone Indapamide	Reduced renal calcium excretion
Lithium		Reduced renal calcium excretion (short term) Parathyroid hyperplasia/adenomas (long term)
Parenteral nutrition		Low bone turnover
Theophylline		Unknown
Foscarnet		Unknown
Growth hormone		Unknown
Omeprazole		Unknown
Aromatase inhibitors		Unknown
Osteoporosis therapies	Denosumab (discontinuation)	Increased bone resorption
	Teriparatide	Increased bone resorption
	Abaloparatide	Increased bone resorption
Hypoparathyroidism replacement therapy	rhPTH(1–84)	Increased bone resorption

Specific Medications Associated with Hypercalcemia

Calcium

Although guidelines have been developed on the recommended daily intake of calcium and vitamin D, in some circumstances, these recommendations would not be appropriate. For example, some patients may require higher doses of calcium and vitamin D intake (e.g., malabsorption disorders, malabsorptive bariatric surgery, and hypoparathyroidism). In the same way, some patients have underlying conditions predisposing them to hypercalcemia where calcium and vitamin D are often restricted: specifically disorders associated with excess 1,25-dihydroxyvitamin D including granulomatous disease such as sarcoidosis and individuals with *CYP24A1* gene mutations associated with 1,25-dihydroxyvitamin D-24-hydroxylase deficiency and reduced ability to degrade 1,25-dihydroxyvitamin D [5]. On the other hand, in primary hyperparathyroidism (PHPT), calcium can be taken and is associated with a reduction in PTH secretion [6, 7].

It is uncommon to see calcium supplements leading to hypercalcemia, especially in the absence of underlying predisposing conditions such as excess 1,25-dihyrodroxyvitamin D, volume depletion, and renal insufficiency. Milk-alkali syndrome (MAS) specifically refers to the triad of hypercalcemia, renal insufficiency, and metabolic alkalosis due to the ingestion of large amounts of calcium and absorbable alkali. MAS is the third most common frequent cause of hospitalization for hypercalcemia after PHPT and malignancy [8]. In the current era of acid-suppressing medications, excess calcium carbonate used for the prevention of bone loss is the primary cause of MAS [9]. In addition to a significant amount of calcium carbonate ingestion (e.g., at least 4 grams daily), there are often contributing conditions such as renal insufficiency, hypochloremia, and dehydration [10]. Other factors that contribute to MAS include alkalosis itself which compromises renal calcium excretion [11] and hypercalcemia which reduces bicarbonate excretion and increases sodium and free water excretion contributing to volume depletion [12]. The diagnosis of MAS should be considered when non-PTH-mediated hypercalcemia is identified in a patient with a history of excessive calcium and absorbable alkali ingestion combined with renal insufficiency and metabolic alkalosis. Discontinuation of the excess calcium and alkali, hydration, and supporting therapies generally lead to rapid improvement of the hypercalcemia with a slower and sometimes incomplete improvement in renal dysfunction [13].

Vitamin D

Vitamin D is a fat-soluble vitamin that is important for skeletal health and calcium homeostasis. Exposure of the skin to UVB radiation (290–315 nm) produces vitamin D3 (cholecalciferol) through photolysis of provitamin D3 into previtamin D3 with subsequent thermal isomerization to vitamin D3 (Fig. 14.1). Vitamin D3 and Vitamin D2 (ergocalciferol) may also be obtained by consuming foods such as fish, eggs, and plants or supplements. Activation of vitamin D into its active form 1,25-dihyroxyvitamin D requires well-regulated steps that require sequential hydroxylation in the liver and kidney, respectively. Vitamin D-binding protein transports vitamin D2 and vitamin D3 to the liver, where it undergoes 25-hydroxylation by 25-hydroxylase to 25-hydroxyvitamin D. 25-Hydroxyvitamin D bound to vitamin D-binding protein is then transported to the kidneys where it is activated by 1-alpha-hydroxylase to its active form 1,25-dihyroxyvitamin D (calcitriol) leading to increased intestinal calcium absorption through the gut, renal tubular calcium reabsorption, and osteoclastic bone resorption [14].

Metabolism and catabolism are regulated via a feedback mechanism where a high level of 1,25-dihyroxyvitamin D inhibits activation of 1-alpha-hydroxylase. In contrast, a high level of PTH in the setting of reduced serum calcium increases the activation of 1-alpha-hydroxylase, thus producing calcitriol (Fig. 14.1). The

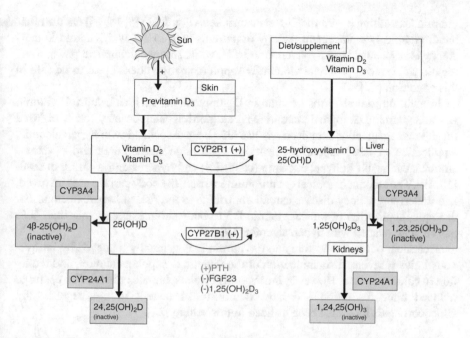

Fig. 14.1 Vitamin D metabolism and catabolism

half-life of the total 25-hydroxyvitamin D is about 1–2 months, whereas the half-life of calcitriol is 15 hours. Thus, depending on the type of vitamin D intoxication, it may take weeks for toxic levels of vitamin D to return to normal. However, with the highly touted nonskeletal benefits of vitamin D such as immune health and cancer prevention, self-supplementation of large doses of supplemental vitamin D is becoming a common practice.

High doses of vitamin D supplementation have been shown to precipitate hypercalcemia, hypercalciuria, and nephrolithiasis. (Also see Chap. 12.) In a 3-year randomized trial of healthy community dwelling adults with serum 25-hydroxyvitamin D levels of 30–125 nmol/L supplemented with 400 IU ($n = 109$), 4000 IU ($n = 100$), or 10,000 IU ($n = 102$) of vitamin D3, 2 participants (1 in 4000 IU group and 1 in 10,000 IU) developed nephrolithiasis. Hypercalciuria was seen in 31% of those on 10,000 IU compared to 17% taking 400 IU, and there were no episodes of hypercalcemia in those taking 400 IU, but mild hypercalcemia was noted in 3% and 9% in the 4000 IU and 10,000 IU groups, respectively [15]. Importantly, reduction in calcium intake improved the hypercalciuria and hypercalcemia suggesting that calcium intake significantly contributes to these conditions. Therefore, although the safe amount of vitamin D intake is unknown, higher doses of vitamin D supplementation can result in hypercalcemia. In addition, it is becoming inherently clear that certain individuals may have genetic variations in the metabolism and catabolism of vitamin D such as mutation of CYP24A1 from the kidney that may predispose them to hypercalcemia and mutation of liver CYP3A4 can accelerate inactivation of vitamin D resulting in vitamin D-resistant rickets (Fig. 14.1) [5, 14, 16] On the other hand, vitamin D replacement therapy in patients with PHPT with vitamin D deficiency is associated with a reduction in PTH, while serum calcium and phosphorus remain stable, so appropriate vitamin D supplementation does appear to be safe in this condition [17].

In addition to oral forms of vitamin D supplements such as calcitriol, vitamin D3, and vitamin D2, topical vitamin D3 (calcipotriol, calcipotriene, calcitriol) used for the management of skin psoriasis has also been associated with hypercalcemia. Application of these topical medications on a large surface area and in excess amounts can result in hypercalcemia (calcitriol) and hypercalciuria (calcipotriene) [18, 19]. The amount of topical cream/ointment used, the body surface area involved, and underlying kidney disease can all contribute to the risk of hypercalcemia. For example, application of topical vitamin D3 to body surface area greater than 40% has been associated with hypercalcemia [19].

Treatment of hypercalcemia due to vitamin D is generally managed by intravenous fluids if severe, discontinuation of the vitamin D supplementation, and reduction in calcium intake. However, intravenous bisphosphonates can also be useful to reduced bone resorption and have demonstrated benefit in this regard [20]. Glucocorticoids have also been utilized in this setting [21].

Vitamin A

Ingestion of excess vitamin A through diet or supplements on a long-term basis can result in hypervitaminosis A. The primary sources of vitamin A are two forms: provitamin A (beta carotene) found in plants (leafy green vegetables, sweet potatoes, and carrots) and preformed vitamin A (retinol) from animal and supplement sources (liver, kidney, egg yolks, and butter). Plant sources of vitamin A (beta carotene) are a provitamin A that requires metabolism to vitamin A for absorption; thus, hypervitaminosis A is not seen in excess beta carotene consumption [22, 23]. In contrast, preformed vitamin A from animal or supplemental sources, however, can be hydrolyzed to active forms of retinoic acid and absorbed into the gut and can result in hypervitaminosis A [22, 24]. Therapeutic use of retinoic acid derivatives for various medical problems such as macular degeneration, acne, and various cancer treatments can also result in hypercalcemia, exacerbated by chronic kidney disease. Hypercalcemia mediated by hypervitaminosis A results from mobilization of calcium from the bone via activation of osteoclasts cells resulting in increased bone resorption [22, 25].

Thiazide Diuretics

Thiazide diuretics are a recognized cause of hypercalcemia that is primarily related to increased renal tubular calcium reabsorption resulting in reduced urinary calcium excretion [26–28]. The increase in serum calcium is independent of PTH [29]. Loop diuretics, on the other hand, induce natriuresis by inhibiting the NA-K-2Cl transporter in the thick ascending limb of the loop of Henle resulting in increased urinary calcium losses and increased PTH levels [26, 29]. Based on a prospective health screening study in adults (66% women) from Sweden, the prevalence of hypercalcemia was 1.9% in those taking thiazides, nearly threefold greater than in the general population (0.6%) [30]. In the only population-based study to date, the incidence of thiazide-associated hypercalcemia was estimated to be 12.2 per 100,000 person-years from 1992 to 2010 in Olmsted County, MN, with an increase in incidence from 1998 and then a decline after 2006 that paralleled the observed incidence seen in PHPT in this community [31]. Hypercalcemia was identified a mean of 5 years after thiazide initiation, and the patients had similar features to patients with PHPT, as they were older (mean age, 67 years), primarily women (86%), and had mild hypercalcemia. Of the patients who discontinued thiazides in this cohort, 71% had persistent hypercalcemia. This data suggests that underlying PHPT is common in patients who develop hypercalcemia while taking thiazide diuretics. Of note, the use of thiazides in patients with PHPT with hypercalciuria has been also been suggested as a clinical consideration since they do not appear to increase serum calcium and are associated with a reduction in PTH and urinary calcium [32], although there are no prospective randomized trials in this regard.

Lithium

Lithium has several adverse effects on the endocrine system, including an association with hypercalcemia and hyperparathyroidism [33]. Shortly after initiation of lithium, an elevation in serum calcium can occur. This appears to be related to an increase in the parathyroid gland calcium set point through the calcium-sensing receptor (CaSR) and a reduction in urinary calcium excretion [34, 35]. Importantly, hypercalcemia with short-term use of lithium usually resolves with its discontinuation. Long-term use of lithium, however, can lead to parathyroid gland hyperplasia or adenomas with persistence of hypercalcemia after its discontinuation in 10–15% of patients [34, 36–38]. Lithium-associated hyperparathyroidism appears to be more common in younger females than patients with classical PHPT [38].

Parenteral Nutrition

Parenteral nutrition is used to provide nutrition in patients who cannot get adequate nutrition by mouth. There are a few reports of an association between total parenteral nutrition (TPN) and hypercalciuria as well as transient hypercalcemia [39, 40]. Pancreatitis related to hypercalcemia has also been reported in patients receiving TPN [41]. PTH was either low or normal in most cases. In those patients with elevated PTH, urinary cyclic AMP was normal, and bone turnover was low suggesting skeletal unresponsiveness to elevated PTH. Transiliac crest bone biopsy identified reduced bone remodeling with decreased bone formation and normal or low bone resorption. Low bone turnover may contribute to the observed hypercalcemia and hypercalciuria due to reduced skeletal calcium uptake, bone pain, and bone loss seen in those patients treated with TPN [40].

Theophylline

Theophylline is a cyclic nucleotide phosphodiesterase inhibitor that is used for respiratory conditions such as asthma. It increases tissue cyclic adenosine monophosphate (cyclic AMP). In one study of 60 patients, 11 out of 60 patients with theophylline toxicity developed hypercalcemia, which resolved after discontinuation of this medication [42]. PTH was unchanged with high or normal serum calcium levels in these subjects. The mechanism by which hypercalcemia occurs is unclear, but the addition of propranolol in those with supratherapeutic theophylline levels appeared to prevent hypercalcemia, suggesting that the hypercalcemia is non-PTH mediated and possibly an adrenergic mechanism is involved [42].

Foscarnet

Foscarnet (phosphonomethanoic acid) is an antiviral medication used to treat human herpesvirus infections. A case series of 2 patients with human immunodeficiency virus (HIV) treated with foscarnet for cytomegalovirus (CMV) reported hypercalcemia that resolved after its discontinuation. Other potential causes of hypercalcemia in the HIV patients were excluded, including lymphoma and immobilization [43]. The mechanism of hypercalcemia is unknown.

Growth Hormone

Human growth hormone (HGH) has been used in critical illness to improve muscle mass and in burn patients to help wound healing and decrease hospital length of stay. Hypercalcemia with normal parathyroid hormone and normal vitamin D has been seen in these patients treated with HGH [44]. Most cases have been seen in conjunction with parenteral feeding and renal insufficiency. Therefore, the potential mechanism may in part be related to increased intestinal calcium absorption combined with reduced renal calcium excretion [44].

Omeprazole

Rare cases of hypercalcemia associated with omeprazole-induced acute interstitial nephritis have been reported. In one case, hypercalcemia was present, along with signs and symptoms of interstitial nephritis. The mechanism by which this occurs is unclear [45].

Aromatase Inhibitors

Anastrozole, an aromatase inhibitor used for managing patients with hormone receptor-positive breast cancer in a setting of mild PHPT, has been associated with worsening of PHPT and severe hypercalcemia [46]. Significant elevation of PTH and serum calcium levels requiring treatment with bisphosphonates and calcitonin has been reported. The mechanism for worsening PHPT is not clear but has been thought to be due to the aromatase inhibitor potentially affecting calcium-sensing receptors (CaSR) resulting in decreased renal calcium clearance and stimulation of endogenous PTH secretion from reduced negative inhibition from serum calcium [46]. It is notable, however, that in postmenopausal women without PHPT, aromatase inhibitors cause a decrease in PTH secretion related to a decrease in systemic estrogen levels and subsequent increase in skeletal calcium efflux [47]. On the other hand, there is a trend toward an increase in PTH with estrogen replacement therapy in postmenopausal women [48, 49] and a reduction in serum calcium in patients with PHPT due to reduced skeletal calcium efflux [50] (Table 14.2).

Parathyroid Hormone

Treatment with recombinant parathyroid hormone 1–34 (rhPTH[1–34]; teriparatide) or parathyroid hormone-related protein analog (PTHrP[1–34]; abaloparatide) for osteoporosis management and recombinant human parathyroid hormone 1–84 (rhPTH[1–84]) for the treatment of hypoparathyroidism can be associated with hypercalcemia. Endogenous 84-amino acid parathyroid hormone (PTH) is the primary regulator of calcium and phosphate metabolism in the bone and kidney. Physiological actions of PTH include regulation of bone metabolism, renal tubular reabsorption of calcium and phosphate, and intestinal calcium absorption.

Teriparatide can increase serum calcium after dosing, with a peak 4–6 hours after injection but returns to normal prior to the next dose. In the pivotal Fracture Prevention Trial [51], 11% of drug-naïve patients treated with teriparatide 20 µg daily (versus 2% placebo) had at least one serum calcium >10.6 mg/dL (> 2.65 mmol/L) at 4–6 hours after the injection, whereas at 16 hours there was no difference from placebo. Importantly, there were no adverse events associated with these transient elevations. Additionally, in patients previously treated with alendronate or raloxifene who were switched to teriparatide 20 µg daily, there was a 0.168 mg/dL (0.042 mmol/L) and 0.216 mg/dL (0.054 mmol/L) increase in predose serum calcium, respectively, which was not clinically meaningful in either group [52]. In the groups adding teriparatide to raloxifene or alendronate there was no significant change in the predose serum calcium. The mechanism of increased serum calcium is likely related to increased bone resorption but may also reflect increased calcium reabsorption in the distal nephron and stimulation of 1,25-dihydroxyvitamin D production [52].

Abaloparatide binds the RG conformation of the parathyroid hormone type 1 (PTH1) receptor. Although abaloparatide can be associated with hypercalcemia, when compared to teriparatide, there is significantly less hypercalcemia with abalo-paratide [53]. This difference may be related to the differential binding of the PTH1 receptor that favors anabolic activity with less stimulation of bone resorption. Of note, in patients treated with osteoporosis therapy who are found to be hypercalce-mic, it is important to consider the possibility of PHPT, since the highest incidence rate is observed in older postmenopausal women, who are also more likely to be on osteoporosis therapy [54].

rhPTH (1–84) is a full amino acid parathyroid hormone used for the treatment of hypoparathyroidism. Doses range from 25 mcg to 100 mcg injected daily. Hypercalcemia can occur using a high dose of rhPHT (1–84) or with concomitant use of other calcium-sustaining medications such as calcium, calcitriol, and thiazide diuretics. Therefore, monitoring serum calcium and patients for signs and symptoms of hypercalcemia is recommended.

Denosumab

Rebound hypercalcemia after discontinuing denosumab has been reported primarily in children and young adults with inherently higher baseline bone remodeling activity, many of whom have conditions that could predispose them to the formation of numerous osteoclasts with denosumab cessation (i.e., Paget's disease of bone, giant cell tumors of the bone, aneurysmal bone cysts) [55–57]. The reported rebound hypercalcemia has occurred 7 weeks to 7 months after the last treatment in the few rare reports of this condition. Treatment with IV fluids and antiremodeling therapy with bisphosphonates or calcitonin have been associated with improvement in the hypercalcemia.

Summary

Medications are an important cause of hypercalcemia that need to be carefully considered in patient evaluations. This includes review of prescription medications, over-the-counter supplements, and medications administered outside of home. Identification of medication-related hypercalcemia can facilitate a correct diagnosis and guide the appropriate evaluation and management of such individuals.

Case

A 77-year-old female was referred for evaluation of hypercalcemia. She had a previous history of hypocalcemia identified 1 year prior when she was hospitalized for congestive heart failure. At that time, her serum calcium was 6.9 mg/dL with an albumin of 2.7 g/dL (albumin correct calcium 7.9 mg/dL). Her 25-hydroxyvitamin D level was normal, and she had evidence of stage 3b chronic kidney disease (CKD). She was placed on calcitriol at that time. She was stable until 8 months later when she developed nausea with a decreased appetite, and her serum calcium was 14.4 mg/dL with a parathyroid hormone (PTH) of 14 pg/mL. At the time of admission, she was taking calcium carbonate with 500 mg elemental calcium twice-daily, calcitriol 0.5 mcg daily, and 5000 IU of vitamin D_3 daily, which were all discontinued upon hospitalization. Normal test results at that time included parathyroid hormone-related peptide (PTHrP), thyroid stimulation hormone (TSH), monoclonal protein studies, and alkaline phosphatase. Her estimated glomerular filtration rate (eGFR) was 13 mL/minute based on cystatin C, and her 25-hydroxyvitamin D level was elevated at 119 ng/mL. She was treated with calcitonin for 3 days without bisphosphonates due to acute worsening of her CKD.

She stabilized rapidly, and at follow-up 2 months later, her serum calcium was 8.7 mg/dL with an albumin of 4.1 g/dL, serum creatinine 2.3 mg/dL (eGFR 20 mL/minute), phosphorus 4 mg/dL, and PTH 158 pg/mL, and her 25-hydroxyvitamin D had decreased to 69 ng/mL. She was diagnosed with non-PTH-mediated hypercalcemia that was multifactorial in nature, including volume depletion, renal insufficiency with acute worsening, and medications (vitamin D_3, calcitriol, and calcium).

The patient presented in this case demonstrates the contribution of medications to the development of hypercalcemia but also highlights some of the complexities, including other factors that can contribute to acute worsening of hypercalcemia including CKD and volume depletion reducing renal calcium excretion.

References

1. Davidge Pitts CJ, Kearns AE. Update on medications with adverse skeletal effects. Mayo Clin Proc. 2011;86(4):338–43. quiz 43
2. Ruppe MD. Medications that affect calcium. Endocr Pract. 2011;17(Suppl 1):26–30.
3. Jacobs TP, Bilezikian JP. Clinical review: rare causes of hypercalcemia. J Clin Endocrinol Metab. 2005;90(11):6316–22.
4. Waghray A, Milas M, Nyalakonda K, Siperstein AE. Falsely low parathyroid hormone secondary to biotin interference: a case series. Endocr Pract. 2013;19(3):451–5.
5. O'Keeffe DT, Tebben PJ, Kumar R, Singh RJ, Wu Y, Wermers RA. Clinical and biochemical phenotypes of adults with monoallelic and biallelic CYP24A1 mutations: evidence of gene dose effect. Osteoporos Int. 2016;27(10):3121–5.
6. Marcocci C, Bollerslev J, Khan AA, Shoback DM. Medical management of primary hyperparathyroidism: proceedings of the fourth international workshop on the Management of Asymptomatic Primary Hyperparathyroidism. J Clin Endocrinol Metab. 2014;99(10):3607–18.
7. Tohme JF, Bilezikian JP, Clemens TL, Silverberg SJ, Shane E, Lindsay R. Suppression of parathyroid hormone secretion with oral calcium in normal subjects and patients with primary hyperparathyroidism. J Clin Endocrinol Metab. 1990;70(4):951–6.
8. Beall DP, Scofield RH. Milk-alkali syndrome associated with calcium carbonate consumption. Report of 7 patients with parathyroid hormone levels and an estimate of prevalence among patients hospitalized with hypercalcemia. Medicine (Baltimore). 1995;74(2):89–96.
9. Medarov BI. Milk-alkali syndrome. Mayo Clin Proc. 2009;84(3):261–7.
10. Wenger J, Kirsner JB, Palmer WL. The milk-alkali syndrome; hypercalcemia, alkalosis and temporary renal insufficiency during milk-antacid therapy for peptic ulcer. Am J Med. 1958;24(2):161–3.
11. Peraino RA, Suki WN. Urine HCO3- augments renal Ca2+ absorption independent of systemic acid-base changes. Am J Phys. 1980;238(5):F394–8.
12. Beck N, Singh H, Reed SW, Davis BB. Direct inhibitory effect of hypercalcemia on renal actions of parathyroid hormone. J Clin Invest. 1974;53(3):717–25.
13. Burnett CH, Commons RR, et al. Hypercalcemia without hypercalcuria or hypophosphatemia, calcinosis and renal insufficiency; a syndrome following prolonged intake of milk and alkali. N Engl J Med. 1949;240(20):787–94.
14. Roizen JD, Li D, O'Lear L, Javaid MK, Shaw NJ, Ebeling PR, et al. CYP3A4 mutation causes vitamin D-dependent rickets type 3. J Clin Invest. 2018;128(5):1913–8.
15. Billington EO, Burt LA, Rose MS, Davison EM, Gaudet S, Kan M, et al. Safety of high-dose vitamin D supplementation: secondary analysis of a randomized controlled trial. J Clin Endocrinol Metab. 2020;105(4):dgz212.
16. Casella A, Long C, Zhou J, Lai M, O'Lear L, Caplan I, et al. Differential frequency of CYP2R1 variants across populations reveals pathway selection for vitamin D homeostasis. J Clin Endocrinol Metab. 2020;105(5):1302–15.
17. Grey A, Lucas J, Horne A, Gamble G, Davidson JS, Reid IR. Vitamin D repletion in patients with primary hyperparathyroidism and coexistent vitamin D insufficiency. J Clin Endocrinol Metab. 2005;90(4):2122–6.
18. Hardman KA, Heath DA, Nelson HM. Hypercalcaemia associated with calcipotriol (Dovonex) treatment. BMJ. 1993;306(6882):896.
19. Braun GS, Witt M, Mayer V, Schmid H. Hypercalcemia caused by vitamin D3 analogs in psoriasis treatment. Int J Dermatol. 2007;46(12):1315–7.
20. Selby PL, Davies M, Marks JS, Mawer EB. Vitamin D intoxication causes hypercalcaemia by increased bone resorption which responds to pamidronate. Clin Endocrinol. 1995;43(5):531–6.
21. Ellis S, Tsiopanis G, Lad T. Risks of the 'Sunshine pill' - a case of hypervitaminosis D. Clin Med (Lond). 2018;18(4):311–3.
22. Haskell MJ. The challenge to reach nutritional adequacy for vitamin A: beta-carotene bioavailability and conversion-evidence in humans. Am J Clin Nutr. 2012;96(5):1193s–203s.

23. Frey SK, Vogel S. Vitamin A metabolism and adipose tissue biology. Nutrients. 2011;3(1):27–39.
24. Conaway HH, Henning P, Lerner UH. Vitamin A metabolism, action, and role in skeletal homeostasis. Endocr Rev. 2013;34(6):766–97.
25. Farrington K, Miller P, Varghese Z, Baillod RA, Moorhead JF. Vitamin A toxicity and hypercalcaemia in chronic renal failure. Br Med J (Clin Res Ed). 1981;282(6281):1999–2002.
26. Grieff M, Bushinsky DA. Diuretics and disorders of calcium homeostasis. Semin Nephrol. 2011;31(6):535–41.
27. Middler S, Pak CY, Murad F, Bartter FC. Thiazide diuretics and calcium metabolism. Metabolism. 1973;22(2):139–46.
28. Brickman AS, Massry SG, Coburn JW. Changes in serum and urinary calcium during treatment with hydrochlorothiazide: studies on mechanisms. J Clin Invest. 1972;51(4):945–54.
29. Rejnmark L, Vestergaard P, Heickendorff L, Andreasen F, Mosekilde L. Loop diuretics alter the diurnal rhythm of endogenous parathyroid hormone secretion. A randomized-controlled study on the effects of loop- and thiazide-diuretics on the diurnal rhythms of calcitropic hormones and biochemical bone markers in postmenopausal women. Eur J Clin Investig. 2001;31(9):764–72.
30. Christensson T, Hellstrom K, Wengle B. Hypercalcemia and primary hyperparathyroidism. Prevalence in patients receiving thiazides as detected in a health screen. Arch Intern Med. 1977;137(9):1138–42.
31. Griebeler ML, Kearns AE, Ryu E, Thapa P, Hathcock MA, Melton LJ 3rd, et al. Thiazide-associated hypercalcemia: incidence and association with primary hyperparathyroidism over two decades. J Clin Endocrinol Metab. 2016;101(3):1166–73.
32. Tsvetov G, Hirsch D, Shimon I, Benbassat C, Masri-Iraqi H, Gorshtein A, et al. Thiazide treatment in primary hyperparathyroidism-a new indication for an old medication? J Clin Endocrinol Metab. 2017;102(4):1270–6.
33. Salata R, Klein I. Effects of lithium on the endocrine system: a review. J Lab Clin Med. 1987;110(2):130–6.
34. Mallette LE, Eichhorn E. Effects of lithium carbonate on human calcium metabolism. Arch Intern Med. 1986;146(4):770–6.
35. McHenry CR, Racke F, Meister M, Warnaka P, Sarasua M, Nemeth EF, et al. Lithium effects on dispersed bovine parathyroid cells grown in tissue culture. Surgery. 1991;110(6):1061–6.
36. Larkins RG. Lithium and hypercalcaemia. Aust NZ J Med. 1991;21(5):675–7.
37. Mallette LE, Khouri K, Zengotita H, Hollis BW, Malini S. Lithium treatment increases intact and midregion parathyroid hormone and parathyroid volume. J Clin Endocrinol Metab. 1989;68(3):654–60.
38. McHenry CR, Lee K. Lithium therapy and disorders of the parathyroid glands. Endocr Pract. 1996;2(2):103–9.
39. Shike M, Sturtridge WC, Tam CS, Harrison JE, Jones G, Murray TM, et al. A possible role of vitamin D in the genesis of parenteral-nutrition-induced metabolic bone disease. Ann Intern Med. 1981;95(5):560–8.
40. de Vernejoul MC, Messing B, Modrowski D, Bielakoff J, Buisine A, Miravet L. Multifactorial low remodeling bone disease during cyclic total parenteral nutrition. J Clin Endocrinol Metab. 1985;60(1):109–13.
41. Izsak EM, Shike M, Roulet M, Jeejeebhoy KN. Pancreatitis in association with hypercalcemia in patients receiving total parenteral nutrition. Gastroenterology. 1980;79(3):555–8.
42. McPherson ML, Prince SR, Atamer ER, Maxwell DB, Ross-Clunis H, Estep HL. Theophylline-induced hypercalcemia. Ann Intern Med. 1986;105(1):52–4.
43. Gayet S, Ville E, Durand JM, Mars ME, Morange S, Kaplanski G, et al. Foscarnet-induced hypercalcaemia in AIDS. AIDS. 1997;11(8):1068–70.
44. Knox JB, Demling RH, Wilmore DW, Sarraf P, Santos AA. Hypercalcemia associated with the use of human growth hormone in an adult surgical intensive care unit. Arch Surg. 1995;130(4):442–5.

45. Wall CA, Gaffney EF, Mellotte GJ. Hypercalcaemia and acute interstitial nephritis associated with omeprazole therapy. Nephrol Dial Transplant. 2000;15(9):1450–2.
46. Yu R. Hypercalcemic crisis associated with anastrozole use in a patient with breast cancer and primary hyperparathyroidism. Endocrine. 2016;53(3):868–9.
47. Heshmati HM, Khosla S, Robins SP, O'Fallon WM, Melton LJ 3rd, Riggs BL. Role of low levels of endogenous estrogen in regulation of bone resorption in late postmenopausal women. J Bone Miner Res. 2002;17(1):172–8.
48. Lufkin EG, Wahner HW, O'Fallon WM, Hodgson SF, Kotowicz MA, Lane AW, et al. Treatment of postmenopausal osteoporosis with transdermal estrogen. Ann Intern Med. 1992;117(1):1–9.
49. Khosla S, Melton LJ 3rd, Riggs BL. The unitary model for estrogen deficiency and the pathogenesis of osteoporosis: is a revision needed? J Bone Miner Res. 2011;26(3):441–51.
50. Marcus R, Madvig P, Crim M, Pont A, Kosek J. Conjugated estrogens in the treatment of postmenopausal women with hyperparathyroidism. Ann Intern Med. 1984;100(5):633–40.
51. Neer RM, Arnaud CD, Zanchetta JR, Prince R, Gaich GA, Reginster JY, et al. Effect of parathyroid hormone (1-34) on fractures and bone mineral density in postmenopausal women with osteoporosis. N Engl J Med. 2001;344(19):1434–41.
52. Wermers RA, Recknor CP, Cosman F, Xie L, Glass EV, Krege JH. Effects of teriparatide on serum calcium in postmenopausal women with osteoporosis previously treated with raloxifene or alendronate. Osteoporos Int. 2008;19(7):1055–65.
53. Miller PD, Hattersley G, Riis BJ, Williams GC, Lau E, Russo LA, et al. Effect of Abaloparatide vs placebo on new vertebral fractures in postmenopausal women with osteoporosis: a randomized clinical trial. JAMA. 2016;316(7):722–33.
54. Griebeler ML, Kearns AE, Ryu E, Hathcock MA, Melton LJ 3rd, Wermers RA. Secular trends in the incidence of primary hyperparathyroidism over five decades (1965-2010). Bone. 2015;73:1–7.
55. Roux S, Massicotte MH, Huot Daneault A, Brazeau-Lamontagne L, Dufresne J. Acute hypercalcemia and excessive bone resorption following anti-RANKL withdrawal: case report and brief literature review. Bone. 2019;120:482–6.
56. Uday S, Gaston CL, Rogers L, Parry M, Joffe J, Pearson J, et al. Osteonecrosis of the jaw and rebound hypercalcemia in young people treated with Denosumab for Giant cell tumor of bone. J Clin Endocrinol Metab. 2018;103(2):596–603.
57. Kurucu N, Akyuz C, Ergen FB, Yalcin B, Kosemehmetoglu K, Ayvaz M, et al. Denosumab treatment in aneurysmal bone cyst: evaluation of nine cases. Pediatr Blood Cancer. 2018;65(4).

Chapter 15
Non-parathyroid Hormone–Mediated Endocrine Causes of Hypercalcemia

Alyyah Malick, Ananya Kondapalli, and Salila Kurra

Epidemiology

Non-parathyroid hormone–mediated hypercalcemia can be seen in endocrinopathies such as thyrotoxicosis, pheochromocytoma, adrenal insufficiency, and acromegaly. Hypercalcemia associated with these endocrine disorders is generally mild and normalizes with treatment of the underlying etiology [1]. Hypercalcemic crisis is rarely seen and when present is usually associated with concurrent comorbidities which can raise serum calcium levels, with the notable exceptions of hyperthyroidism and Addison's disease [2–5]. Thyrotoxicosis is the most common non-parathyroid endocrine cause of hypercalcemia [1]. Prevalence of hypercalcemia in thyrotoxicosis has been reported to range from 17 to 50% [6, 7], with an asymptomatic serum calcium elevation seen in up to 23% of hyperthyroid patients [8]. Adrenal insufficiency, pheochromocytoma, and acromegaly are rarer, but well recognized, causes of hypercalcemia. In a study of 27 patients with acromegaly, 10% were found to have mild hypercalcemia [9]. In a series of 108 patients with Addison's disease, approximately 6% of patients presented with hypercalcemia; the prevalence of hypercalcemia in secondary adrenal insufficiency is unknown, but a few case reports have described isolated adrenocorticotropic hormone (ACTH) deficiency associated with hypercalcemia [10]. Hypercalcemia in pheochromocytoma has largely been described only in case reports [11–15].

A. Malick
Columbia University, Vagelos College of Physicians and Surgeons, New York, NY, USA
e-mail: am5106@cumc.columbia.edu

A. Kondapalli · S. Kurra (✉)
Division of Endocrinology, Department of Medicine, Columbia University Irving Medical Center, New York, NY, USA
e-mail: ak4576@cumc.columbia.edu; Sk850@columbia.edu

M. D. Walker (ed.), *Hypercalcemia*, Contemporary Endocrinology,
https://doi.org/10.1007/978-3-030-93182-7_15

223

Causes

Thyrotoxicosis

Thyrotoxicosis is caused by excess thyroid hormone levels and can occur due to primary hyperthyroidism from overproduction (autoimmune disease, hyperfunctioning nodules), thyroiditis, or overtreatment with levothyroxine. Graves' disease is an autoimmune disorder in which stimulating antibodies increase production of thyroid hormone. Autonomous production of thyroid hormone is also seen with single toxic adenomas or toxic multiple nodular goiters. Thyroiditis refers to a condition in which inflammation of the thyroid gland leads to release of preformed thyroid hormone and transient thyrotoxicosis typically occurring due to viral or bacterial infections, radiation, medications, postpartum, or autoimmune diseases. Overtreatment with levothyroxine can be seen in hypothyroid patients receiving replacement therapy or thyroid cancer patients requiring suppressive therapy [16, 17].

Pathophysiological Mechanism

Two mechanisms have been proposed for the development of hypercalcemia in thyrotoxicosis: increased bone turnover and increased catecholamine levels. In hypercalcemic hyperthyroid patients, bone biopsies have shown higher appositional rate, reflecting cortical bone formation and more active resorptive surfaces. These increases are correlated with levels of free thyroxine (FT4) [18]. Thyroid hormone weights the balance in favor of resorption: osteoclasts mobilize calcium from the skeleton, resulting in an overall increase of bone cortical porosity in hyperthyroidism [19, 20]. Thyroid hormone likely mediates these bone metabolic changes through alterations in cytokine signaling. Hyperthyroidism is associated with increased levels of interleukin-6 and its soluble receptor [21–24]. Triiodothyronine (T3) increases the sensitivity of bone to interleukin-6, which may stimulate differentiation of osteoclasts from their precursor cells [25, 26]. T3 also increases the expression of receptor activator of nuclear factor-κβ ligand (RANKL) in osteoblasts, which activates RANK in osteoclast precursors, contributing to osteoclastogenesis [27]. Increased calcium levels from bone mobilization suppress parathyroid hormone (PTH), which in turn decreases renal tubular reabsorption of calcium and increases urinary calcium excretion [28]. Some have proposed that increased adrenergic tone is responsible for hypercalcemia associated with hyperthyroidism [29]. This theory is controversial as catecholamine levels have been shown to be normal in some hyperthyroid patients [30]. However, it may account for resolution of hypercalcemia in some patients with propranolol treatment alone and explain how increased bone turnover can continue long after the resolution of hypercalcemia [31].

Presentation

Females are more frequently affected with hypercalcemia in association with thyrotoxicosis than males, likely due to the higher prevalence of thyroid diseases in women [17]. The most common cause of hypercalcemia due to thyrotoxicosis is Graves' disease [17]. Weight loss and nausea/vomiting are the most common symptoms seen in thyrotoxic patients with hypercalcemia; other symptoms include palpitations, heat intolerance, and tremors, which are the symptoms typically seen in thyrotoxic patients [17]. Hypercalcemia due to thyrotoxicosis may present with or without hyperthyroid symptoms [17, 32]. Most instances of hypercalcemia are mild and asymptomatic. Four cases of hyperthyroidism complicated by hypercalcemic crisis have been reported. In two cases, hypercalcemic crisis occurred in conjunction with primary hyperparathyroidism or central diabetes insipidus [2, 3]. In the others, it was attributed to hyperthyroidism alone [33, 34].

Clinical and Biochemical Patterns

Both low-normal and suppressed intact parathyroid hormone (PTH) levels can be seen in hypercalcemia due to thyrotoxicosis [28, 32]. Serum calcium levels are increased in a mild to moderate range, rarely exceeding 12 mg/dL or 3.0 mmol/L. Alkaline phosphatase (ALP) may be normal or elevated, and serum phosphorus is mildly elevated [17, 28, 32, 35]. 1,25-Dihydroxyvitamin D $(1,25(OH)_2D)$ may be suppressed with no change in 25-hydroxyvitamin D (25(OH) D), but as with PTH, this does not hold true in all patients [18, 19, 35]. Changes in $1,25(OH)_2D$ levels are likely mediated by hypercalcemia and decreased parathyroid hormone, which regulate renal 1-alpha-hydroxylase, rather than by thyroid hormone [35, 36]. The biochemical patterns of hypercalcemia associated with thyrotoxicosis are shown in Table 15.1.

Table 15.1 Biochemical Patterns of Non-Parathyroid Endocrine Causes of Hypercalcemia

Condition	PTH	PTHrP	Calcium	Phosphorus	Alkaline phosphatase	1,25-$(OH)_2D_3$	25-(OH)D
Thyrotoxicosis	––/↓	∅	↑	↑	––/↑	↓	––
Pheochromocytoma	↓ or ↑	↑ or ↓	↑	––/↓	↑	––	––
Adrenal insufficiency	––/↓	∅	↑-↑↑	––/↑	––	↓	––/↓
Acromegaly	––	∅	↑	––/↑	↑	↑	––/↓

PTH parathyroid hormone, *PTHrP* parathyroid hormone-related peptide, *1,25-(OH)₂D₃* 1,25-dihydroxyvitamin D₃, *25-(OH)D* 25-hydroxyvitamin D

Diagnostic Testing

Diagnostic testing involves checking thyroid function tests and assessing for causes of thyrotoxicosis. The initial test in patients with a clinical suspicion for hyperthyroidism is thyroid-stimulating hormone (TSH), followed by free T4 and total T3 if TSH is suppressed. Typically, TSH is low, and free T4 and total T3 are elevated, although this can vary based on the clinical situation, critical illness, and medications. T3 is checked to rule out T3 thyrotoxicosis and if significantly high compared to free T4 can also suggest Graves' disease or nodular goiter. TSH receptor antibody and thyroid-stimulating immunoglobulin should be checked to evaluate for Graves' disease, and a 24-hour radioactive iodine uptake and scan of the thyroid can help differentiate between Graves' disease, which has increased diffuse uptake; toxic nodules, which have single or irregularly increased uptake; and thyroiditis, which has decreased uptake [32, 37].

Treatment

The mainstay of treatment is to address the underlying thyroid disorder. Thionamides, including methimazole and propylthiouracil, radioactive iodine (RAI) ablation, and surgery are the primary treatments for hyperthyroidism. RAI ablation causes serum calcium and free T4 levels to decrease in parallel, while intact PTH and $1,25(OH)_2D$ concentrations normalize over the course of 6 to 12 weeks [32, 37, 38]. In some cases, radioiodine treatment worsens sympathetic symptoms and raises serum calcium levels temporarily. In patients with severe hypercalcemia and Graves' disease, surgery should be considered given risk of relapse with thionamides and worsening symptoms and hypercalcemia with RAI [17]. Beta blockers which alleviate adrenergic symptoms were also found to decrease calcium levels [17, 32]. Calcitonin and bisphosphonates are also effective at controlling calcium levels (see Chap. 5) [17]. After definitive treatment of hyperthyroidism, patients may frequently become hypothyroid and can receive thyroid replacement therapy without recurrence of hypercalcemia [32]. While the biochemical changes are reversible with anti-thyroid treatment [39], bone metabolism does not normalize for almost a year after and thus may increase future risk for fracture [38, 40].

Pheochromocytoma

Pheochromocytomas are catecholamine-producing tumors that arise from chromaffin cells of sympathetic ganglia in the adrenal medulla. The majority of pheochromocytomas are sporadic; however, a small subset can be found in patients with hereditary diseases such as multiple endocrine neoplasia 2 or von Hippel-Lindau syndrome [14].

Pathophysiological Mechanism

In cases of hereditary pheochromocytomas, hypercalcemia is typically explained by a concomitant primary hyperparathyroidism or renal cell carcinoma. In sporadic cases [14], four mechanisms have been proposed for the pathogenesis of hypercalcemia by pheochromocytomas: stimulation of bone resorption by catecholamines [41], stimulation of PTH secretion from the parathyroid gland by catecholamines [42], ectopic production of PTH by the tumor, and production of parathyroid hormone-related peptide (PTHrP) by the tumor. The latter two mechanisms are supported by most evidence, with production of PTH or PTHrP by pheochromocytoma documented in several case reports [11–14, 43]. Alpha adrenergic signaling may be involved in the release of PTHrP from pheochromocytomas [13]. PTHrP produced by pheochromocytomas causes hypercalcemia in a similar fashion to humoral hypercalcemia of malignancy [12] (please see Chap. 9 for more information).

Hypercalcemia associated with pheochromocytoma in the absence of elevated PTH or PTHrP has been described in a case report, suggesting that alternative mechanisms remain to be elucidated [15]. Mouse models suggest a direct effect of catecholamines could be responsible. Murine work has demonstrated that activation of β_2-adrenergic receptors on osteoblasts decreases osteoblast proliferation, differentiation, and bone formation by increasing expression of circadian rhythm genes and decreasing cell cycle regulators [44]. Additionally, β_2-adrenergic receptor activation results in increased osteoclastic bone resorption indirectly by increasing osteoblast expression of RANKL [45]. Thus an excess of catecholamines, as seen in pheochromocytoma, might lead to an excess of bone resorption relative to formation that could predispose to hypercalcemia.

Presentation

Pheochromocytomas classically present with episodic hypertension, tachycardia, headache, and diaphoresis. Nonspecific signs such as fatigue, abdominal pain, nausea, and loss of appetite or weight loss can also be present, either due to pheochromocytoma or hypercalcemia [14, 15, 46]. Pheochromocytomas are often found incidentally on abdominal imaging [46].

Clinical and Biochemical Patterns

PTH and PTHrP are low except in cases of pheochromocytoma with ectopic PTH or PTHrP production. Calcium levels may be on the high end of normal or mildly elevated (from 10 to 14 mg/dL or 2.5 to 3.5 mmol/L). Serum phosphorus is typically low to normal. ALP is elevated. $1,25(OH)_2D$ and $25(OH)D$ levels are both normal [11–15].

Diagnostic Testing

Biochemical testing is recommended in patients with clinical suspicion for pheo-chromocytoma with paroxysmal symptoms, adrenal nodule, and/or family history. Plasma free metanephrines and 24-hour urinary fractionated metanephrines have higher sensitivity and specificity compared to other tests and are considered first line. Elevated levels confirm the diagnosis; however, false positives may occur in setting of acute critical illness and stress. Plasma and urinary catecholamines, uri-nary total metanephrines, and urinary vanillylmandelic acid have lower sensitivity and specificity making them second-line alternatives [45]. Once biochemical testing indicates pheochromocytoma, imaging studies should be done to locate the tumor. Imaging options include CT (first line), MRI, and 123-I MIBG scintigraphy [14, 15]. Adrenalectomy with histology is used to confirm the presence of pheochromo-cytoma [11–15].

Treatment

The mainstay of treatment is surgical removal of the pheochromocytoma. Hypercalcemia can be controlled with IV saline and bisphosphonates. Therapy with an alpha-adrenoreceptor antagonist, such as phenoxybenzamine or doxazosin, is started prior to surgery and may help to decrease calcium levels by decreasing PTHrP levels [13]. Adrenalectomy is subsequently performed a few weeks later [15]. Calcium levels return to normal within a year after adrenalectomy [11, 15], sometimes immediately after surgery [14].

Adrenal Insufficiency

Adrenal insufficiency is caused by decreased glucocorticoid production due to either adrenal gland destruction (primary) or ACTH deficiency (secondary). The most common cause of adrenal insufficiency is exogenous steroid use leading to suppression of ACTH secretion. Primary adrenal insufficiency, Addison's disease, is most frequently due to 21-hydroxylase antibodies in developed countries. In developing countries, it is most commonly due to tuberculosis, human immunode-ficiency virus, and disseminated fungal infections. In addition to exogenous ste-roids, secondary adrenal insufficiency can also occur due to pituitary dysfunction, infiltrative diseases, immunotherapy, and head trauma [50].

Pathophysiological Mechanism

Adrenal insufficiency causes hypovolemia and reduction in glomerular filtration rate (GFR), leading to decreased calcium filtration and increased calcium reabsorp-tion in the proximal renal tubule [47]. Rehydration with normal saline normalizes

GFR and calcium excretion [48]; however, hypercalcemia may persist, indicating that hemoconcentration is not the sole cause of hypercalcemia [47]. Adrenal insufficiency increases calcium mobilization from the bone; however, the mechanism remains incompletely understood. Bone biopsies in patients with Addison's disease and hypercalcemia did not show increased osteoclast activity. In fact, both bone formation and resorption were found to be decreased in trabecular bone suggesting either increased osteoclast activity is occurring at nontrabecular sites or bone resorption is not the major driver of calcium release from the bone [46]. Studies suggest that increased active transport of calcium out of interstitial bone fluid by osteocytes and decreased levels of circulating stanniocalcin, a paracrine hormone produced by the adrenal glands that regulates calcium and phosphate, contribute to calcium mobilization [46, 48, 49].

Lastly, increased absorption of intestinal calcium via a $1,25(OH)_2D$-mediated process has been proposed; however, this remains controversial as levels of $1,25(OH)_2D$ are typically low in adrenal insufficiency, and estimated calcium influx into the extracellular space was found to be unresponsive to changes in dietary calcium intake [47, 48].

Presentation

Adrenal insufficiency commonly presents with weight loss, anorexia, nausea, vomiting, lethargy, and fatigue. In primary adrenal failure, skin hyperpigmentation, postural hypotension, muscle cramps, abdominal discomfort, and salt craving may also be seen due to mineralocorticoid deficiency. Other signs include hypoglycemia and loss of axillary and pubic hair. Acute adrenal insufficiency or adrenal crisis is a medical emergency and presents with hypotension, tachycardia, and hypovolemia often in conjunction with altered mental status [49]. Hypercalcemia can be seen in both primary and secondary adrenal insufficiency, due to various causes including isolated ACTH deficiency, pituitary apoplexy or atrophy, glucocorticoid withdrawal, opioid-induced adrenal insufficiency (which can occur with both acute and chronic exposure), tuberculous adrenal insufficiency, and adrenal hemorrhage [50–56]. It is often seen in conjunction with acute kidney injury or chronic renal failure [51, 57]. In adrenal crisis due to Addison's disease, hypercalcemia can reach severe levels [4, 5].

Clinical and Biochemical Patterns

Both low-normal or suppressed PTH levels can be seen in hypercalcemia due to adrenal insufficiency. Serum calcium levels are increased, ranging from mildly elevated to severe (11.5–16 mg/dL or 2.87–3.99 mmol/L). Serum phosphorus is normal to mildly elevated, and ALP is within normal range. $1,25(OH)_2D$ is decreased and $25(OH)D$ can be either decreased or normal [4, 5, 47, 48, 50, 52, 54, 57–60].

Diagnostic Testing

Cortisol secretion has a circadian rhythm, so the time of sampling affects results. A random serum cortisol greater than 500 nmol/L (18 mcg/dL) at any time makes adrenal insufficiency unlikely, while a morning (8 am) cortisol of less than 100 nmol/L (~3 mcg/dL) suggests adrenal failure. ACTH is normally measured concurrently, and a low cortisol with low or normal ACTH is indicative of secondary adrenal insufficiency, while low cortisol with elevated ACTH suggests primary adrenal insufficiency. For equivocal cortisol levels, ACTH stimulation testing is done whereby 250 μg of ACTH is administered parenterally and serum cortisol is measured 30 and/or 60 minutes later. If cortisol levels exceed 500 nmol/L (18 mcg/dL), response is considered normal, and primary adrenal insufficiency and chronic secondary adrenal insufficiency is ruled out. If cortisol levels do not rise appropriately, adrenal insufficiency is likely [49].

Treatment

The mainstay of treatment is glucocorticoid replacement. While rehydration with isotonic fluids helps stabilize patients, as discussed above it does not fully address hypercalcemia [48]. Treatment with glucocorticoids such as hydrocortisone, prednisone, or prednisolone returns serum calcium levels to normal in 1 to 5 days [47, 48, 50, 57, 58]. Long-term treatment with steroids is necessary in some cases and may lead to decreased bone density and increased risk of fractures long term [57].

Acromegaly

Pathophysiological Mechanism

Acromegaly results from excessive growth hormone (GH) production, which in turn leads to increased secretion of insulin-like growth factor (IGF-1). Hypercalcemia in patients with acromegaly is rare and typically due to co-existent primary hyperparathyroidism from parathyroid adenomas, often in the context of multiple endocrine neoplasia type 1 syndrome [61–64]. Less commonly, hypercalcemia can be due to a parathyroid-independent $1,25(OH)_2D$-mediated process, GH-mediated parathyroid hyperplasia, or increased bone turnover. IGF-1 may increase renal 1-alpha-hydroxylase activity and subsequent conversion of $25(OH)D$ to $1,25(OH)_2D$ in a dose-dependent fashion. This leads to increased absorption of calcium and phosphorus in the duodenum and reabsorption of calcium in the distal renal tubule. IGF-1 also increases phosphate reabsorption in the proximal tubule [61, 62]. In one study, serum $1,25(OH)_2D$ levels and urinary calcium levels in acromegalic patients were significantly elevated compared to normal subjects and both decreased after surgical treatment [69]. GH injections in rats led to increased parathyroid gland weight and secretion suggesting GH hypersecretion can lead to parathyroid hyperplasia and increased PTH and calcium levels. This may account for the lack of complete suppression of PTH during hypercalcemia in acromegaly. Increased bone turnover, evidenced by elevated serum osteocalcin, bone-specific alkaline phosphatase and urinary n-terminal telopeptide, c-terminal telopeptide, and hydroxyproline in patients with acromegaly, may also contribute, though it is not the dominant mechanism [61, 63]. Five to seven percent of pituitary adenomas co-secrete GH and prolactin; as a result some patients with acromegaly and hypercalcemia have shown hyperprolactinemia as well. Prolactin has been hypothesized to contribute to hypercalcemia through an unclear mechanism, perhaps hypogonadism leading to increased bone resorption [61, 62].

Presentation

Clinical symptoms of acromegaly can occur due to pituitary tumor mass effect or systemic effects from GH and IGF-1 hypersecretion. Given the slow progression and insidious nature of this disease, diagnosis can be delayed up to more than 10 years from onset of symptoms. Classic symptoms of acromegaly related to GH and IGF-1 secretion include acral growth (increase in ring and shoe size), enlarged or coarsened facial features, jaw prognathism, macroglossia, hyperhidrosis, hypertension, and impaired glucose tolerance. Headaches and temporal visual field defects can be seen with expansion of the pituitary mass [61, 62, 65].

Hypercalcemia tends to present late in the course of acromegaly, 5 to 10 years after onset [62]. Hypercalciuria is also common and may result in recurrent urolithiasis [66, 67].

Clinical and Biochemical Patterns

PTH level is typically normal or low normal, and serum calcium levels are mildly elevated from 10 to 11 mg/dL. Phosphorus is normal to high and ALP is high. $1,25(OH)_2D$ levels are increased and $25(OH)D$ can be either normal or low [61–63, 68].

Diagnostic Testing

Biochemical testing confirms a clinical diagnosis of acromegaly. The initial screening test is measurement of a serum IGF-1 level. Random serum GH levels are not used for diagnosis due to pulsatile release, rapid clearance, and stimulation from a variety of activities including sleep, exercise, stress, and fasting. Serum IGF-1 reflects the integral growth hormone secretion over the course of a day or longer. An elevated serum IGF-1 level in a patient with clinical signs of acromegaly confirms the diagnosis. If serum IGF-1 level is equivocal, an oral glucose tolerance test

(OGTT) must be performed. In an OGTT, serum GH is measured before and 2 hours after a glucose load, and a serum GH level that is not suppressed (<1 ng/mL) is diagnostic of acromegaly. Imaging is then used to determine the source of growth hormone secretion. MRI of the pituitary is the initial imaging of choice as somatotroph adenomas of the pituitary gland are the most common cause of acromegaly. If pituitary MRI is negative, additional imaging including computed tomography of the chest, abdomen, and pelvis or positron emission tomography (PET) DOTATATE scan can be considered [69].

Treatment

Transsphenoidal tumor resection is the primary treatment modality for majority of patients with acromegaly [69]. In poor surgical candidates, medical therapy with a somatostatin analog, dopamine agonist, or pegvisomant can be considered based on the clinical situation. Biochemical remission of acromegaly, with normalized growth hormone and IGF-1, is associated with normalized calcium and $1,25(OH)_2D$ levels [61]. Both surgical treatment and medical treatment with bromocriptine have been shown to decrease $1,25(OH)_2D$ levels [70, 71]. Calcium levels tend to normalize by 2 weeks post-tumor resection [62]. No data are available on the use of medical treatment to reduce serum calcium levels. Patients with acromegaly continue to be at long-term risk for fractures despite achieving biochemical control [63].

Case
A 64-year-old woman presented with weight loss of 30 pounds over the last 6 months, increased frequency of bowel movements, palpitations, tremor, and insomnia. Her symptoms had begun about 7 months ago and gradually increased in intensity, prompting her to seek medical care. Her medical history was significant only for osteoporosis, a history of appendectomy, and cholecystectomy. She took no medications. On exam, she was overweight, hyperkinetic, and anxious. Her thyroid was symmetrically enlarged, nontender, and without nodules. A thyroid bruit was audible. She had no proptosis or exophthalmos. She was mildly tachycardic. Her skin was smooth. She had a fine bilateral intention tremor and was hyper-reflexic. Her exam was otherwise normal. Laboratory testing revealed TSH <0.01 (normal 0.5–4.5 mIU/L), free T4 4.2 ng/dl (0.7–1.7 ng/dL), total T4 24.1 ug/dL (5–12 ug/dL), and T3 484 (76–181 ng/dL). Thyrotropin receptor antibody (Trab) levels were elevated. Calcium was 11.1 mg/dL (normal 8.5–10.2 mg/dL). Liver function tests revealed a mildly elevated alkaline phosphatase 135 U/L (40–129 U/L) and alanine aminotransferase 35 U/L with normal aspartate transaminase and bilirubin levels. Her renal function and complete blood counts were normal. She denied symptoms of hypercalcemia. She had an I-123 uptake and scan that indicated homogenously increased uptake consistent with Graves'

disease. She was started on methimazole and propranolol. Her calcium was repeated with PTH and found to be 10.4 mg/dl with PTH 12 pg/dL (normal 15–65 pg/dL). 25-Hydroxyvitamin D was 44 ng/dL (normal 20–50 ng/dL), and her phosphate was 4.6 mg/dl (normal 2.5–4.5 mg/dl). About 8 weeks later, her thyroid function tests had improved (TSH <0.01 mIU/L, free T4 1.0 ng/dL, T4 8.7ug/dL), and her calcium normalized (ca 9.9 mg/dl), but her alanine aminotransferase and alkaline phosphatase were higher, and she had developed pruritis. She was unable to tolerate methimazole. One month later, she underwent thyroidectomy. Post-thyroidectomy, she was started on levo-thyroxine, and her calcium remained normal. One year later, her bone mineral density improved, but her scores remained in the osteoporotic range.

This patient has Graves' disease, and this case illustrates that hypercalce-mia can be observed in patients with thyrotoxicosis. In this case, the hypercal-cemia was mild and asymptomatic, which is most typical when seen in patients with hyperthyroidism. Her calciotropic profile is consistent with the pattern described in patients with Graves' disease (mildly increased calcium and phosphate with low PTH). Additionally her alkaline phosphatase was elevated which may be due to increased bone resorption or alternatively to Graves' disease itself. The hypercalcemia was transient and resolved with treatment of her hyperthyroidism. Improvement in bone mineral density has been described in some patients with treatment of Graves' disease, as was observed in this patient.

References

1. Bollerslev J, Pretorius M, Heck A. Parathyroid hormone independent hypercalcemia in adults. Best Pract Res Clin Endocrinol Metab. 2018;32(5):621–38.
2. Yokomoto M, Minamoto M, Utsunomiya D, Umakoshi H, Fukuoka T, Kondo S. Hypercalcemic crisis due to primary hyperparathyroidism occurring concomitantly with Graves' Disease. Intern Med. 2015;54(7):813–8.
3. Endo A, Shigemasa C, Kouchi T, Taniguchi S, Ueta Y, Yoshida A, et al. Development of hyper-calcemic crisis in a Graves' hyper thyroid patient associated with central diabetes insipidus. Intern Med. 1995;34(9):924–8.
4. Miell J, Wassif W, McGregor A, Butler J, Ross R. Life-threatening hypercalcaemia in associa-tion with Addisonian crisis. Postgrad Med J. 1991;67(790):770–2.
5. Downie W, Gunn A, Paterson C, Howie G. Hypercalcaemic crisis as presentation of Addison's disease. Br Med J. 1977;1(6054):145.
6. Mosekilde L, Eriksen EF, Charles P. Effects of thyroid hormones on bone and mineral metabo-lism. Endocrinol Metab Clin N Am. 1990;19(1):35–63.
7. Gordon D, Suvanich S, Erviti V, Schwartz M, Martinez C. The serum calcium level and its significance in hyperthyroidism: a prospective study. Am J Med Sci. 1974;268(1):31–6.
8. Baxter JD, Bondy PK. Hypercalcemia of thyrotoxicosis. Ann Intern Med. 1966;65(3):429–42.
9. Ezzat S, Melmed S, Endres D, Eyre DR, Singer FR. Biochemical assessment of bone forma-tion and resorption in acromegaly. J Clin Endocrinol Metabol. 1993;76(6):1452–7.

10. Nerup J. Addison's disease–clinical studies. A report of 108 cases. Eur J Endocrinol. 1974;76(1):127–41.
11. Bernini M, Bacca A, Casto G, Carli V, Cupisti A, Carrara D, et al. A case of pheochromocytoma presenting as secondary hyperaldosteronism, hyperparathyroidism, diabetes and proteinuric renal disease. Nephrol Dial Transplant. 2011;26(3):1104–7.
12. Kimura S, Nishimura Y, Yamaguchi K, Nagasaki K, Shimada K, Uchida H. A case of pheochromocytoma producing parathyroid hormone-related protein and presenting with hypercalcemia. J Clin Endocrinol Metabol. 1990;70(6):1559–63.
13. Mune T, Katakami H, Kato Y, Yasuda K, Matsukura S, Miura K. Production and secretion of parathyroid hormone-related protein in pheochromocytoma: participation of an alpha-adrenergic mechanism. J Clin Endocrinol Metabol. 1993;76(3):757–62.
14. Takeda K, Hara N, Kawaguchi M, Nishiyama T, Takahashi K. Parathyroid hormone-related peptide-producing non-familial pheochromocytoma in a child. Int J Urol. 2010;17(7):673–6.
15. Edafe O, Webster J, Fernando M, Vinayagam R, Balasubramanian SP. Phaeochromocytoma with hypercortisolism and hypercalcaemia. Case Reports. 2015;2015:bcr2014208657.
16. Endres DB. Investigation of hypercalcemia. Clin Biochem. 2012;45(12):954–63.
17. Zhang Y, Gao Y, Zhang J, Gao Y, Guo X, Shi B. Thyrotoxicosis and concomitant hypercalcemia. Chin Med J. 2014;127(4):796–8.
18. Jastrup B, Mosekilde L, Melsen F, Lund B, Lund B, Sørensen O. Serum levels of vitamin D metabolites and bone remodelling in hyperthyroidism. Metabolism. 1982;31(2):126–32.
19. Mosekilde L, Melsen F, Bagger JP, Myhre-Jensen O, Sørensen NS. Bone changes in hyperthyroidism: interrelationships between bone morphometry, thyroid function and calcium-phosphorus metabolism. Eur J Endocrinol. 1977;85(3):515–25.
20. Mundy GR, Shapiro J, Bandelin J, Canalis E, Raisz L. Direct stimulation of bone resorption by thyroid hormones. J Clin Invest. 1976;58(3):529–34.
21. Akalin A, Colak Ö, Alatas Ö, Efe B. Bone remodelling markers and serum cytokines in patients with hyperthyroidism. Clin Endocrinol. 2002;57(1):125–9.
22. Salvi M, Girasole G, Pedrazzoni M, Passeri M, Giuliani N, Minelli R, et al. Increased serum concentrations of interleukin-6 (IL-6) and soluble IL-6 receptor in patients with Graves' disease. J Clin Endocrinol Metabol. 1996;81(8):2976–9.
23. Lakatos P, Foldes J, Horvath C, Kiss L, Tatrai A, Takacs I, et al. Serum interleukin-6 and bone metabolism in patients with thyroid function disorders. J Clin Endocrinol Metabol. 1997;82(1):78–81.
24. Salvi M, Pedrazzoni M, Girasole G, Giuliani N, Minelli R, Wall JR, et al. Serum concentrations of proinflammatory cytokines in Grave's disease: effect of treatment, thyroid function, ophthalmopathy and cigarette smoking. Eur J Endocrinol. 2000;143(2):197–202.
25. Kurihara N, Bertolini D, Suda T, Akiyama Y, Roodman GD. IL-6 stimulates osteoclast-like multinucleated cell formation in long term human marrow cultures by inducing IL-1 release. J Immunol. 1990;144(11):4226–30.
26. Tarjan G, Stern PH. Triiodothyronine potentiates the stimulatory effects of interleukin-1β on bone resorption and medium interleukin-6 content in fetal rat limb bone cultures. J Bone Miner Res. 1995;10(9):1321–6.
27. Nicholls JJ, Brassill MJ, Williams GR, Bassett J. The skeletal consequences of thyrotoxicosis. J Endocrinol. 2012;213(3):209–21.
28. Mosekilde L, Christensen MS. Decreased parathyroid function in hyperthyroidism: interrelationships between serum parathyroid hormone, calcium-phosphorus metabolism and thyroid function. Eur J Endocrinol. 1977;84(3):566–75.
29. Skrabanek P. Catecholamines cause the hypercalciuria and hypercalcaemia in phaeochromocytoma and in hyperthyroidism. Med Hypotheses. 1977;3(2):59–62.
30. Levey GS, Klein I. Catecholamine-thyroid hormone interactions and the cardiovascular manifestations of hyperthyroidism. Am J Med. 1990;88(6):642–6.
31. Cardoso LF, Maciel LM, de Paula FJ. The multiple effects of thyroid disorders on bone and mineral metabolism. Arquivos Brasileiros de Endocrinologia & Metabologia. 2014;58(5):452–63.

32. Iqbal AA, Burgess EH, Gallina DL, Nanes MS, Cook CB. Hypercalcemia in hyperthyroidism: patterns of serum calcium, parathyroid hormone, and 1, 25-dihydroxyvitamin D3 levels during management of thyrotoxicosis. Endocr Pract. 2003;9(6):517–21.
33. Chen K, Xie Y, Zhao L, Mo Z. Hyperthyroidism-associated hypercalcemic crisis: a case report and review of the literature. Medicine. 2017;96(4):e6017.
34. Suzuki H, Kondo K, Saruta T. A case of hypercalcemic crisis with resistant hypertension due to hyperthyroidism. Jpn J Med. 1983;22(2):137–9.
35. Bouillon R, De Moor P. Influence of thyroid function on the serum concentration of 1, 25-dihydroxyvitamin D3. J Clin Endocrinol Metabol. 1980;51(4):793–7.
36. Kumar R. Metabolism of 1, 25-dihydroxyvitamin D3. Physiol Rev. 1984;64(2):478–504.
37. Alikhan Z, Singh A. Hyperthyroidism manifested as hypercalcemia. South Med J. 1996;89(10):997–8.
38. Pantazi H, Papapetrou PD. Changes in parameters of bone and mineral metabolism during therapy for hyperthyroidism. J Clin Endocrinol Metabol. 2000;85(3):1099–106.
39. Mosekilde L, Christensen MS, Melsen F, Sørensen NS. Effect of antithyroid treatment on calcium-phosphorus metabolism in hyperthyroidism I: chemical quantities in serum and urine. Eur J Endocrinol. 1978;87(4):743–50.
40. Mosekilde L, Melsen F. Effect of antithyroid treatment on calcium-phosphorus metabolism in hyperthyroidism. II: Bone histomorphometry. Acta endocrinologica. 1978;87(4):751–8.
41. Finlayson JF, Casey JH. Hypercalcaemia and multiple Pheochrcmocytomas. Ann Intern Med. 1975;82(6):810–1.
42. Kukreja SC, Hargis GK, Rosenthal IM, Williams GA. Pheochromocytoma causing excessive parathyroid hormone production and hypercalcemia. Ann Intern Med. 1973;79(6):838–40.
43. Shanberg AM, Baghdassarian R, Tansey LA, Bacon D, Greenberg P, Perley M. Pheochromocytoma with hypercalcemia: case report and review of literature. J Urol. 1985;133(2):258–9.
44. Takeda S, Elefteriou F, Levasseur R, Liu X, Zhao L, Parker KL, et al. Leptin regulates bone formation via the sympathetic nervous system. Cell. 2002;111:305–17.
45. Elefteriou F, Ahn JD, Takeda S, Starbuck M, Yang X, Liu X, et al. Leptin regulation of bone resorption by the sympathetic nervous system and CART. Nature. 2005;434:514–20.
46. Kopetschke R, Slisko M, Kilisli A, Tuschy U, Wallaschofski H, Fassnacht M, et al. Frequent incidental discovery of phaeochromocytoma: data from a German cohort of 201 phaeochromocytoma. Eur J Endocrinol. 2009;161(2):355–61.
47. Montoli A, Colussi G, Minetti L. Hypercalcemia in Addison's disease: calciotropic hormone profile and bone histology. J Intern Med. 1992;232(6):535–40.
48. Muls E, Bouillon R, Boelaert J, Lamberigts G, Van Imschoot S, Daneels R, et al. Etiology of hypercalcemia in a patient with Addison's disease. Calcif Tissue Int. 1982;34(1):523–6.
49. Pazderska A, Pearce SH. Adrenal insufficiency–recognition and management. Clin Med. 2017;17(3):258.
50. Harano Y, Kitano A, Akiyama Y, Kotajima L, Honda K, Arioka H. A case of isolated adrenocorticotropic hormone deficiency: a rare but possible cause of hypercalcemia. Int Med Case Rep J. 2015;8:77.
51. Sakao Y, Sugiura T, Tsuji T, Ohashi N, Yasuda H, Fujigaki Y, et al. Clinical manifestation of hypercalcemia caused by adrenal insufficiency in hemodialysis patients: a case-series study. Intern Med. 2014;53(14):1485–90.
52. Lee AS, Twigg SM. Opioid-induced secondary adrenal insufficiency presenting as hypercalcaemia. Endocrinol Diabetes Metab Case Rep. 2015;2015(1):150035.
53. Glémarec J, Varin S, Rodet D, Guillot P, Prost A, Maugars Y, et al. Hypercalcemia in a patient with tuberculous adrenal insufficiency. Joint Bone Spine. 2002;69(1):88–91.
54. Sharma A, Subhash MJ, Pandit A, Bhan S, Bhatnagar S. Hypercalcemia due to methadone-induced adrenal insufficiency in a case of oral cancer. Palliat Support Care. 2020;18(6):751–3.
55. Isaia GC, Pellissetto C, Ravazzoli M, Tamone C. Acute adrenal crisis and hypercalcemia in a patient assuming high liquorice doses. Minerva Med. 2008;99(1):91–4.

56. Pieters T, Devogelaer J-P, Meunier H. Nagant de Deuxchaisnes C. Hypercalcaemia in acute adrenal insufficiency a case report. Acta Clin Belg. 1990;45(1):42–6.
57. Ahn SW, Kim TY, Lee S, Jeong JY, Shim H, Min Han Y, et al. Adrenal insufficiency presenting as hypercalcemia and acute kidney injury. Int Med Case Rep J. 2016;9:223.
58. Siegler D. Idiopathic Addison's disease presenting with hypercalcaemia. Br Med J. 1970;2(5708):522.
59. Kato A, Shinozaki S, Goga T, Hishida A. Isolated adrenocorticotropic hormone deficiency presenting with hypercalcemia in a patient on long-term hemodialysis. American Journal of Kidney Diseases. 2003;42(2):e10. 1-e. 5.
60. Bhatti RS, Flynn MD. Adrenal insufficiency secondary to inappropriate oral administration of topical exogenous steroids presenting with hypercalcaemia. Case Rep. 2012;2012:bcr0320125983.
61. Shah R, Licata A, Oyesiku NM, Ioachimescu AG. Acromegaly as a cause of 1, 25-dihydroxyvitamin D-dependent hypercalcemia: case reports and review of the literature. Pituitary. 2012;15(1):17–22.
62. Manroa P, Kannan S, Hatipoglu B, Licata A. Hypercalcemia and acromegaly-clarifying the connections: a case report and review of the literature. Endocr Pract. 2014;20(5):e86–90.
63. Anthony JR, Ioachimescu AG. Acromegaly and bone disease. Curr Opin Endocrinol Diabetes Obes. 2014;21(6):476–82.
64. Ueda M, Inaba M, Tahara H, Imanishi Y, Goto H, Nishizawa Y. Hypercalcemia in a patient with primary hyperparathyroidism and acromegaly: distinct roles of growth hormone and parathyroid hormone in the development of hypercalcemia. Intern Med. 2005;44(4):307–10.
65. Vilar L, Vilar CF, Lyra R, Lyra R, Naves LA. Acromegaly: clinical features at diagnosis. Pituitary. 2017;20(1):22–32.
66. Pines A, Olchovsky D. Urolithiasis in acromegaly. Urology. 1985;26(3):240–2.
67. Tsuchiya H, Onishi T, Takamoto S, Morimoto S, Fukuo K, Imanaka S, et al. An acromegalic patient with recurrent urolithiasis. Endocrinol Jpn. 1985;32(6):851–61.
68. Halupczok-Żyła J, Jawiarczyk-Przybyłowska A, Bolanowski M. Patients with active acromegaly are at high risk of 25 (OH) D deficiency. Front Endocrinol. 2015;6:89.
69. Katznelson L, Laws ER Jr, Melmed S, Molitch ME, Murad MH, Utz A, et al. Acromegaly: an endocrine society clinical practice guideline. J Clin Endocrinol Metabol. 2014;99(11):3933–51.
70. Takamoto S, Tsuchiya H, Onishi T, Morimoto S, Imanaka S, Mori S, et al. Changes in calcium homeostasis in acromegaly treated by pituitary adenomectomy. J Clin Endocrinol Metabol. 1985;61(1):7–11.
71. Lund B, Eskildsen PC, Lund B, Norman AW, Sørensen OH. Calcium and vitamin D metabolism in acromegaly. Eur J Endocrinol. 1981;96(4):444–50.

Chapter 16
Rare and Other Causes of Hypercalcemia

Angela L. Carrelli

Immobilization

Immobilization is a rare cause of hypercalcemia [1, 2]. It is a non-PTH-mediated hypercalcemia driven by increased bone resorption, in particular in patients with underlying high bone turnover from other conditions [1, 2]. Albright et al. authored a case report in 1941 that was considered the first description of a case of hypercalcemia from immobilization [3]. They described a 14-year-old male who developed hypercalcemia and hypercalciuria while immobilized following a fracture. The authors used the term osteoporosis of disuse to refer to the changes in bone that occurred in the setting of immobilization and led to the development of hypercalcemia and hypercalciuria [3]. The authors reported that similar cases of immobilization-associated hypercalcemia were seen in young children with paralysis due to polio. In considering why hypercalcemia only occurs in some cases of immobilization, the authors noted a young patient who was previously active was likely at greater risk due to a larger release of calcium from the skeleton. They did also note that associated renal insufficiency can exacerbate this condition as it limits calcium excretion [3].

An early study by Stewart et al. explored the pathophysiology of calcium balance in immobilization in patients after spinal cord injury [4]. This study concluded that bone resorption during immobilization is the central process and leads to a mean serum calcium in the high-normal range, increased 24-hour urine calcium excretion, and suppression of the PTH and 1,25-dihydroxyvitamin D levels [4]. The authors described this process as a resorptive hypercalciuria. They suggested that when there is increased calcium resorption from a higher skeletal load or there is a

A. L. Carrelli (✉)
Division of Endocrinology, Columbia University Irving Medical Center, New York, NY, USA
e-mail: Ac2482@cumc.columbia.edu

© The Author(s), under exclusive license to Springer Nature
Switzerland AG 2022
M. D. Walker (ed.), *Hypercalcemia*, Contemporary Endocrinology,
https://doi.org/10.1007/978-3-030-93182-7_16

237

reduction in renal function that limits calcium excretion, immobilization-associated hypercalcemia can occur [4].

In understanding immobilization hypercalcemia, it is helpful to review what is known about the changes in bone metabolism in this setting. In the case of immobilization from spinal cord injury, the changes in bone remodeling are evident soon after injury. Within 1 week post-injury, an increase in bone resorption markers has been reported, with highest values at 10–16 weeks post-injury [5]. The changes in bone formation markers are not as clear, with some studies showing they remain normal and others showing a possible small increase or decrease in bone formation markers [5–7]. For example, in one study of bone turnover following spinal cord injury, a small increase in bone formation markers was reported [5]. However, this was accompanied by a significant increase in bone resorption markers up to 10 times the upper limit of normal [5]. The important process appears to be the resultant mismatch or uncoupling that occurs between bone formation and the significantly increased bone resorption in immobilization [2, 6, 7]. While evidence suggests bone resorption persists for years in the setting of immobilization from spinal cord injury [6], when hypercalcemia of immobilization does occur, it is usually in the earlier phase of within a year following spinal cord injury [7]. One study found that 50% of patients developed hypercalcemia of immobilization in the first year post-spinal cord injury [8].

While other factors specific to spinal cord injury may affect changes in calcium balance and bone metabolism from immobilization in this setting [7], studies of patients with immobilization from other causes have noted similar patterns. For example, a 12-week study of normal subjects placed on bed rest used bone biopsy and bone turnover markers to better understand the impact of immobilization [9]. Immobilization led to a significant increase in urinary calcium, an increase in serum calcium with the mean remaining in the normal range, and declines in both PTH and 1,25-dihydroxyvitamin D levels with mean values also remaining in the normal range [9]. The bone turnover markers showed bone formation did not significantly change, but markers of bone resorption significantly increased during immobilization. Bone biopsy data confirmed an increase in bone resorption. Of note, when ambulation resumed, markers of bone resorption and urinary calcium then declined [9].

While immobilization leads to these alterations in calcium balance and bone turnover, immobilization remains an uncommon cause of hypercalcemia. It appears immobilization-associated hypercalcemia can occur in patients with underlying high bone turnover, as may be seen for example in young patients or patients with Paget's disease of the bone or hyperparathyroidism [1, 2]. The larger calcium load from bone in these settings can lead to immobilization-associated hypercalcemia [2]. One of the more commonly reported settings for hypercalcemia of immobilization remains patients with spinal cord injury as discussed above. Hypercalcemia has been reported in a study of immobilized trauma patients, and the risk of developing hypercalcemia in this setting was related to the number of fractured bones or the number of immobilized limbs; however, PTH and vitamin D levels were not measured in this study [10]. There is a report of immobilization hypercalcemia developing in patients with prolonged immobilization in the setting of sepsis [11]. The authors proposed that the inflammatory cytokines may have contributed to the increased bone resorption that led to hypercalcemia from immobilization in these patients [11]. The risk of immobilization hypercalcemia appears to be increased in the setting of chronic kidney disease due to a limited ability to excrete calcium as discussed earlier. There are case reports of immobilization hypercalcemia developing in patients with chronic kidney disease or end-stage renal disease during immobilization while hospitalized or in a skilled nursing facility [12–14]. Hypercalcemia has been reported in a patient with hypophosphatasia and chronic renal failure on hemodialysis during immobilization following fractures [15]. Hypercalcemia from immobilization has also been reported in patients with extensive burns, and the risk of developing hypercalcemia was associated with longer duration in the hospital and reduced creatinine clearance; however, only one patient in this study had evaluation that included measurement of PTH and vitamin D metabolites to rule out other causes of hypercalcemia [16].

Immobilization remains a rare cause of hypercalcemia and is a non-PTH-mediated process driven by increased bone resorption [1, 2]. This remains a diagnosis of exclusion and in particular may be seen in patients with underlying high bone turnover as discussed above. The treatment of hypercalcemia is discussed in detail elsewhere (Chap. 5), but it is important to note that resumption of normal weight bearing can reverse the changes described in calcium metabolism [2].

Rhabdomyolysis

Acute kidney injury (AKI) is associated with changes in mineral metabolism, and when serum calcium is impacted in acute kidney injury, it is typically hypocalcemia that occurs in this setting [17, 18]. However, acute kidney injury may sometimes be associated with hypercalcemia. When hypercalcemia is seen in acute kidney injury, it is important to consider that the AKI may be caused by the hypercalcemia, as discussed in Chap. 2, or that another process is contributing to the AKI that can cause acute kidney injury and also hypercalcemia, like concurrent multiple myeloma or sarcoidosis [18]. In addition, it is important to consider rhabdomyolysis, as the recovery phase from AKI in this setting can be associated with hypercalcemia [2].

Rhabdomyolysis is associated with electrolyte abnormalities including hypocalcemia in the oliguric phase of acute renal failure, which is thought to be due in part to calcium entry into the damaged muscle cells, calcium phosphate deposition in muscle, and possibly a decrease in responsiveness of bone to parathyroid hormone [19–21]. However, hypercalcemia can then occur during the phase of recovery from rhabdomyolysis-induced acute kidney injury. The pathophysiology of this process is not entirely clear. 1,25-dihydroxyvitamin D may play a role in mediating this hypercalcemia [20, 21]. An early study of calcium metabolism in the setting of acute kidney injury from rhabdomyolysis found that the hypercalcemia in the recovery phase was associated with elevated PTH and 1,25-dihydroxyvitamin D levels

[21] A subsequent study of 4 patients that developed hypercalcemia during the recovery of renal function after rhabdomyolysis also confirmed elevated 1,25-dihydroxyvitamin D levels, but the PTH levels were undetectable [20]. It was proposed that 1,25-dihydroxyvtitamin D plays a role in mediating hypercalcemia in this setting and the increased levels may possibly be from extrarenal production [20]. However, other studies have found low 1,25- dihydroxyvitamin D levels and PTH levels during hypercalcemia in the recovery phase, suggesting that the hypercalcemia is not driven by PTH or 1,25-dihydroxyvitmamin D [22–25]. Based on these findings, the impression was that the hypercalcemia is primarily being driven by mobilization of the calcium deposits in tissue from the earlier phase of rhabdomyolysis and that the PTH is suppressed and 1,25-dihdroxyvitamin D levels are low in the setting of this hypercalcemia [22–25]. When measured, 24-hour urine calcium was significantly elevated during the hypercalcemic phase [23]. Case reports have included whole-body bone scintigraphy, which confirmed the presence of calcium deposits in the muscle [23, 24]. Another study also used technetium-99 m pyrophosphate whole-body scans during the hypercalcemic phase and found increased uptake in muscle corresponding to the calcium deposits. Serial scans then showed a gradual decline in the increased uptake in muscles, which supported the impression that mobilization of these calcium deposits is contributing to the hypercalcemia [26].

In 2015, a retrospective review of 295 cases of rhabdomyolysis from two US hospitals in the Midwest found a prevalence of hypercalcemia in the setting of rhabdomyolysis of 9.2% [27]. This is significantly lower than reported in older literature, which typically quoted around a 30% incidence of hypercalcemia in this setting [20]. In this more recent review, they noted the hypercalcemia in rhabdomyolysis developed around day 3 to day 11 of the oliguric phase and proposed that the lower reported prevalence in their study may be due to the role of shorter hospital stays now than in the past [27].

In summary, hypercalcemia from rhabdomyolysis is a known complication of rhabdomyolysis [2] though the exact mechanism is not clear. It remains important to consider the risk for hypercalcemia in rhabdomyolysis and in particular that this occurs in later phase during recovery of renal function.

Paget's Disease of the Bone

The serum calcium is typically normal in Paget's disease of the bone, and when hypercalcemia occurs, further evaluation is needed [28, 29]. It appears that when hypercalcemia occurs in the setting of Paget's disease, it is due to the presence of a concurrent condition, like immobilization in the setting of a fracture [30] or immobilization from other causes [31, 32], underlying malignancy [33], fracture of a bone with Paget's disease [34], or primary hyperparathyroidism [35]. For example, a population based study from Minnesota of 236 patients with Paget's disease found hypercalcemia occurred in 5.2% of the patients (12 patients) [35]. The hypercalcemia was due to likely primary hyperparathyroidism in ten patients, one patient had tertiary hyperparathyroidism in the setting of kidney disease, and in one patient the hypercalcemia was only noted once and no cause reported [35]. In the past a potential link between Paget's disease of the bone and primary hyperparathyroidism was considered; however, it does not appear there is an increased risk of primary hyperparathyroidism in Paget's disease [33]. A study from 1999 included assessment of 184 consecutive patients with Paget's disease of the bone presenting to endocrinology at a hospital in Australia and found 21 patients had hypercalcemia [33]. The hypercalcemia was due to multiple myeloma in one patient and a malignancy in another patient, and in the other 19 patients, the hypercalcemia was due to primary hyperparathyroidism. Based on their estimation of the prevalence of primary hyperparathyroidism in Paget's disease, which they estimated was 2.2–6% based on a literature review, versus that in elderly in the general population, and the typical distribution of cases between females versus males, the authors concluded the association of primary hyperparathyroidism and Paget's disease could potentially be explained by chance association [33]. A thorough evaluation for an underlying cause is needed when hypercalcemia is found in Paget's disease.

Advanced Chronic Liver Disease

Another rare cause of hypercalcemia can be advanced chronic liver disease, though the mechanism of this form of hypercalcemia is not known [1]. This association was first reported in 1987 in a review of 16 patients with advanced chronic liver disease and hypercalcemia evaluated at a liver transplantation program [36] Five of these patients were subsequently found to have underlying malignancy (hepatocellular carcinoma or cholangiocarcinoma), and one patient had suspected primary hyperparathyroidism. However, the remaining 10 patients did not have a clear cause of hypercalcemia identified [36]. The PTH levels were low or normal range, and impression was the hypercalcemia was non-PTH mediated. The 25-hydroxyvitamin D and 1,25-dihydroxyvitamin D levels were normal or low when measured [36]. The authors did note that most of the patients included had renal insufficiency and some degree of immobilization due to their chronic liver disease, which may have contributed to the observed hypercalcemia [36]. Another case report noted hypercalcemia in the setting of advanced liver disease due to chronic hepatitis [37]. The hypercalcemia in this case was associated with a low PTH and normal 25-hydroxyvitamin D and 1,25-dihydroxyvitamin D levels and persisted over 2 years of follow-up with no other cause identified. Another report of 2 cases of hypercalcemia in advanced chronic liver disease reported low normal PTH levels and normal 1,25-dihydroxyvitamin D levels and noted that the hypercalcemia in these cases was transient [38]. More recently, a retrospective review of patients presenting with hypercalcemia to a tertiary care center in India found that advanced chronic liver disease was considered the etiology of hypercalcemia in 8.9% of patients presenting with PTH-independent hypercalcemia (34 out of 380 patients), which is higher than would be expected for this rare cause of hypercalcemia [39]. However, the authors did note the limitations of this data, in particular given the high volume of liver patients seen there and that a full workup was not available for all patients in this retrospective review [39].

Hypercalcemia attributed to advanced chronic liver disease is uncommon and remains a diagnosis of exclusion [38]. The etiology of hypercalcemia in chronic liver disease is not clear; it appears to be non-PTH mediated with normal or low 25-hydroxyvitamin D and 1,25-dihydroxyvitamin D levels [36].

Paraffin Granulomatosis

Another rare cause of non-PTH-mediated hypercalcemia is paraffin granulomatosis from paraffin oil injections for cosmetic purposes [1, 40–42]. Recent data suggests this hypercalcemia is in part mediated by 1,25-dihydroxyvitamin D production from the foreign body granulomas that form due to the paraffin oil injections [40]. The mechanism of this hypercalcemia is not entirely clear, in part because case reports have shown normal 1,25-dihydroxyvitamin D levels [42]. One case report found hypercalcemia in a male with history of paraffin oil injections with low PTH levels and initially a high-normal 1,25-dihydroxyvitamin D level; however, on repeat measurements, the 1,25-dihydroxyvitamin D level was later elevated [41] . Imaging suggested granulomatous inflammation in the pectoralis muscles in the areas of prior paraffin oil injections; these granulomas are sometimes referred to as paraffinomas [41]. A more recent report of 88 males with history of paraffin oil intramuscular injections 5–6 years earlier found that 34% developed hypercalcemia, which was associated with suppressed PTH levels and hypercalciuria [40]. Only some of the men in this study had elevated levels of 1,25-dihydroxyvitamin D [40]. However, through the ex vivo study of granuloma tissue samples from 3 patients, they concluded that ectopic production of 1,25-dihydroxyvitamin D by the granulomas does likely contribute to the hypercalcemia [40]. Hypercalciuria was noted in the patients with hypercalcemia and those with normal serum calcium levels but a suppressed PTH. A high prevalence (47–48%) of nephrolithiasis was also noted in both the group with hypercalcemia and the group with normal serum calcium levels but a suppressed PTH [40]. The authors identified the patient reported volume of oil injected as a potential risk factor for the development of hypercalcemia in this setting [40]. It is important to note that hypercalcemia from paraffin oil injections appears to be a late complication; another case series of 12 men with history of paraffin oil injections found hypercalcemia occurred an average of 5 years (range 1–8 years) after the injections [42].

PTHrP-Associated Hypercalcemia in Benign Disease

Humoral hypercalcemia of benignancy is a term sometimes applied to the rare cause of hypercalcemia due to PTHrP secretion from benign tumors [1, 43]. For example, there are case reports of PTHrP-associated hypercalcemia in nonpregnant women with leiomyomas where surgical removal of the leiomyoma resulted in normalization of the serum calcium and PTHrP levels [44, 45]. There is also a case report of PTHrP-associated hypercalcemia due to a benign ovarian tumor where hypercalcemia and elevated PTHrP resolved following surgery; analysis of the tumor suggested it did produce PTHrP [43]. Hypercalcemia due to PTHrP secretion from benign pheochromocytoma has also been reported [46, 47]. There are other rare causes of PTHrP-mediated hypercalcemia in benign diseases. For example, there is a case report of hypercalcemia in the setting of massive mammary hyperplasia during pregnancy, which resolved following mastectomy. Immunohistochemical studies on the excised breast tissue were later done, and the authors concluded the hypercalcemia was due to PTHrP production from the breast tissue [48].

Conclusions

In conclusion, this chapter discussed some of the uncommon causes of hypercalcemia that need to be considered when more typical causes have been excluded. In addition, the importance of evaluating for underlying causes of hypercalcemia in certain cases like Paget's disease of the bone was reviewed.

References

1. Jacobs TP, Bilezikian JP. Clinical review: rare causes of hypercalcemia. J Clin Endocrinol Metab. 2005;90(11):6316–22.
2. Horwitz MJ. Non-parathyroid hypercalcemia. Primer on the metabolic bone diseases and disorders of mineral metabolism. Wiley-Blackwell, Hoboken, NJ, 2018. p. 639–45.
3. Albright F, Burnett CH, Cope O, Parson W. Acute atrophy of bone (osteoporosis) simulating hyperparathyroidism12. J Clin Endocrinol Metabol. 1941;1(9):711–6.
4. Stewart AF, Adler M, Byers CM, Segre GV, Broadus AE. Calcium homeostasis in immobilization: an example of resorptive hypercalciuria. N Engl J Med. 1982;306(19):1136–40.
5. Roberts D, Lee W, Cuneo RC, Wittmann J, Ward G, Flatman R, et al. Longitudinal study of bone turnover after acute spinal cord injury. J Clin Endocrinol Metab. 1998;83(2):415–22.
6. Reiter AL, Volk A, Vollmar J, Fromm B, Gerner HJ. Changes of basic bone turnover parameters in short-term and long-term patients with spinal cord injury. Eur Spine J. 2007;16(6):771–6.
7. Maimoun L, Fattal C, Sultan C. Bone remodeling and calcium homeostasis in patients with spinal cord injury: a review. Metabolism. 2011;60(12):1655–63.
8. Zehnder Y, Luthi M, Michel D, Knecht H, Perrelet R, Neto I, et al. Long-term changes in bone metabolism, bone mineral density, quantitative ultrasound parameters, and fracture inci-

dence after spinal cord injury: a cross-sectional observational study in 100 paraplegic men. Osteoporos Int. 2004;15(3):180–9.

9. Zerwekh JE, Ruml LA, Gottschalk F, Pak CY. The effects of twelve weeks of bed rest on bone histology, biochemical markers of bone turnover, and calcium homeostasis in eleven normal subjects. J Bone Miner Res. 1998;13(10):1594–601.

10. Yusuf MB, Akinyoola AL, Orimolade AE, Idowu AA, Badmus TA, Adeyemi TO. Determinants of hypercalcemia and hypercalciuria in immobilized trauma patients. Bonekey Rep. 2015;4:709.

11. Gallacher SJ, Ralston SH, Dryburgh FJ, Logue FC, Allam BF, Boyce BF, et al. Immobilization-related hypercalcaemia–a possible novel mechanism and response to pamidronate. Postgrad Med J. 1990;66(781):918–22.

12. Gopal H, Sklar AH, Sherrard DJ. Symptomatic hypercalcemia of immobilization in a patient with end-stage renal disease. Am J Kidney Dis. 2000;35(5):969–72.

13. Prince RL, Eisman JA, Simpson RW. Hypercalcaemia in association with renal failure: the role of immobilisation. Aust NZ J Med. 1983;13(1):8–10.

14. Booth KA, Hays CI. Using denosumab to treat immobilization hypercalcemia in a post-acute care patient. J Clin Endocrinol Metab. 2014;99(10):3531–5.

15. Whyte MP, Leelawattana R, Reinus WR, Yang C, Mumm S, Novack DV. Acute severe hypercalcemia after traumatic fractures and immobilization in hypophosphatasia complicated by chronic renal failure. J Clin Endocrinol Metab. 2013;98(12):4606–12.

16. Sam R, Vaseemuddin M, Siddique A, Haghighat L, Kazlauskaite R, An G, et al. Hypercalcemia in patients in the burn intensive care unit. J Burn Care Res. 2007;28(5):742–6.

17. Waikar SS, Bonventre JV. Acute kidney injury. In: Jameson JL, Fauci AS, Kasper DL, Hauser SL, Longo DL, Loscalzo J, editors. Harrison's principles of internal medicine. 20th ed. New York: McGraw-Hill Education; 2018.

18. Leaf DE, Christov M. Dysregulated mineral metabolism in AKI. Semin Nephrol. 2019;39(1):41–56.

19. Bosch X, Poch E, Grau JM. Rhabdomyolysis and acute kidney injury. N Engl J Med. 2009;361(1):62–72.

20. Akmal M, Bishop JE, Telfer N, Norman AW, Massry SG. Hypocalcemia and hypercalcemia in patients with rhabdomyolysis with and without acute renal failure. J Clin Endocrinol Metab. 1986;63(1):137–42.

21. Llach F, Felsenfeld AJ, Haussler MR. The pathophysiology of altered calcium metabolism in rhabdomyolysis-induced acute renal failure. Interactions of parathyroid hormone, 25-hydroxycholecalciferol, and 1,25-dihydroxycholecalciferol. N Engl J Med. 1981;305(3):117–23.

22. Hadjis T, Grieff M, Lockhat D, Kaye M. Calcium metabolism in acute renal failure due to rhabdomyolysis. Clin Nephrol. 1993;39(1):22–7.

23. Hechanova LA, Sadjadi SA. Severe hypercalcemia complicating recovery of acute kidney injury due to rhabdomyolysis. Am J Case Rep. 2014;15:393–6.

24. Mirza ZB, Hu S, Amorosa LF. Bone scintigraphy of severe hypercalcemia following simvastatin induced rhabdomyolysis. Clin Cases Miner Bone Metab. 2016;13(3):257–61.

25. Shrestha SM, Berry JL, Davies M, Ballardie FW. Biphasic hypercalcemia in severe rhabdomyolysis: serial analysis of PTH and vitamin D metabolites. A case report and literature review. Am J Kidney Dis. 2004;43(3):e31–5.

26. Lane JT, Boudreau RJ, Kinlaw WB. Disappearance of muscular calcium deposits during resolution of prolonged rhabdomyolysis-induced hypercalcemia. Am J Med. 1990;89(4):523–5.

27. Wilczynski C, Emanuele MA. Prevalence of hypercalcemia associated with rhabdomyolysis: a dual-center case series. Am J Kidney Dis. 2015;65(4):632.

28. Charles JF, Siris ES, Roodman GD. Paget disease of bone. In: Primer on the metabolic bone diseases and disorders of mineral metabolism. Hoboken, NJ: Wiley-Blackwell. 2018. p. 713–20.

29. Singer FR, Bone HG 3rd, Hosking DJ, Lyles KW, Murad MH, Reid IR, et al. Paget's disease of bone: an endocrine society clinical practice guideline. J Clin Endocrinol Metab. 2014;99(12):4408–22.
30. Nathan AW, Ludlam HA, Wilson DW, Dandona P. Hypercalcaemia due to immobilization of a patient with Paget's disease of bone. Postgrad Med J. 1982;58(685):714–5.
31. Ralston SH, Langston AL, Reid IR. Pathogenesis and management of Paget's disease of bone. Lancet. 2008;372(9633):155–63.
32. Fuss M, Bergans A, Corvilain J. Hypercalcaemia due to immobilisation in Paget's disease of bone. Lancet. 1978;2(8096):941.
33. Gutteridge DH, Gruber HE, Kermode DG, Worth GK. Thirty cases of concurrent Paget's disease and primary hyperparathyroidism: sex distribution, histomorphometry, and prediction of the skeletal response to parathyroidectomy. Calcif Tissue Int. 1999;65(6):427–35.
34. Bannister P, Roberts M, Sheridan P. Recurrent hypercalcaemia in a young man with monoostotic Paget's disease. Postgrad Med J. 1986;62(728):481–3.
35. Wermers RA, Tiegs RD, Atkinson EJ, Achenbach SJ, Melton LJ 3rd. Morbidity and mortality associated with Paget's disease of bone: a population-based study. J Bone Miner Res. 2008;23(6):819–25.
36. Gerhardt A, Greenberg A, Reilly JJ Jr, Van Thiel DH, Hypercalcemia. A complication of advanced chronic liver disease. Arch Intern Med. 1987;147(2):274–7.
37. Cadranel JF, Cadranel J, Buffet C, Ink O, Pelletier G, Bismuth E, et al. Hypercalcaemia associated with chronic viral hepatitis. Postgrad Med J. 1989;65(767):678–80.
38. Kuchay MS, Mishra SK, Farooqui KJ, Bansal B, Wasir JS, Mithal A. Hypercalcemia of advanced chronic liver disease: a forgotten clinical entity! Clin Cases Miner Bone Metab. 2016;13(1):15–8.
39. Kuchay MS, Kaur P, Mishra SK, Mithal A. The changing profile of hypercalcemia in a tertiary care setting in North India: an 18-month retrospective study. Clin Cases Miner Bone Metab. 2017;14(2):131–5.
40. Eldrup E, Theilade S, Lorenzen M, Andreassen CH, Poulsen KH, Nielsen JE, et al. Hypercalcemia after cosmetic oil injections: unraveling etiology, pathogenesis, and severity. J Bone Miner Res. 2021;36(2):322–33.
41. Khanna P, Khatami A, Swiha M, Rachinsky I, Kassam Z, Berberich AJ. Severe hypercalcemia secondary to paraffin oil injections in a bodybuilder with significant findings on scintigraphy. AACE Clin Case Rep. 2020;6(5):e234–e8.
42. Solling ASK, Tougaard BG, Harslof T, Langdahl B, Brockstedt HK, Byg KE, et al. Non-parathyroid hypercalcemia associated with paraffin oil injection in 12 younger male bodybuilders: a case series. Eur J Endocrinol. 2018;178(6):K29–37.
43. Knecht TP, Behling CA, Burton DW, Glass CK, Deftos LJ. The humoral hypercalcemia of benignancy. A newly appreciated syndrome. Am J Clin Pathol. 1996;105(4):487–92.
44. Dagdelen S, Kalan I, Gurlek A. Humoral hypercalcemia of benignancy secondary to parathyroid hormone-related protein secreting uterine leiomyoma. Am J Med Sci. 2008;335(5):407–8.
45. Bilici A, Doventas A, Karadag B, Hekim N, Tezcan V. Hypercalcemia associated with a uterine leiomyoma: a case report and review of the literature. Gynecol Oncol. 2004;93(1):269–71.
46. Kimura S, Nishimura Y, Yamaguchi K, Nagasaki K, Shimada K, Uchida H. A case of pheochromocytoma producing parathyroid hormone-related protein and presenting with hypercalcemia. J Clin Endocrinol Metab. 1990;70(6):1559–63.
47. Mune T, Katakami H, Kato Y, Yasuda K, Matsukura S, Miura K. Production and secretion of parathyroid hormone-related protein in pheochromocytoma: participation of an alpha-adrenergic mechanism. J Clin Endocrinol Metab. 1993;76(3):757–62.
48. Khosla S, van Heerden JA, Gharib H, Jackson IT, Danks J, Hayman JA, et al. Parathyroid hormone-related protein and hypercalcemia secondary to massive mammary hyperplasia. N Engl J Med. 1990;322(16):1157.

Index

Printed in the United States
by Baker & Taylor Publisher Services